Midwifery and Sexuality

Sam Geuens • Ana Polona Mivšek
Woet L. Gianotten
Editors

Midwifery and Sexuality

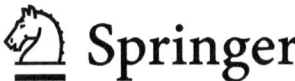 Springer

Editors
Sam Geuens ⓘ
Department of Healthcare - Midwifery
PXL University of Applied Arts and Science
Hasselt, Belgium

Outpatient Center for Sexual Health
Saint Franciscus Hospital
Heusden-Zolder, Belgium

Ana Polona Mivšek ⓘ
Faculty of Health Studies
University of Ljubljana
Ljubljana, Slovenia

Woet L. Gianotten ⓘ
Univ. Medical Center Utrecht
Erasmus University Medical Center
Rotterdam, The Netherlands

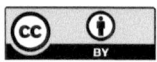

This book is an open access publication.

ISBN 978-3-031-18431-4   ISBN 978-3-031-18432-1   (eBook)
https://doi.org/10.1007/978-3-031-18432-1

Actual Society Midwifery & Sexuality

This Springer imprint is published by the registered company Springer Nature Switzerland AG
The registered company address is: Gewerbestrasse 11, 6330 Cham, Switzerland

Preface

Every year 140 million children are born around the globe, and the great majority of those mothers and newborns receive care from maternity service providers, professions with a wide range of status and training. Their background varies from traditional birth attendants (TBAs), who frequently learned the job through experience, to highly specialised midwives with a complete university education. There is a wide variety in their responsibilities and daily practices. In some countries, the midwife will hand over the woman in labour to the gynaecologist/obstetrician, whereas in other countries, that only takes place in case of complications. In some countries, midwives are responsible for a good percentage of home deliveries, which is, on the other hand, illegal in some other countries. While male midwives are nearly lacking in many countries, they make up one-fifth of the midwife workforce in other countries. Many midwives only deal with pregnancy and labour, for some with and for others without additional postpartum counselling and contraception care. A minor part is also involved in adolescent sexuality education, PAP smears, breast examination, menopausal care and other elements of the wide range of women's reproductive health. The primary task of the midwife is to optimally guide the woman (and her partner) through the period of an active child wish until well after birth. That period is characterised by many sexual worries, sexual questions, sexual changes and sexual insecurities.

The World Health Organization and the International Confederation of Midwives recognise the vital role the midwife can play in empowering women and adolescent girls, and they acknowledge the midwife's role in sexual counselling and sexual and reproductive health issues. For instance, think that most first-time parents of small children experience a drop in the quality of their relationship, with a decrease in sexual satisfaction in the first 4 years after birth. In some cases, even after 8 years, that drop is not yet wholly restored. The low sexual satisfaction found in many young fathers can easily threaten the stability of the relationship and the well-being of the parents and, thus, the child. In this stage of life, the midwife is directly involved with the physical, emotional and social changes, worries, and problems of both the woman and the couple.

As mentioned above, that clearly makes the midwife the right professional for targeted education and prevention of those sexual and relationship issues. Studies indeed suggest that sexuality education provided during pregnancy by well-educated and trained midwives can improve the couple's sexual well-being. The midwife can achieve this by enhancing communication between partners and by emphasising the role of intimacy and sexuality during the transition into young parenthood. Needed for this is a pro-active approach by midwives and other healthcare professionals and the skill *'to answer the often not-asked questions'* about sexuality and intimacy. However, in midwifery practice, this often does not happen. It is fair to recognise that this is the same for almost all medical and paramedical professions.

The great majority of midwives don't address sexuality and intimacy. One important reason is that the woman and her partner won't spontaneously share their worries or ask questions about sexuality and intimacy. But even more important is the straightforward reason that midwives neither have been educated to talk about sex with their clients nor know how to do that, let alone to inquire about sexual well-being pro-actively. It is a sad reality, but sexuality and intimacy are often only briefly mentioned or even totally absent from the midwifery textbooks, journals and the midwifery curriculum.

This absence from the midwifery curriculum became the primary argument to start this book. Therefore the editors set themselves the goal to create a midwifery textbook that systematically addresses the issue of sexuality and intimacy within the midwifery scope of practice. The book addresses various knowledge, skills and professional behaviour concerning sexuality and sexual well-being. We aimed to build on the recommended competencies for midwives and expand them when it comes to their roles concerning sexual health and well-being.

As (co-)authors for crucial midwifery chapters, we have tried to attract midwives with additional sexological expertise. The book combines the expertise of some 35 authors from 14 countries. To guarantee maximal dissemination of the book's contents, the editors decided to publish Open Access.

The book is composed of five modules. Module 1 deals with sexuality and sexual well-being in healthcare. Module 2 deals with the sexual aspects of the various phases and parts of the physiological, uncomplicated pregnancy, starting with preconception and getting pregnant, pregnancy, childbirth, postpartum and young parenthood, breastfeeding, with the last chapter focusing on pelvic floor function. Module 3 follows the same structure but focuses on the sexual aspects of the non-physiological course, with fertility disturbances, high-risk pregnancy, labour-induced trauma, difficult postpartum period and early parenthood. It also has additional chapters on sexual aspects of difficult breastfeeding, pelvic floor disturbances, mental health disturbances, physical health disturbances and side effects of common pregnancy-related medication. Module 4 addresses sexual aspects of 'special topics' with chapters on contraception, lesbian pregnancy, male experiences of pregnancy, birth and young fatherhood, cultural differences, trauma experience and female genital mutilation (FGM). Module 5 finishes the textbook with chapters on skills, including 'talking sexuality', teaching and learning about sexuality, the sexual consequences of daily midwifery practice and management of sexual problems by sexology professionals. The module ends with a vision of the future, outlining sexuality-integrated midwifery, showcasing how midwifery can comprehensively integrate sexuality into high-quality care for women's health.

The book is primarily geared to midwives and midwifery students in middle-income and high-income countries, although much information is similarly applicable to midwives and TBAs working in the urban areas of low-income countries.

The book is equally helpful for other professionals working in this field like lactation specialists, pelvic floor physiotherapists, gynaecologists in training, GPs dealing with childbirth, and doulas. We believe that any sexologist who counsels couples during these periods could greatly benefit from this book's information.

Finally, our aim is that all women and couples receive sexuality-integrated and intimacy-integrated care in their reproduction phase of life.

For us, editors and authors, this book was a work in progress and, as such, a very educational process. We hope that it progressively will contribute to the integration of sexuality in pregnancy and postpartum care. We hope it will instigate a step towards better sexual health, sexual pleasure, sexual rights, and sexual justice for women, their partners, and in some way also their children—because if we show women that speaking of sexuality is natural, they will also pass this message to the future generations.

With a sense of optimism, let's hope that midwives and other maternity service providers will make sexual health a more prominent public health priority.

Hasselt, Belgium   Sam Geuens
Ljubljana, Slovenia   Ana Polona Mivšek
Rotterdam, The Netherlands   Woet L. Gianotten

The original version of this book has been revised. A correction to this book can be found at https://doi.org/10.1007/978-3-031-18432-1_31

Contents

Editors and Contributors

About the Editors

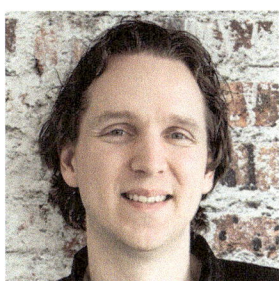

Sam Geuens became a clinical sexologist by chance. He started his University career studying Moral Sciences with a particular interest in semantics—the way people use words and play with their meaning. Realising that sexuality and intimacy are full of semantic pitfalls and miscommunication, he moved to clinical sexology after finishing his ethics degree. He added psychotherapy and started working with people and couples experiencing various relationship and sexual difficulties. He practised in the Netherlands and Wales before settling in Flemish institutionalised healthcare.

Ever since he has been practising medical sexology within hospital settings. Many hospitals did and do not yet have departments focused on treating sexual difficulties. So he started outpatient sexology clinics at the hospitals in Herentals, Hasselt and Heusden-Zolder. In this last one, he is still counselling patients/couples with various sexual problems.

Working in this intersection of gynaecology, urology, psychiatry and endocrinology has convinced him that our healthcare systems have a long way to go before taking people's sexual health and well-being seriously. Wanting to contribute to such a brighter sexual health future, Sam is active as a board member for both the Flemish Society for Sexology and the European Federation for Sexology, helping to get sexology and sexual health the attention it deserves in Flanders and the rest of Europe.

Ten years ago, he entered midwifery in a rather suiting way. He was standing in the hallway of his hometown's maternity ward, having just become a father for the second time, when getting a phone call from the University's head of midwifery announcing that he got a job lecturing their midwifery bachelor students.

Since then, his primary focus has been training aspiring midwives at the PXL University College in Hasselt, Belgium, teaching them psychology and mental health related to reproduction and early childhood development, sexual health and well-being, communication and counselling skills, and deontology and clinical ethics. Aspiring midwives are always a thrilling and engaging bunch of students, eager to learn and develop themselves.

He hopes this new textbook on Sexuality and Midwifery can help colleagues to integrate sexuality into their midwifery programmes, help practising midwives to take up the sexual well-being of their clients and educate his fellow sexologists on all matters regarding sexuality and childwish, pregnancy and young parenthood.

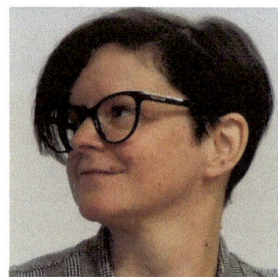

Ana Polona Mivšek At age 5, when her brother was born, Ana Polona Mivšek decided to become a midwife when she had the privilege of meeting her mother's birthing assistant. It was precisely the year when midwifery education was abolished in Slovenia. Without the opportunity to fulfil that dream, she went to the gymnasium. In the last year, when she was deciding on her professional future, the government revived midwifery education, and the University of Ljubljana was accepting its first generation of midwifery students. It felt as if she was called to become a midwife.

In 2000 she graduated as the first bachelor of midwifery in Slovenia. Though she got a job in the delivery room of a maternity hospital in Ljubljana, her curiosity was not yet satisfied, and she applied for an MSc in midwifery. Since this was impossible in Slovenia, she headed to Scotland, where she met her mentor, an aspiring midwifery researcher who became her role model.

A few years later, she began to teach at the University of Ljubljana, Faculty of Health Sciences, in the Department of Midwifery. The following 10 years were a hectic time—she became the head of the midwifery department, was the only midwifery teacher in Slovenia, was doing her PhD alongside her job, and in all this chaos, had a daughter.

In her midwifery practice, she became increasingly aware that sexuality doesn't get adequate attention. After completing her doctorate in 2012, with her daughter growing up, her thirst for knowledge was reawakened, which led her to take a course in sexology and establish a subject, 'Sexology in midwifery', as part of the undergraduate midwifery study programme.

In 2016, at the European Federation of Sexology conference in Dubrovnik, she spoke about the need for sexology in midwifery education and shared her experiences teaching this subject as an essential part of the midwifery curriculum. There, meeting the co-editors, the seed of an idea for this book was planted. It took a while—in midwifery terminology: during this 'birthing process', the editing team several times faced dystocia. But midwives are patient and do not easily lose faith. They are aware that good things take time to grow. Now, this book is sent out among midwives, to those who teach and those in practice. The editors hope they are planting a seed that can improve midwifery care.

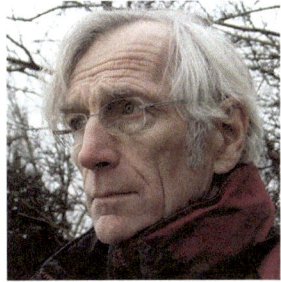

Woet L. Gianotten is a Dutch retired physician and registered psychotherapist. His dream was to be a tropical doctor in Africa. After graduating from Utrecht in 1967 as a physician, he spent a year in surgery and the tropical medicine course and moved to Gabon, West Africa, to work in a refugee camp with Biafran children. His next job was in obstetrics in Rotterdam, where he, for several months, replaced the practice of a midwife in the Red Light district. He then moved for 3 years to be the single doctor in a 110-bed upcountry mission hospital in Rubya, Tanzania.

In addition to much work in surgery and obstetrics, he built a maternity unit and a mother and child clinic. When asked to lecture in the school for nurses and midwives, he discovered the joy of teaching, which he has done ever since. With the help of a midwife student, he assisted his wife, Erna, at the birth of their second child. Their third and last child was born in their home with nobody else.

He started training in gynaecology back in the Netherlands, hoping to return to Africa as a medical specialist. However, after a year and a half, he had become so fascinated by the new fields of sexology and contraception that he quit gynaecology, a decision supported by his severe colour blindness. Not being able to see someone turning pale or blue and not making a correct Apgar Score is a real handicap for a gynaecologist. For a sexologist, however, it proved to be an asset since not being able to see the client blushing, one easily can continue asking difficult questions.

With Africa still pulling, he moved again to Tanzania to work in medical care and public health at Kilombero hospital. He built and started a family planning clinic and taught the midwives to insert IUDs and run that clinic independently.

Back in the Netherlands, he combined several jobs. For 20 years, he worked in contraception and abortion care. For 25 years, he worked in common sexology (where sexuality is not primarily influenced by disease or medical interventions). He enrolled in psychotherapy training to better understand the non-physical connections and gradually 'crossed the blood-brain barrier'. For 15 years, he was intensely involved in sexual abuse in care and in an advisory role to the Dutch Ministry of Health.

His third job was as a senior lecturer in Medical Sexology at the Rotterdam and Utrecht University Hospitals. In medical sexology, cancer, chronic diseases, physical impairment or medical interventions play an important role in sexual disturbances. Having an extra eye for 'unmet needs', he was part of the development of oncosexology and gerontosexology and being under the wings of gynaecology naturally introduced him to reproduction sexology.

In 2006, when obliged to retire from his University appointments, he was asked to continue in physical rehabilitation sexology. Gradually he became a freelance national and international teacher and trainer in sexology.

Contributors

Suaad Abdulrehman, MD, NVVS Parnassia Groep IPSY/Psyq Almere, Almere, The Netherlands

Sandrine Atallah, MD, FECSM, ECPS Women Health Center, American University of Beirut Medical Center, Beirut, Lebanon

Erna Beers, MD, PhD Pharmacosexology, SUNSCKS, Hilversum, The Netherlands

Johannes Bitzer, MD, PhD Department of Obstetrics and Gynecology, University Hospital Basel, Basel, Switzerland

Ruth Borms Sensoa vzw, Antwerp, Belgium & Private Practice, Willebroek, Belgium

Bente Dahl, PhD, RM, RN Faculty of Health and Social Sciences, University of South-Eastern Norway, Kongsberg, Norway

Serena Debonnet Federal Public Service: Public Health, Brussels, Belgium

Maaike Fobelets, RM, MSc, PhD Department of Public Health, Biostatistics and Medical Informatics Research Group, Faculty of Medicine and Pharmacy, Vrije Universiteit Brussel (VUB), Brussels, Belgium

Department of Teacher Education, Vrije Universiteit Brussel (VUB), Brussels, Belgium

Sam Geuens, MA, MSc, PG Department of Healthcare - Midwifery, PXL University College of Applied Arts and Sciences, Hasselt, Belgium

Woet L. Gianotten, MD-Psychotherapist Department of Gynaecology and Obstetrics, Erasmus University Medical Center, Rotterdam, The Netherlands

Els Hendrix, MSc, BSc Department of Healthcare - Midwifery, PXL University College of Applied Arts and Sciences, Hasselt, Belgium

Agnes Higgins, RPN, RGN, BNS, RNT, MSc, PhD School of Nursing and Midwifery, University of Dublin, Trinity College, Dublin, Ireland

Astrid Ditte Højgaard, MD, FECSM Sexological Centre, Aalborg University Hospital, Aalborg, Denmark

Marjolijn Lutke Holzik-Mensink, MSc, Specialised Physiotherapy Bekkenfysi otherapie Twente, Expertise Center for Pelvic Floor Physiotherapy, Enschede, The Netherlands

SOMT University of Physiotherapy, Master Pelvic Physiotherapy, Amersfoort, The Netherlands

Annelies Jaeken, BSc, RN, RM PXL University College of Applied Arts and Sciences, Healthcare Department, Midwifery, Hasselt, Belgium

Mijke Lambregtse-van den Berg, MD (Psy in Child&adolescent),Phd Department of Psychiatry/Child & Adolescent Psychiatry, Erasmus University Medical Center, Rotterdam, The Netherlands

Evelien Luts, MSc Sexology Department of Health Care, Brussels Centre for Healthcare Innovation, Erasmus Brussels University of Applied Sciences and Arts, Brussels, Belgium

Sexologist, Antwerp, Belgium

Deirdre O'Malley, RN, RM, PhD Department of Nursing, Midwifery and Early Years, Dundalk Institute of Technology, Dundalk, Co Louth, Ireland

Patrícia M. Pascoal, PhD CICPSI, Faculdade de Psicologia, Universidade de Lisboa, Lisbon, Portugal

HEI-Lab: Digital Human-Enviroment Interation Lab, Lusófona University, Lisbon, Portugal

Hester Pastoor, MSc, ECPS, PhD Division Reproductive Endocrinology and Infertility, Department of Obstetrics and Gynaecology, Erasmus MC, Rotterdam, The Netherlands

Petra Petročnik, MSc Faculty of Health Sciences, University of Ljubljana, Ljubljana, Slovenia

Ana Polona Mivšek, PhD Faculty of Health Sciences, University of Ljubljana, Ljubljana, Slovenia

Catarina F. Raposo, PhD Faculty of Psychology and Education Sciences, University of Porto, Porto, Portugal

Center for Psychology, University of Porto, Porto, Portugal

Aida Martín Redón, RN, RM, MSc Department of Obstetrics and Gynaecology, BovenIJ Hospital, Amsterdam, The Netherlands

Gabrijela Simetinger, MD, PhD, FECSM Department of Gynaecology and Obstetrics, General Hospital Novo mesto, Novo mesto, Slovenia

Tanja Repič Slavič, PhD Marital and Family Therapist at Franciscan Family Institute, University of Ljubljana, Ljubljana, Slovenia

Valerie Smith, PhD, RM, RGN School of Nursing and Midwifery, University of Dublin, Trinity College, Dublin, Ireland

Xuan-Hong Tomai, MD, PhD Department of Obstetrics and Gynecology, University of Medicine and Pharmacy, Ho Chi Minh City, Vietnam

Dilek Uslu, MD-gynaecologist, PhD, FECSM Doctor's Center, Nisantasi, Istanbul, Turkey

Minke van der Velde, MSc Seksuologiepraktijk Twente, Center for Sexology, Enschede, The Netherlands

Rik H. W. van Lunsen, MD, PhD Department of Sexology and Psychosomatic Gynaecology (Retired), Amsterdam University Medical Center, Independent Sexual Health Expert, Amsterdam, The Netherlands

Joeri Vermeulen, RM, MSc Department of Public Health, Free University of Brussel (VUB), Brussels, Belgium

Midwifery Department, Erasmus Brussels University of Applied Sciences and Arts, Brussels, Belgium

Department of Health Care, Brussels Centre for Healthcare Innovation, Erasmus Brussels University of Applied Sciences and Arts, Brussels, Belgium

Department of Public Health, Biostatistics and Medical Informatics Research Group, Faculty of Medicine and Pharmacy, Vrije Universiteit Brussel (VUB), Brussels, Belgium

Eva Wendt, RN, RM, Dr. Med. Sciences , Halland, Sweden

Liesbeth Westerik-Verschuuren, MSc, Specialised Physiotherapy Bekkenfysio therapie Twente, Center of Expertise for Pelvic Floor Physiotherapy, Enschede, The Netherlands

SOMT University of Physiotherapy, Master Pelvic Physiotherapy, Amersfoort, The Netherlands

Marleen Wieffer-Platvoet, MSc, Specialised Physiotherapy Bekkenfysiotherap ie Twente, Centre of Expertise for Pelvic Floor Physiotherapy, Enschede, The Netherlands

Z. Burcu Yurtsal, RM, PhD, Ass professor Midwifery Department, Faculty of Health Science, Sivas Cumhuriyet University, Sivas, Turkey

Endorsing Organisations

Midwifery and Sexuality, the textbook on sexual health and well-being for midwives and other related health care providers, is fully endorsed by several leading professional organisations worldwide:

EMA	**European Midwife Association**	
ISSM	**International Society for Sexual Medicine**	
WAS	**World Association for Sexual Health**	
ESSM	**European Society for Sexual Medicine**	
EFS	**European Federation of Sexology**	
ESCRH	**European Society of Contraception and Reproductive Health**	
AFSHR	**African Federation for Sexual Health and Rights**	

Substantial Donors Who Made Open Access Publication Possible

We, editors, hope that *Midwifery and Sexuality* will positively impact the midwifery practice and education today and, by extension, the sexual health and well-being of women and couples. To maximise that effect, we decided to publish *Midwifery and Sexuality* Open Access. In other words, freely available for anyone, anywhere in the world, with an internet connection.

Open Access publication is not possible without costs. Below is a list of professional organisations that have endorsed our project and, in addition, made a financial contribution. We, editors, are deeply grateful for all who contributed to improving the sexual health and well-being of women worldwide.

We received substantial donations from (in random order):

- Foundation for Disease and Sexuality, Hilversum, Netherlands
- Department of Obstetrics and Gynaecology, Erasmus University Medical Centre, Rotterdam, Netherlands
- Austrian Society for the Promotion of Sexual Medicine and Health, Vienna, Austria
- Department of Sexology and Psychosomatic Gynaecology, UMCG, University Medical Centre Groningen, Netherlands
- Kinderwunschzentrum Heinsberger Höfe (Centre for Childwish), Heinsberg, Germany
- Department of Healthcare – Midwifery and Nursing Science, PXL University College of Applied Arts & Sciences, Hasselt, Belgium
- Midwifery Department, Faculty of Health Sciences, University of Ljubljana, Ljubljana, Slovenia
- School of Nursing and Midwifery, Trinity College Dublin, Ireland
- IOSS, International Online Sexology Supervisors
- ASSM, African Society for Sexual Medicine
- BSSM, British Society for Sexual Medicine, Great Britain
- NVVS, Dutch Scientific Society for Sexology, Netherlands
- VVS, Flemish Society for Sexology, Belgium
- Soroptimist International; Club Bennekom & Beekdal, Netherlands; Club Hilversum, Netherlands
- Individual donations arrived from Armenia, the Netherlands, Norway, Slovenia, South Africa, and Türkiye

Part I

Introduction to the Book and Module 1

Woet L. Gianotten, Sam Geuens, and Ana Polona Mivšek

General Introduction

Over the last decades, the topic of sexuality has come far more into the open in affluent Western societies. However, that is not the case in healthcare, with a few exceptions. Most healthcare professionals (HCPs), on the one hand, avoid that theme. The great majority of patients, on the other hand, do not address sexuality, even when having extensive sexual problems and questions. They hope that the HCP will start that conversation [1].

Combining the expertise of HCPs in midwifery/sexology and advanced teaching, the editors of this book realized the same reality in current midwifery practice. There is nearly no attention to sexuality and intimacy in midwifery textbooks, journals, and curricula [2]. That is somewhat surprising since precisely this phase of pregnancy and transition to parenthood is associated with many sexual and relationship changes, questions, uncertainties, and problems.

Some midwives seem comfortable accepting sex as just the means to get pregnant. Then they focus on women's general physical and psychological well-being during pregnancy and postpartum. On the other hand, research gradually informs about the general importance of sexuality for people's physical and mental well-being [3]. So, before starting with the practicalities of the outline, modules, and chapters, we pause and take a closer look at the arguments why attention to sexuality and intimacy is essential. Below, we will give some arguments for the importance of healthy sexuality as part of a woman's and couple's well-being.

- Sexuality is an integral part of people's quality of life and relationships.
- Pregnancy changes a woman's sexual physiology. It can be responsible for less desire (and sometimes more), more arousal (and sometimes less), and changes in orgasm.
- Nearly all first-time fathers-to-be experience emotional and physical changes. Even his gonadal hormones (and their influence on sexuality) change during the pregnancy.

- The first pregnancy significantly impacts the romantic and sexual relationship of the parents-to-be. Loss (or increase) of sexual desire can occur in each. Real troubles can develop when these changes go in opposite directions and the couple doesn't successfully deal with those changes.
- Pregnant women and their partners can be scared if sexual activity can impact the pregnancy, even fearing miscarriage or premature birth. Without being well explained, such worries will not disappear.
- Regular sexual activity and orgasm appear to promote the proper duration of pregnancy.
- 'Birth is un-coupling!'. Many young parents experience sexual problems post-partum. For some of them, this seriously impacts their relational happiness.
- Approximately 5% of young parents get divorced within 2 years after the first childbirth [4].
- When the baby has far too low weight, this percentage can go up to 15%. Problems with sexuality and intimacy are significant reasons for such young parenthood disasters.
- Addressing sexuality is, for many HCPs, 'a touchy topic'. However, addressing this area will improve the HCP's relationship with the woman/couple, which may enhance compliance with treatment and lifestyle recommendations [1].
- Given the intimate nature of the relationship with their clients, there is no other group of HCPs that has such perfect opportunities to promote sexual health as midwives.

All arguments together could be translated into the slogan:

Midwifery care is only good care
when sexuality and intimacy have been adequately addressed.

Some authors sidestepped broader aspects of women's health. Through their role in the frontline of women's healthcare, midwives and other maternity professionals have ample opportunities to empower women with their education and approach. Significant elements to strive for are sexual satisfaction for all women and couples, comprehensive sexuality education, safe and legal abortion, and the right and power to make autonomous decisions about their bodies, sexuality, and reproduction [5].

The Structure of the Book

The book consists of five modules. The first one starts with general information on sexuality. The following two modules cover the phases of reproduction. Each phase has its typical bio-psycho-social influence on sexuality. Granting them a separate chapter enables the reader to concentrate on that specific stage. Module 2 will focus on those phases in the natural, physiological, 'healthy' development and Module 3 will focus on the problematic developments. The fourth module will address general themes (such as the male partner; and other cultures) and some relevant sidelines. The last module will focus on how to learn and integrate the topic of sexuality into midwifery practice and education.

Introduction to Module 1

This first module intends to familiarize the reader with some general aspects of sexuality and intimacy, preparing them to grab the next modules' information fully.

The module will offer a mixture of philosophical discourse (Chap. 1), 'technical' aspects (Chap. 2), 'sexology' with practical insight into aspects of sexual function and sexual dysfunction (Chap. 3), and the preventive health aspects of sexuality (Chap. 4).

Especially for the midwifery student, who uses this book as a textbook, the editors recommend starting with Chap. 26, dealing with how to communicate sexuality with clients, an essential skill.

Chapter 1: Sexuality Redefined

People have many different ideas about what sexuality is. This chapter explores the concept of 'sex' itself, looking at people's views on what sex is, broadening the concept way beyond intercourse and masturbation. We will examine why people have sex, broadening our ideas of sexual contexts beyond romance and intimacy.

This model provides a means of understanding sexual behaviour, sexual functioning, and dysfunctioning. The model will explore each dimension concerning sexuality and also examine its interdependency. And this chapter will provide a larger framework for a holistic approach to sexuality, namely the bio-psycho-social perspective.

Chapter 2: Relevant Sexual Anatomy, Physiology, and Endocrinology

This chapter will give more insights into the anatomical, endocrinological, and physiological aspects of (female) sexual functioning. And, although less extensively, also on aspects of relevant male sexual functioning. There are many similarities between (elements of) sexuality and pregnancy. The physical expressions of female sexual arousal resemble the circulatory changes that occur in pregnancy. And orgasm contractions resemble, in many ways, labour contractions.

The chapter will address relevant physiological and anatomical changes over the stages of pregnancy, and it will give a detailed overview of the relevant aspects of the changes in endocrinology during pregnancy and the postpartum period.

So, this chapter lays the necessary foundation for understanding the rest of the book.

Puberty and menopause are two other relevant transition phases in the woman's life, with extensive hormonal changes and sexual implications. We have decided not to include these topics in this book and limit ourselves to the entire reproduction width.

We know that midwifery has integrated these topics in some countries in their daily practice. Chapter 30 gives some information on the approach in Sweden, where the midwife has a much broader range of tasks, including care of the women from puberty to menopause.

Chapter 3: How Sex Works (and When it's not Working)

For a sexual encounter or masturbating, one doesn't need to know 'how sex works'. Moreover, the more you think about it at that moment, the greater is the risk that it might not 'work'. However, such knowledge is relevant and essential in the daily practice of the HCP.

This chapter will describe the various stages of the sexual process, from sexual desire, via sexual arousal to orgasm, then resolution (and the range of variety). It will indicate some of the changes that will occur during the various stages of pregnancy.

The majority of the content will focus on female sexuality, but the sexual functioning of males will get some attention as well. Also, common relevant gender differences will be highlighted.

Further, this chapter explores the types and reasons for sexual problems or dysfunctions. Understanding how things can go wrong would help HCPs provide care for women and couples struggling with sexual problems. The chapter highlights the common problems with sexual desire (not enough, too much or difference between partners), difficulties with arousal (lack of lubrication, erectile failure), sexual pain problems, including vaginismus, etc. Sexual problems are relevant to midwifery practice because they can negatively impact the couple's or the woman's general well-being and because they can be a reason for impaired fertility or they can complicate the quality of care.

A simple diagnostic tool will be presented to help midwives and other non-sexologist-HCPs to structure their clinical reasoning about their client's sexual problems.

The chapter will not cover treatment aspects since they will get attention in Chap. 29 so that the HCP will understand what will happen after referring a couple.

Chapter 4: The Health Benefits of Sexual Expression

Next to the procreative benefits of sexual intercourse, at least three valuable arguments include attention to sexuality and intimacy in good care: (1) For many people, sexuality is highly relevant for their quality of life in general and thus deserves attention from their care providers. (2) Attention to sexuality and intimacy appears to improve the contact between HCP and the couple. (3) Because sexual activities have direct physical and mental health benefits. This chapter concentrates on those health benefits.

Having sex for better health will seem like a strange fact for some people. Some might think it is nothing more than just another transient media trend. For others, it might be an attractive idea. Although it is an infrequent research topic, there is gradually more information about the various health benefits of sexual expression. This chapter will focus on those health benefits, especially regarding fertility and pregnancy.

Recommended Books for Further Reading on Sexuality

Here we give a small note on additional books for further reading. We don't mean the books for the sexology and sexual medicine professionals. We focus on relevant sexuality books written by devoted professionals and useful for HCPs. We'll mention three of the relevant English ones.

- Meston CM, Buss DM. *Why women have sex: Understanding sexual motivation from adventure to revenge (and everything in between).* London, The Bodley Head, 2009.
- Winston S. *Women's anatomy of arousal. Secret maps to buried pleasure.* Mango Garden Press, 2010.
- Nagoski E. *Come as you are.* Simon & Schuster Paperbacks. 2015.

References

1. Gianotten WL, Bender J, Post M, Höing M. Training in sexology for medical and paramedical professionals. A model for the rehabilitation setting. Sex Relat Ther. 2006;21:303–17.
2. Percat A, Elmerstig E. "We should be experts, but we are not!"; sexual counseling at the antenatal care clinic. Sex Reprod Health. 2017;14:85–90.
3. Gianotten WL, Alley JC, Diamond LM. The health benefits of sexual expression. Int J Sex Health. 2021;33:478–93.
4. Swaminathan S, Alexander GR, Boulet S. Delivering a very low birth weight infant and the subsequent risk of divorce or separation. Matern Child Health J. 2006;10:473–9. https://doi.org/10.1007/s10995-006-0146-3.
5. Forum Generation Equality. https://forum.generationequality.org/sites/default/files/2021-06/UNW%20-%20GAP%20Report%20-%20EN.pdf.

Sexuality Redefined

1

Sam Geuens ⓘ and Els Hendrix ⓘ

1.1   A History of Defining Sexuality

Over the last decades, sexuality has been constantly redefined. Sexual practices, sexual identities, sexual norms and sexual values all seem to be in flux.

When we want to define sexuality to make it a tangible and usable concept within midwifery practice, we have to start by adopting a broad perspective on sex itself. Over the past three decades, numerous studies have been looking into how people of all genders and sexual identities interpret 'having sex'.

In 1999, Sanders and Reinisch published an early and influential study, giving insights into how young adults view having sex [1]. Since then, numerous studies have explored the same question in different cultural settings. In a recent survey, Horowitz and Bedford showed that the view of young adults on sex has changed over the past decades [2]. From this 2016 study, they stated that definitions of sex are better viewed as categorizations exhibiting a graded structure, in stead of fixed categories (moving beyond 'yes it's sex', or 'no it's not sex') This is illustrated by our own findings where 4% of young adults indicate that deep kissing can also qualify as 'having sex' and 3% do not necessarily feel they had sex, even when they experienced penile-vaginal penetration [3]. This clarifies that there is not one single definition covering all people's views of having sex.

S. Geuens (✉)
Department of Healthcare - Midwifery, PXL University College of Applied Arts and Sciences, Hasselt, Belgium

Outpatient Center for Sexual Health, Saint Franciscus Hospital, Heusden-Zolder, Belgium
e-mail: sam.geuens@pxl.be

E. Hendrix
Department of Healthcare - Midwifery, PXL University College of Applied Arts and Sciences, Hasselt, Belgium

S. Geuens et al. (eds.), *Midwifery and Sexuality*,
https://doi.org/10.1007/978-3-031-18432-1_1

The majority of this research is geared towards sexual risk behaviour. However, we can use it also to better understand the complexities of sexual interaction, both pre- and post-natal, and during the period of trying to conceive. Overall it is safe to say that people's ideas on having sex differ widely, which is relevant knowledge for practicing midwives.

For example, a couple consults the midwife because they have an active child wish but are still not pregnant after 12 months of trying. When you ask 'if they have sex frequently' and they answer: 'We're having loads of sex', this does not necessarily mean that the woman is frequently experiencing intra-vaginal ejaculations.

Another example: At the exit consultation when going home after childbirth, the couple gets a well-intended message to 'better refrain from having sex for a period of 6 weeks'. Such a strict, medically focussed recommendation might seem wise in light of minimising infection risk and giving the vulva and vagina enough time to heal. But, unintended, this advice often leads to couples not having the satisfying sexual experiences without vaginal penetration they can perfectly engage in, risk free, during this periode. Healthcare professionals (HCPs) need to be very clear in communicating what they mean, paying attention to the language they use. If the take-home message for couples is '*Beware of vaginal infection when having intercourse before the vagina is fully recovered from childbirth!*', then the HCP should clearly state that the couple should refrain from any form of vaginal penetration. Preferably this is followed up by equally explicitly addressing which sexual behaviour will not cause problems: '*All other forms of intimate and sexual behaviour, such as kissing, cuddling, stimulation of the breasts or the clitoris are perfectly safe!*' Those are important messages, as research points out that these intimate and sexual moments are a way of finding connection during the start of young parenthood, a period that can be very stressful for some couples.[1]

A broader idea of what sex can be for a wide variety of couples can help the practicing midwife give more clear informational messages to clients, but it can also make it easier to think of possible solutions for the clients' sexual distress. If you think back on the new parents who just left the maternity ward after having their baby, the couple that always viewed vaginal intercourse as a way to keep connected might struggle these first weeks after the advice not to do so for a while. When one's idea of having sex also includes, for example, connected masturbation, in other words, both or one partner masturbating while in physical, intimate contact with each other, switching to connected masturbation for a while might be helpful advice for such a couple. Looking back at the research on definitions of sexuality, few people tend to view connected masturbation as 'having sex'. A Canadian study [4] found that only 3.7% of individuals view masturbating in each other's presence to orgasm as 'having sex'. Imagine the couple looking for a way to be sexually active when their usual sexual script has become difficult to maintain, for instance, shortly after vaginal birth when experiencing painful penetration. Then being advised by a

---

[1] More detailed information on post-partum sexuality can be found in Chaps. 8 and 14.

midwife, whose frame of reference on sex is broader than 'just penetration' and has an open view on numerous other forms of sexually stimulating activities, could be a huge advantage. Midwives with such a broader view on sex and sexuality will be more inclined to ask for clinically relevant details, and by doing so, they will more easily connect to the couple's actual needs and practices instead of unknowingly making assumptions based on their own frame of reference. Think, for instance, of the woman divulging pain during intercourse, telling the midwife that they engage in foreplay before starting intercourse. Foreplay can mean many things, ranging from mood lighting, romantic music and back rubs to manual or oral stimulation of the genitals. With such a broad frame of reference, the midwife will ask what the woman means when she says 'foreplay', knowing that lack of physical arousal and lubrication might be causing her sexual pain. Although such mood lighting, romantic music and a back rub can be adequate ways to start up intimacy and sexuality in a couple, they will not automatically cause high physical arousal and lubrication in all women. Often more sexually focussed activities and even direct genital stimulation are needed.

1.2 Why People Want 'Sex' and What They Actually Want in Practice

When addressing sexuality during consultation, we should use clear/explicit language.[2] Knowing that even 'having sex' can have so many different meanings in people's minds, one can imagine that using even more abstract terms like *'being intimate'* or *'having relations'* are a sure way to create misunderstanding between the HCP and the woman or couple. So the clinical implications of the term 'sex' covering such a broad range of actual practices and behaviours that might or might not imply health risks are numerous. Besides, even within couples, people's ideas on sex can vary regarding the emotional meaning and importance they attribute to their sexual practices. It can vary, for instance, because of the context. Where people might see a sexual one-night-stand as *'just having fun'*, having sex in a committed relationship will almost always carry additional meanings like expressing feelings of love, searching for comfort, etc. Research has shown that people have sex for various reasons ranging from 'wanting to experiece the physical pleasure' and *'wanting to conceive'* to *'wanting to relieve menstrual cramps'* and *'wanting to be popular/boost my social status'* [5].

Concerning the importance of sex during pregnancy, a recent study indicated that partners do differ in the importance they attach to remaining sexually active [6]. In case of such differences between the partners, keeping a positive attitude towards sexuality as a couple seems to be the most relevant factor to address for the practicing midwife, who wants to help this couple remain sexually satisfied and happy during pregnancy.

---

[2] More detailed information on 'Talking sexuality' with clients can be found in Chap. 26.

1.3   Sexual Health and Its Place Within Midwifery Care

An excellent professional approach to sexuality within midwifery (and health care in general) thus needs to be a broad approach. An overarching framework for such a broad approach was provided by the World Health Organisation in 2006 when they proposed their definition of sexual health [7].

> *Sexual health is a state of physical, mental, and social wellbeing in relation to sexuality. It requires a positive and respectful approach to sexuality and sexual relationships and the possibility of having pleasurable and safe sexual experiences, free of coercion, discrimination, and violence [7].*

So, the WHO globally recognises sexuality as an integral part of people's overall health and wellbeing. Building on this theoretical framework, the WHO defines several necessary parameters to ensure people's sexual health: Among them are:

> *The ability of men and women to achieve sexual health and wellbeing depends on:*

- *Their access to comprehensive, good-quality information about sex and sexuality*
- *Knowledge about the risks they may face and their vulnerability to adverse consequences of unprotected sexual activity*
- *Ability to access sexual health care*
- *Living in an environment that affirms and promotes sexual health*

> *Sexual health-related issues cover a wide range, encompassing sexual orientation, gender identity, sexual expression, relationships, and pleasure. They also include negative consequences or conditions such as infections with human immunodeficiency virus (HIV), sexually transmitted infections (STIs), reproductive tract infections (RTIs), and their adverse outcomes (such as cancer and infertility); unintended pregnancy and abortion; sexual dysfunction; sexual violence; and harmful practices (such as female genital mutilation, FGM) [7].*

When looking at this definition, one realises its far-reaching consequences if fully applied in practice. First, we need to realise that sexual health is more than maintaining a level of physical health that enables people to have sexual experiences. Sexual health is not just a physical affair, aimed at being free from infections, disabilities or dysfunctions that could harm one's potential for sexual expression. Next to the physical aspect of sexual health, we recognise the psychological and social dimensions of sexual health as equally crucial for attaining sexually healthy people. The biopsychosocial model, one of today's leading models for understanding health in general, clearly echoes that philosophy [8].

The biopsychosocial approach to health emphasises that we should see health as a constant search for balance between the physical, psychological and social dimensions of someone's being. Only when these three equally important aspects of a person's self are in harmony, the person is 'healthy'. This approach also highlights that these three dimensions are overlapping and intertwined. This means that when one of these dimensions, e.g. the physical, gets out of balance, for instance, by hyperemesis, this could sooner or later affect both the psychological and the social dimensions. As a result, people will become unbalanced, e.g. depressed mood, unable to contribute to household chores, experiencing less or no sexual desire, possibly impacting the partner relationship, etc. The same applies to sexual health: the physical, psychological and social dimensions need to be in balance, both individually and mutually, to enable them to have pleasurable sexual experiences. Only then can we genuinely say people are in a state of optimal sexual health.[3] That reality also implies that any sexual problem can have root causes in these three dimensions or even in all three simultaneously. When left unchecked for too long, sexual problems will evolve. Even when the original cause has already abided (e.g. an old episiotomy scar that used to induce pain during penetration), maintaining factors (e.g. a fear-response causing high pelvic floor tension) can arise because the original problem was not addressed in due time. When given time, problems stemming from one dimension of our health can begin to impact possibly all three dimensions of our being. Sadly, due to social stigma, people tend to wait very long before consulting a health care professional about sexual problems. For example, in Flanders, researchers found 7 years as the mean time between the first experience of a sexual problem and consulting a health professional [9].

Next to the realisation that sexual health requires a balance between people's physical, mental and social wellbeing, the WHO's definition of sexual health declares that sexual health can only be attained if people have safe and pleasurable sexual experiences. In short: if we want our patients to be sexually healthy, it is our responsibility to ensure that they can enjoy their sexuality. For midwives, this means actively stimulating couples to keep sexuality pleasurable when trying to conceive (no matter how long this might take) and during pregnancy and young parenthood. If we take a broader approach, we have to make sure that when patients, even those admitted to health care institutions, wish to have pleasurable sexual experiences, we need to enable them to do so, despite their current physical or mental state and their limited social environment.

Think, for instance, about the women admitted at 10 weeks of pregnancy because of hyperemesis. An extended stay in a hospital environment makes it challenging for the couple to retain a certain level of intimacy, let alone sexuality. Still, the same view on sexual health applies. They should be able to eg. lay together, cuddle, kiss, ... during the hospital stay. This is even more so for this couple, as we know that keeping intimacy and sexuality alive during pregnancy is a critical factor in preventing possible sexual problems post-partum and in young parenthood. Within this broad approach, one quickly realises that we still have a long way to go to bring the WHO's vision on sexual health into practice.

---

[3] Be aware: People can find balance even when they have physical, psychological or social problems and have learned to deal with them in such a way that it does not impact their daily lives.

Picking up the WHO's message, in 2019, the World Association for Sexual Health (WAS) published its Declaration on Sexual Pleasure [10].

Sexual pleasure is the physical and psychological satisfaction and enjoyment derived from shared or solitary erotic experiences, including thoughts, fantasies, dreams, emotions, and feelings. Self-determination, consent, safety, privacy, confidence, and the ability to communicate and negotiate sexual relations are key enabling factors for pleasure to contribute to sexual health and wellbeing. Sexual pleasure should be exercised within sexual rights, particularly the rights to equality and non-discrimination, autonomy and bodily integrity, the right to the highest attainable standard of health, and freedom of expression. The experiences of human sexual pleasure are diverse and sexual rights ensure that pleasure is a positive experience for all concerned and not obtained by violating other people's human rights and wellbeing. WAS [10].

The WAS tried to bridge the gap between theory and practice. To implement their vision of sexual pleasure, WAS stated: 'The programmatic inclusion of sexual pleasure to meet individuals' needs, aspirations, and realities ultimately contributes to global health and sustainable development, and it should require comprehensive, immediate, and sustainable action'.

For example, practicing midwives might scan the general information leaflets they use. Do they include sexuality? For the midwifery tutor, that could mean reviewing their course material. Does it link to sexuality (e.g. when teaching about breastfeeding, do we also address the effects of breastfeeding on sexuality)? Etc.

Following these frameworks, one can summarise the following key elements for sexual-health-sensitive midwifery practice:

1. Sexual health is an integral part of general health and wellbeing and requires a biopsychosocial approach.
2. Sexual satisfaction is a necessary component of healthy sex life.
3. Midwives have a professional and moral obligation to promote the sexual health of their patients by both disseminating accurate information and if needed, guidance on sexuality-related issues.
4. Midwives' responsibilities to address sexuality issues apply to all levels: on a micro-level (in relationship with the client/couple), meso-level (within their broader scope of practice, among colleagues and within professional organisations) and macro-level (diminishing the taboo around sexuality in the society, thus further deconstructing the myths surrounding sexuality and influencing local and global policies).

In conclusion, the only good midwifery practice is sexual health-sensitive midwifery practice.

References

1. Sanders SA, Reinisch JM. Would you say you "had sex" if . . . ? JAMA. 1999;281:275–7.

2. Horowitz A, Bedford E. Graded structure in sexual definitions: categorizations of having "had sex" and virginity loss among homosexual and heterosexual men and women. Archives of Sexual Behavior. 2016;46:1653–65.
3. Geuens S, Willems L, Nuyts E. What is sex? exploring the links between students definitions of sex and their safe-sex behavior., Own data, What is sex? (2018). https://www.researchgate.net/publication/366465249_Findings_descriptive_stats.
4. Randall HE, Byers ES. What is sex? Students' definitions of having sex, sexual partner, and unfaithful sexual behaviour. Can J Hum Sexuality. 2003;12:87–96.
5. Meston CM, Buss DM. Why humans have sex. Arch Sex Behav. 2007;36:477–507.
6. Tavares IM, Barros T, Rosen NO, et al. Is expectant couples' similarity in attitudes to sex during pregnancy linked to their sexual wellbeing? A dyadic study with response surface analysis. J Sex Res. 2021;58:1–13.
7. World Health Organisation. Sexual health. 2020. https://www.who.int/teams/sexual-and-reproductive-health-and-research/key-areas-of-work/sexual-health/defining-sexual-health.
8. Bolton D, Gillett G. The biopsychosocial model of health and disease, new philosophical and scientific developments. Cham: Springer Nature; 2019.
9. Buysse A, Caen M, Dewaele A, et al. Sexual health in flanders: [sexpert]. Gent: Academia Press; 2013.
10. World Association for Sexual Health. Declaration on sexual pleasure. 2019. https://worldsexualhealth.net/declaration-on-sexual-pleasure/.

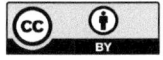

Relevant Sexual Anatomy, Physiology and Endocrinology

2

Gabrijela Simetinger (ID)

2.1 Introduction

To understand the physiology of sexual response, it is essential to have some basic knowledge of the genitals and other body parts associated with human sexual response. Since midwives and obstetric HCPs will be familiar with most of the anatomy and physiology of this area, this chapter will mainly focus on the aspects relevant to sexuality. Addressing the physiology and anatomy of 'the female sexual machinery' in detail is extra appropriate because of the many similarities between sexuality and reproduction. Sexual arousal resembles, in many ways, the circulatory changes of pregnancy. For example, childbirth, orgasm and breastfeeding have much in common, including hormonal control and being able 'to let go'.

The chapter will look at the various elements of anatomy and its changes over the different stages of pregnancy, including the relevant aspects and changes in physiology and endocrinology.

A great deal of the knowledge in this chapter is extracted from the books by Masters and Johnson and Bancroft. So no additional references to that information are given [1–3].

2.2 Female Anatomy

Female genitalia can be subdivided into the internal genitalia (vagina, cervix, uterus, fallopian tubes and the ovaries) and the external genitalia (vulva), including mons pubis, clitoris, the labia majora and minora which are the structures surrounding the urogenital cleft [4].

G. Simetinger (✉)
Department of Gynaecology and Obstetrics, General Hospital Novo mesto,
Novo mesto, Slovenia
e-mail: gabrijela.simetinger@sb-nm.si

© The Author(s) 2023
S. Geuens et al. (eds.), *Midwifery and Sexuality*,
https://doi.org/10.1007/978-3-031-18432-1_2

Mons pubis is the hair-covered area over the pubic bone which forms the antero-superior limit of the urogenital cleft and ends posteriorly at the anterior margin of the perineal body. Labia majora, called the outer lips, are the two prominent, fatty lateral boundaries of the urogenital cleft. Anteriorly they meet, creating the anterior commissure in front of the glans of the clitoris, posteriorly forming the posterior commissure. On the lateral surface, the outer lips have pigmented hairy, slightly wrinkled skin, and on the vaginal side, a smooth surface lined with multiple sebaceous glands. The outer labia often meet and close the vaginal introitus. Labia minora, here called the inner lips, can be smaller (or bigger) and may vary in size (length 61 ± 17 mm, width 22 ± 9 mm, range 7–50 mm). Anteriorly, they split into two layers forming the clitoral prepuce and the clitoral frenulum. They have no subcutaneous fat or hairs, contain elastic skin and erectile tissue with an appearance between smooth and extensively corrugated.

The gross clitoral structure is like an iceberg. A tiny part—the glans—is visible while the rest is hidden beneath the skin and deep. It is a three-dimensional complex of erectile and spongious tissues [5]. The best known is the midline shaft with glans (5–10 mm long) and clitoral body (10–60 mm long). It divides into two crura (25–70 mm long), bending sideways and laying close to the ischiopubic rami. From the clitoral shaft, the clitoral bulbs, also called vestibular bulbs (15–70 mm), bend on both sides around the vulvar entrance, under the outer lips.

The clitoral body and crura contain cavernous tissue (as in the male corpus cavernosum). The clitoral body can erect and bring the clitoris more in view when fully aroused. Just as in the male corpus spongiosum, the vestibular bulbs and the glans contain spongious tissue. The swollen bulbs softly narrow the vulvar entrance. A suspensory ligament connects the clitoral body to the symphysis.

Bilaterally, the ischiocavernosus muscles originate from the ischiopubic rami and insert onto the clitoral crura.

Although the clitoral hood or prepuce (comparable to the male foreskin) can be retracted, it usually covers the glans, preventing pain. Directly touching the very densely innervated glans tends to cause too much sensation.

The 'periurethral glans' is the triangular part of the vaginal vestibule that surrounds the urinary meatus, extending from below the clitoral glans to the vaginal introitus and laterally to the beginning of the inner lips. The vulvar vestibule includes the vulvar area between the inferior part of the clitoris, the medial aspect of the inner lips and the fourchette (the fold posteriorly connecting the inner lips) [4].

The hymen forms the boundary between the vulva and vagina. This usually thin (but sometimes thick) layer of tissue has mostly a crescent shape in young girls, but it can have many different forms. At puberty, the circumferential elasticity increases [6]. The hymen is the subject of much confusion and fear. It can be difficult to ascertain if penetration has taken place in children. From puberty, it is even for an experienced physician very difficult 'to prove virginity'. The first sexual intercourse/penetration is called defloration. That is usually not accompanied by blood loss, but it sometimes does, depending on the variety in anatomy. In the well-lubricated vulva, defloration is usually also not accompanied by pain (but sometimes it does). Most defloration pain results from a combination of fear and lack of lubrication.

The vagina is a tube collapsed in the non-aroused state, with an H-shaped cross-section. It is usually 10–11 cm in length to the depth of the posterior fornix. The deeper parts are more sensitive than the superficial parts [7], and the anterior wall is more sensitive than the posterior wall.

The pelvic floor is neither flat nor horizontal. It is called the levator ani muscle and consists of several distinct muscle groups, of which the iliococcygeus and pubococcygeus are the most important ones. In the resting state, they both support the vagina and rectum, and together with the presacral fascia, they form the levator plate.

The female genitals have a rich arterial blood supply. The internal pudendal artery and the superficial branch of the femoral artery supply the labia/lips. The clitoris receives its blood supply from the terminal part of the internal iliac artery, the common clitoral artery, which branches into the clitoral cavernosal and dorsal clitoral arteries. The uterine and hypogastric arteries supply the inner part of the vagina, and the clitoral and middle haemorrhoidal arteries the outer part [2, 4].

2.3   Male Anatomy

A rigid fibrous cylinder, the tunica albuginea, encapsulates a fused pair of corpora cavernosa. These sponge-like vascular spaces of erectile tissue form the shaft or body of the penis. See Fig. 2.1.

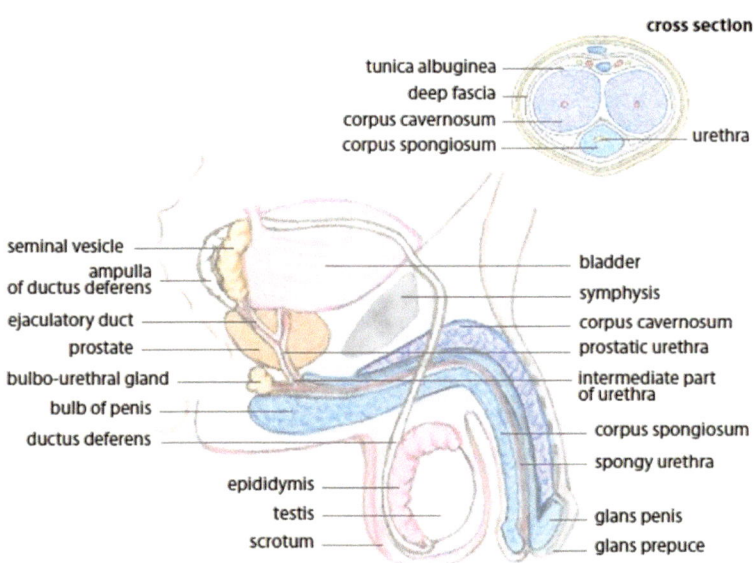

Fig. 2.1 The male anatomy. (Illustration composed by Gabrijela Simetinger and Helena Černej)

That cylinder combines an inner space that can fill up with blood (like an inner tube) and a robust outside enclosure (like a tyre), making the critical structure for a rigid, fully erect penis. The root of the penis is attached to a muscular layer, the bulbospongiosus and ischiocavernosus muscles. They contract voluntarily and semi-voluntarily during the development of erection and also rhythmically during orgasm. Beneath the two fused corpora cavernosa lies the corpus spongiosum, which envelops the urethra in its course along the lower surface of the penis. Near the tip of the penis, the corpus spongiosum expands into the glans.

In the uncircumcised male, a hood of lax skin, the prepuce or foreskin, covers the glans. A longitudinal fold of skin, the frenulum, attaches the prepuce to the glands on the lower surface. Beyond the dilated urethral bulb and before its junction with the urinary bladder, the male urethra transverses the prostate gland, a firm fibromuscular structure with glands contributing accessory fluid to the ejaculate. The penis receives its blood supply from the internal pudendal artery, one of the terminal branches of the internal iliac artery.

The testicles/male gonads lie in the scrotum, a superficial pouch of skin and muscle. Within the scrotum, the position of the testicles is controlled by the cremaster and dartos muscles, responsible for keeping the testis at a lower body temperature by actively changing their distance to the body. A long, convoluted tubule, the epididymis, bends over the testis and ends in the ductus deferens leading to the prostate gland. The final maturation of the sperm cells takes place in the epididymis. Behind the bladder and the prostate gland lie the seminal vesicles, elongated sacs that secrete accessory fluid needed for sperm viability.

2.4   The Nerve Supply to the Genitalia in Men and Women

The genitalia and pelvic floor muscles are regulated by the sympathetic and parasympathetic nervous system (pelvic nerves, hypogastric nerve, paravertebral sympathetic chains) and by the (somatic) pudendal nerve. These nerves convey impulses from the brain and spinal cord to control motor, secretory and vascular functions or mediate pleasurable or painful sensations. The autonomic nerves regulate blood flow and the involuntary smooth-muscle contractions that may accompany arousal, while the somatic nerves control the voluntary or striated muscle responses that often occur during orgasm. Sensory input from the genitalia or brain can facilitate arousal and orgasmic responses. Both somatic and autonomic systems mediate these processes. The pelvic and pudendal nerves convey the afferent (sensory) and efferent (motor) information during the urogenital reflexes. The pudendal (somatic) nerve conveys sensory stimuli from the perineum, penis, clitoris, urethra and pelvic floor musculature. The dorsal nerve of the clitoris is tiny and the most distal branch of the pudendal nerve. It terminates in a plexus of nerve endings within the substance of the glans and the corpora cavernosa.

2.5   Endocrinology of Sexual Response

Pre-pubertal boys and girls differ in their behaviour. Culture and education can explain that, but only for a minor part. Hormones form the more significant part of the explanation. However, before puberty, neither boys nor girls have gonadal hormones. The explanation lies at a much earlier moment, during intra-uterine life. The default is the development of a female baby. At ±8 weeks of pregnancy, an XY chromosome pattern encourages the cells that have to become the testes producing testosterone (T). That T is responsible for the male anatomy and different connections in the brain [1]. This neural development during intra-uterine life, called 'the dimorphic wiring of the brains', is responsible for many female-male differences in behaviour.

Despite much research, we still do not fully understand the influence of the various hormones, neuropeptides and neurotransmitters on sexual activity. The information is more evident in male sexuality than in female sexuality. And more evident in the non-pregnant woman than during pregnancy.

Testosterone ('T') appears to be the most important hormone for sexual activity, directly influencing desire and indirectly via mood and energy. Higher T-levels increase arousability, sexual fantasies and sexual activity. Sexual activity (f.i. intercourse) also increases the T-levels in men and women. In women who are not using hormonal contraception, sexual thoughts also increase their T-levels [8].

Oxytocin, well-known in obstetrics, has a relevant role in sexuality, with the levels increasing during sexual arousal and at orgasm.

Prolactin, a peptide hormone with an important role in lactation, also appears to have a role in sexuality. After orgasm, there is a rise in prolactin level, reducing sexual desire. The same happens during the high prolactin levels in the lactating woman. That 'sexual inhibition' of prolactin is supposed to act via inhibition of dopaminergic activity.

Men and women differ very much in hormonal fluctuations over time. Both have a diurnal fluctuation with the highest level of gonadal hormones in the morning. Otherwise, the male hormone levels are very predictable/stable (or dull), which is one reason why most medical research is done on men.

On the other hand, women experience significant changes in gonadal hormone levels between puberty and menopause every month, eventually interspersed by extensive periods of pregnancy and breastfeeding and contraceptive use, all influencing body and mind. That makes women far more complex (or exciting) and less predictable, with more significant risks of depression and less reliability for research.

2.5.1   Women

Testosterone   Compared to male sexuality, the influence of T on female sexuality is less clear. One explanation is that women appear far more influenced by context and co-existing psychological and affective factors and partly by the wide individual variation in sensitivity to testosterone. In women, higher T-levels are linked to more solitary desire and higher masturbation frequency and less dyadic desire (but that is only when controlled for cortisol and perceived social stress). Besides, testosterone has a relevant influence on mood, energy and arousability.

Estradiol is essential for vaginal health. Whereas the levels are very high during pregnancy, they decrease sharply after the birth, especially when the woman is breastfeeding. The resulting vaginal atrophy is comparable to the vaginal atrophy of many women during menopause. It is tempting to explain that atrophy responsible for dyspareunia (pain at intercourse). However, dyspareunia usually results from insufficient lubrication, caused by lower arousability, poor couple communication and poor sexual stimulation.

Oxytocin, one of the peptides, has multiple reproductive roles. During lactation, it facilitates the milk ejection reflex. During parturition, it stimulates uterine contractions. On the other hand, oxytocin levels increase at high arousal and during orgasm in several inter-related ways. An example is sexual stimulation during parturition enhancing uterine contractions. Whereas an orgasm in the lactating woman can give milk outflow, breastfeeding can create pleasurable sensations in the uterine area and sometimes even orgasm.

Intra-partum pressure on the cervix and vaginal wall (by the penis, the examining fingers or the fetal head) causes an increase in oxytocin levels (the 'Ferguson reflex'), enabling bearing down.

Beta-endorphin, another neuropeptide with pain-reducing properties, has relations to birth and sexuality. Higher oxytocin levels appear to provoke ß-endorphin release, increasing the pain threshold. Outside and during pregnancy and labour, stimulation of the clitoris and anterior vaginal wall increases the pain threshold, especially when accompanied by orgasm.

2.5.2   Men

Testosterone plays a vital role in men, both for sexual desire, arousability (the ability to become 'horny'), sexual fantasy and spontaneous (nocturnal and early morning) erections.

Male T-levels appear influenced by reproduction and fatherhood. When a couple tries to conceive, the man will develop a monthly T-increase towards the middle of the woman's hormonal cycle.

In the second half of pregnancy, the male T-level will decrease (and in some men, the oestrogen level will increase), which can be a reason for lower sexual desire.

After the (first) birth, the T-level stays lower than before pregnancy, possibly making the man react better when the baby cries. So, male T-levels differ depending on the man's social role, being the lowest in young fathers, higher in childless partnered men and the highest in single men.

2.6   Sexual Response and Sexual Function

When Masters and Johnson started their research on sexuality in the laboratory, they described the visible sexual responses of the body in a model with arousal, plateau phase, orgasm and resolution [1]. Later, researchers added the phase of sexual desire. In common sexology, the plateau phase and resolution phases are rarely relevant, so one tends to use the model with desire-arousal-orgasm for sexual function. However, in pregnancy, the resolution phase is relevant because it coincides with the increasing genital hypercongestion.

Sexology defines physiological sexual arousal in humans as increased autonomic activation that prepares the body for sexual activity. It includes parasympathetic blood flow to genital and erectile tissues, particularly the clitoris, labia, vaginal epithelium and penis, and sympathetic blood flow from the heart to various striated and smooth muscles that participate in the sexual response [2].

Sexual arousal also includes a central component that increases neural 'tone' or preparedness to respond to sexual incentives. This is also called 'the arousability of the sexual system'. The person can perceive peripheral and central arousal as subjective sexual arousal, which can enhance the responsiveness of the genital tissues and influence specific copulatory responses, such as the latency to orgasm or ejaculation. In other words, more arousal, faster orgasm or ejaculation [4].

Between women and men, there are several apparent differences.

Desire   Being relatively strongly determined by hormones, sexual desire tends to be higher in men (with their far higher T-levels).

Arousal   Male genital arousal (erection) is unmistakable visible (present or absent), whereas many women even do not know if they are lubricated (wet) or not.

That corresponds with the erection as an essential part of the male identity. Having no erection 'when needed' makes many men insecure. Having no lubrication is, for women, far less critical. It can be remedied by saliva or another lubricant and usually does not impair her female identity. It can also cause pain, but that does not pose a significant problem if it does not become part of a vicious pain circle.

Orgasm in men is accompanied by a refractory period after which he cannot restart immediately, whereas an estimated 50% of women can have more than one orgasm in a short period.

Male orgasm easily happens premature ('too fast'), which, in women, is very exceptional.

2.6.1   Female Genital Sexual Response

Physiologic changes during sexual activity start with increased blood flow ('engorgement') to the genitals, causing vaginal lubrication (=lubrification or 'getting wet'). The vagina lengthens and dilates due to smooth muscle relaxation. The increased blood flow to the clitoris increases intra-cavernous pressure, tumescence and protrusion of the glans clitoris, next to unfolding ('eversion') and congestion of the inner lips.

Outer lips When arousal in the nulliparous woman increases, the outer lips thin out and flatten against the perineum. The anatomic displacement of the outer lips is caused by a protrusion of the rapidly engorging inner lips and vasocongestion of the external third of the vagina. At orgasm, there is no change in the outer lips. After orgasm, involution of the outer lips occurs rapidly, returning them to their standard thickness and midline positioning. When arousal is maintained longer, the outer lips can become severely engorged with venous blood and sometimes even develop oedema, which may persist for several hours after cessation of all sexual stimulation. The outer lips react to arousal in the multiparous woman and become distended with venous blood. They increase 2–3× in diameter and hang swollen as a partial curtain to the vaginal outlet.

Inner lips At genuine arousal, they increase at least 2–3 times in diameter, adding to the clinical length of the vaginal cylinder. With increasing arousal, the colour of the inner lips changes from pink to bright red or a deep vine colour. This florid colouration diffuses along both sides of the vaginal outlet, usually including the clitoral hood area. The more intense the degree of pelvic and labial hypercongestion, the darker the colour. Short before orgasm, the inner lips form a turgid cuff, which narrows and elongates the outer third of the vaginal canal. The change of both lips results in opening the vaginal outlet by removing the natural anatomic protection of the vaginal orifice. The skin colouration signifies intense sexual arousal, clinically a sign of impending orgasm. After orgasm, the intense colouration of the skin returns from deep or bright red to light pink in 10–15 s. If the woman does not 'reach' orgasm, the colouration of the inner lips will fade rapidly, long before the resolution of the vasocongestive diameter increase.

The clitoris This is probably the only organ in the human body with the generation of pleasure as its only function (see Fig. 2.2). During sexual arousal, the central

Fig. 2.2 The clitoris in the female anatomy. (Illustration composed by Gabrijela Simetinger and Helena Černej)

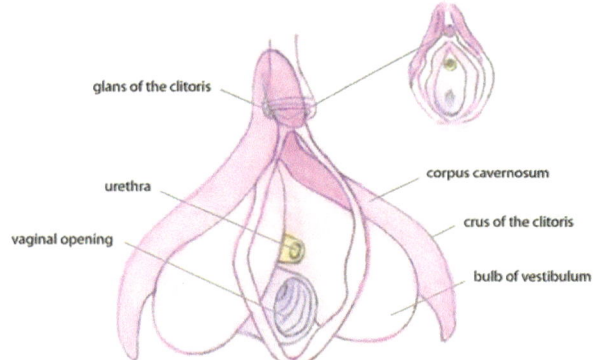

glans of the clitoris

urethra

vaginal opening

corpus cavernosum

crus of the clitoris

bulb of vestibulum

reduction of sympathetic tone and the release of vasodilator neurotransmitters increase the blood flow to the clitoris and relax the smooth muscles of the clitoral cavities, by which they are filled with blood. Sexual stimulation will cause the clitoral glans to become tumescent, with a speed depending on the intensity of whatever sexual stimulation is experienced. Once observable tumescence develops, the engorgement persists as long as any significant degree of sexual stimulation is maintained. Short before orgasm (in the plateau phase), the entire clitoral body (shaft and glans) retracts from its normal pudendal overhanging positioning. After orgasm, the clitoris returns to its normal position within 5–10 s.

The vagina Within 10–30 s after any sexual stimulation, the vagina produces lubricating fluid. Sexual stimulation causes the capillaries of the micro-circulation in the vaginal wall to fill with blood. The increased hydrostatic pressure forces plasma to transudate into the interstitial space around the blood vessels, causing the fluid passing through and between the cells of vaginal epithelium and leaking through the surface of the vaginal wall as vaginal lubrication ('getting wet'). With increasing sexual arousal, the inner two-thirds of the vaginal cylinder lengthens and distends, and the surface changes into a darker, purplish colour. During orgasm, the outer third of the vagina, pelvic muscles and anal sphincter contract powerfully in a regularly recurring (clonic) pattern. After orgasm, the vasocongestion disperses rapidly, and all the other changes disappear within 15 min.

The uterus In the late-excitement phase, the uterus and cervix are elevated upwards, away from the posterior floor of the vagina. This phenomenon, called 'tenting', is supposed to have a function in conception since in the ordinary ('missionary') intercourse position, it removes the cervix away from the expected 'sperm pool', which should prevent too early contact of the cervix with the not-yet-liquefied semen [9].

2.6.2 Male Genital Sexual Response

The penis, scrotum and rectum are very sensitive and respond to effective sexual stimulation by vasoconstriction and elevated muscle tone. During arousal, secretion comes from the bulbourethral (Cowper's) glands, which lie on each side of the urethra, and from the urethral glands, along the penile part of the urethra. This fluid lubricates the glans and can show (as 'pre-cum') before ejaculation occurs. Living sperm is regularly found in this fluid, making the withdrawal method of contraception (coitus interruptus) risky.

In the uncircumcised man, the foreskin can, during erection, become partially retracted along the elongated penile shaft, exposing the tip of the glans and urethral orifice. During penetrating, the foreskin of the uncircumcised penis usually glides backwards, allowing the slippery glans to enter without pain for both woman and man.

Erection Sexual stimuli cause parasympathetic signals to the muscular fibres in the cavernous body. Their relaxation causes engorgement with blood that first creates fullness and then hardness due to the tight encapsulation of the tunica albuginea and the compression of the veins.

Ejaculation This occurs under sympathetic control. The sperm starts from the epididymis, gets supporting additions from the seminal vesicles (alkaline) and the prostate, and is forcefully expelled to and through the urethral meatus. Regularly recurring contractions take place in the bulbospongiosus, ischiocavernosus and transverse superficial and deep perineal muscles and the urethral sphincter, with ejaculatory contractions involving the entire length of the penile urethra. After ejaculation, penile detumescence occurs. After ejaculation follows a refractory period, which is needed for restoring the supporting fluids for the sperm cells.

Orgasm For experiencing orgasm, a signal is sent from the centres in the spinal cord to the brain. Though most men consider orgasm and ejaculation identical, they are not. A few men can have several orgasms in a row as long as there is no ejaculation.

Semen An average ejaculation is 5 mL (i.e. two teaspoons) and contains 20–150 million sperm cells per mL. Yet ±70% comes from the seminal vesicles and ±30% from the prostate. That is why, after vasectomy, the man does not have less semen.

2.6.3 Extragenital Sexual Response

The human physiologic response to sexual stimulation involves many areas other than the primary or secondary organs of reproduction. Physical signs of sexual arousal occur in the entire body, with superficial and deep vasocongestion and generalised and specific myotonia. Generalised muscle tension appears in the hands, feet and abdomen, and specific muscle tension in the bulbospongiosus and ischiocavernosus muscles and the rectal sphincter.

The female breasts The first sign of arousal is the erection of the nipple (in full arousal, an increase of 5–10 mm) and an increase in venous flush, shown as a skin rash. Later in arousal, the areola becomes swollen, by which the nipple erection seems to diminish. With full arousal, the breast volume can increase by 20–25%. After having breastfed one baby, that increase in volume during arousal is less. After having nursed two babies, there is no more arousal-related volume increase. Before orgasm, a maculopapular rash appears over the epigastrium and the breast surface. After orgasm, the skin rash quickly disappears, just as the areolar swelling, by which the nipple erection seems to return.

The male breasts In part of the males, nipple erection and tumescence can happen. In half of the men, stimulation of the nipples increases their arousal.

In both sexes, the superficial vasocongestive reaction is called sex flush. This sex flush can spread over the breast, lower abdomen, shoulders and even the inner skin of the elbows (antecubital fossa) when sexual arousal mounts. After orgasm, it disappears.

High muscular tension (myotonia) is seen late in the arousal phase, both generalised and specific. Various muscles contract with regularity or involuntary spasms, but the contractions are frequently also voluntary, depending on the coital position.

In women, the external meatus of the urethra can show occasional involuntary widening during orgasm. Due to the nulliparous structures (firm perineum and constriction of the vaginal outlet), the posterior wall of the urinary bladder can be irritated by penile thrusting, causing postcoital dysuria, a complication sometimes known as 'honeymoon cystitis'.

During the arousal phase, voluntary contractions of the external rectal sphincter are visible in women and involuntary contractions in men. Involuntary contraction of the rectum occurs during orgasm and ejaculation in both sexes.

Hyperventilation, tachycardia and elevation of systolic blood pressure increase directly when sexual arousal increases. Involuntary perspiration may develop during the post-orgasmic phase independent of the degree of physical activity.

2.7 Sexual Response in Pregnancy

Pregnancy markedly increases the vascularity of the pelvic organs. The fetal support system creates gross vasodilatation in the female pelvis. Any physiologic response to sexual stimulation on top of that further increases the massive pelvic vasocongestion. That superposition of sexual arousal on top of pregnancy hypercongestion can reach high levels during the second and can continue well into the third trimester. During the second trimester, part of the pregnant women has an increase in sexual drive, with more need for coital and other sexual stimulation and sometimes intense orgasmic experiences. The female reproductive organs alter significantly during pregnancy. Those changes are predominantly related to intense generalised pelvic vasocongestion. Therefore, the vasocongestive response is a much more significant factor in pregnancy than the development of myotonia. During arousal, both inner and outer lips become very engorged, with the outer lips even becoming edematous. Towards the end of the first trimester, there is a definitive increase in the production of vaginal lubrication, which continues throughout pregnancy. After elevation of the uterus into the abdomen, sexual stimuli cause the same vaginal expansion and distension as in the non-pregnant state. The further pregnancy develops, the more severe the venous engorgement of the entire vaginal barrel becomes, and the more advanced the secondary development of the orgasmic platform in response to sexual stimulation. It can develop to such an extent that the lateral vaginal walls meet in the midline in severe vasocongestive response to high sexual excitement, with the entrance sometimes becoming completely anaesthetic or painful.

One can observe orgasmic platform contractions as specific physiologic evidence of orgasm during the first and the second trimester of pregnancy. During the third trimester, one can barely observe them because of the vasocongestion of the vulvar entrance, although the woman subjectively feels the contractions.

Whereas regular, clonic contractions typically accompany an orgasm, the contraction pattern can change into one long-lasting tonic contraction during the last trimester. Spastic contraction may occasionally cause fetal heart tones to become slower, but this reaction is transitory. No further evidence of fetal distress has been demonstrated.

After orgasm, the pelvic vasocongestion is not entirely relieved (in other words: there is no complete resolution). The pregnant women who is in the Masters and Johnson laboratory study repeatedly got an orgasm did not get complete relief from their sexual arousal levels for a significant time, although their orgasms were objectively most intense and subjectively quite satisfying [1].

In the second and third trimester, residual pelvic vasocongestion and the high 'pelvic pressure' (of the heavy uterus) may cause maintained high levels of sexual arousal in part of the women.

2.7.1 The Breasts

During the first trimester, the breasts rapidly increase in size due to the developing vascular and glandular beds. When the nulliparous woman responds to sexual stimuli in the first trimester of her pregnancy, venous congestion of the breasts is more evident than in a non-pregnant state. This superposition of sexual arousal and pregnancy can cause pain frequently localised in turgid nipples and engorged areolar elements. During the second and third trimesters of pregnancy, there is less reduction in breast tenderness. Reactions of nipple erection and areolar tumescence remain constant through all three trimesters of pregnancy.

2.8 Post-partum Physiology and Sexual Response

Immediately post-partum, many changes occur with critical roles for uterine involution and hormonal switches and, in addition, many hormonal consequences for the breastfeeding woman.

The weight of the uterus decreases from 1.000 g immediately after birth to 500 g after 1 week and back to 60 g in 6 weeks. Extensive venous congestion accompanies that process, responsible for the 'full feeling' comparable to the hypercongestion in the second and third trimester. For some women, this appears to promote sexual feelings [1].

The high levels of oestrogen and progesterone during pregnancy decrease towards the end of pregnancy to drop sharply after birth. With expelling the placenta, the placental hormones disappear, causing a steep increase in prolactin levels, which, without breastfeeding, will be back to pre-pregnancy levels in one week. For the other women, breastfeeding will cause high prolactin levels. Prolactin directly diminishes sexual desire. It keeps the oestrogen levels low, causing vaginal atrophy and the T-levels low, causing low desire and arousability, fatigue and low mood.

Although this sounds rather bleak for part of the breastfeeding mothers, the outcome is more favourable for others. Breastfeeding has a dual effect on sexuality, causing for some an increase in sexual sensations and even orgasm, or an increased sense of femininity and partner contact. Other women can be so absorbed by the intimacy with the baby that sexuality seems forgotten. The outcome can be somewhat problematic when that gets combined with vaginal atrophy and low arousability and a partner who needs penetration sex to solve his internal tensions.

2.9   Conclusion

One can read this extensive explanation of anatomy, physiology and endocrinology just as an additional technical package of knowledge for reproduction healthcare professionals. However, this chapter also intends to increase awareness of the simultaneous multitude of influences these processes can have on sexuality and intimacy. Sexuality and reproduction are, after all, very strongly intertwined.

The choreography of birth, a female sexual encounter and breastfeeding have many aspects in common. It is not surprising that some women experience birth (nearly) as an orgasm, some women have experienced an orgasm just because of breastfeeding and breasts can start leaking during sexual arousal. In the same way, it is not surprising that oxytocin, the essential 'bonding hormone' in breastfeeding, also increases during sexual play and orgasm.

Thus, adequate knowledge of the sexual system's functioning seems relevant for midwives and obstetric HCPs to adequately address the sexual health needs of the woman and the couple from pre-conception through young parenthood.

References

1. Masters HW, Johnson VE. Human sexual response. Boston: Little, Brown and Company; 1966.
2. Bancroft J. The endocrinology of sexual arousal. J Endocrinol. 2005;186:411–27.
3. Bancroft J. Human sexuality and its problems. 3rd ed. Edinburgh: Churchill Livingstone; 2009.
4. Montorsi F, Basson R, Adaikan G, et al., editors. Sexual medicine, sexual dysfunction in men and women. Paris: Edition; 2010.
5. Jackson LA, Hare AM, Carrick KS, et al. Anatomy, histology, and nerve density of clitoris and associated structures: clinical applications to vulvar surgery. Am J Obstet Gynecol. 2019;221(519):e1–9.

6. Pokorny SF, Murphy JG, Preminger MK. Circumferential hymen elasticity. A marker of physi-
    ologic maturity. J Reprod Med. 1998;43:943–8.
7. Bronselaer G, Callens N, De Sutter P, et al. Self-assessment of genital anatomy and sexual
    function within a Belgian, Dutch-speaking female population: a validation study. J Sex Med.
    2013;10:3006–18.
8. Goldey KL, van Anders SM. Sexy thoughts: effects of sexual cognitions on testosterone, corti-
    sol, and arousal in women. Horm Behav. 2011;59:754–64.
9. Levin RJ. Can the controversy about the putative role of the human female orgasm in
    sperm transport be settled with our current physiological knowledge of coitus? J Sex Med.
    2011;8:1566–78.

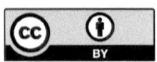

How Sex Works (and When it's not Working)

3

Sam Geuens ⓘ and Ana Polona Mivšek ⓘ

Sex is one of the central aspects of the human condition and one of the driving factors of our evolution as a species. It is a necessary element of midwifery because, aside from modern medical-assisted reproduction techniques, there will be no pregnancies without sex.

Various publications have clarified that midwives need expertise—both skills and knowledge—concerning human sexuality. This chapter will broadly focus on how sex works and when sex is not working, both on an individual and couple level. Other chapters of this book will tackle sexuality and sexual health from a more biological, psychological or social perspective, concerning different parts of the midwife's field of practice—from pre-conception to young parenthood.

What makes sex work? Can we define parameters for promoting satisfying sexual experiences or understanding how sexual experiences can be disappointing or frustrating, e.g. when sex does not work?

This chapter strives to go beyond the mere description of models of sexual response [1] and aims to outline a simple to use '3-Conditions Framework', describing the necessary conditions that sexual experiences have to meet to be 'good'. 'Good' meaning pleasant, satisfying, fulfilling, bonding, fun or whatever one wants it to be.

S. Geuens (✉)
Department of Healthcare - Midwifery, PXL University College of Applied Arts and Sciences, Hasselt, Belgium

Outpatient Center for Sexual Health, Saint Franciscus Hospital, Heusden-Zolder, Belgium
e-mail: sam.geuens@pxl.be

A. Polona Mivšek
Faculty of Health Studies, University of Ljubljana, Ljubljana, Slovenia
e-mail: polona.mivsek@zf.uni-lj.si

3.1   The 3-Conditions Framework for satisfying sexual experiences

We propose a simple framework for how sex works, outlining three more or less essential requirements for a satisfying sexual experience: (1) a sufficiently intact and functioning sexual system; (2) 'good enough' sexual stimuli and (3) a 'comfortable' context.

When one fully understands these three conditions, it enables the HCP to translate them towards diverse human sexual practices. They then can serve as a framework for exploring clients' sexual problems in counselling (e.g. by actively exploring these three conditions), as a mini-diagnostical tool (e.g. helping to understand which condition(s) are likely causing/maintaining the sexual problems) and as a framework for promoting sexual wellbeing (e.g. as a psycho-education tool).

This chapter will first explain the '3-conditions framework' and then successively address its use as a counselling tool, diagnostic tool and psycho-educational tool.

3.1.1   What Makes for Good Sex?

What does one need for good sex? What is the right way to stimulate women/men sexually? What is required to be sexually satisfied? If one tries to answer these questions factually, the result would likely be a useless list of sexual practices that might work for a given woman, her partner or a given couple. If we were to ask 100 people what they would need to have a good sexual experience, we would wind up with 100 personal sexual guide books. At best, one could read someone else's guide as a source of inspiration. In the margin of this chapter, this might be a personally enlightening exercise for each HCP in a committed relationship.

The question then becomes: what are the conditions for people to have pleasurable sexual experiences? We recommend approaching this on a meta-level to understand what is needed to make any sexual experience satisfying. The three most relevant conditions are the sexual system, the stimuli and the context.

3.1.2   An Intact and Functioning Sexual System

Sex requires activity in multiple brain regions. The hippocampus, hypothalamus and amygdala play a central role in routing and rerouting signals related to sexuality [2]. These signals travel through nerve bundles, connecting the brain with relevant erogenous zones (genitals, breasts, nipples, mouth, skin, neck, ears, feet, etc.) [3]. If one of the links in this chain of information-sharing is malfunctioning, the entire system can become stressed, sometimes even making certain aspects of sexual experiences impossible. A person's nervous system, endocrine system, genitalia, sensory organs, skin, hands, lips, tongue, etc. need to be intact and functioning, at least up to a certain level. In other words: one needs to be able to register internal and external sexual stimuli (fantasies or desires, seeing a beautiful man/woman, feeling someone lightly brush your neck, etc.) and all internal systems and organs that play a part in the elicited sexual response need to be functioning enough.

One can immediately understand that any pathology or medical intervention that can impact the normal functioning of the nervous system, endocrine system or senses can influence how we experience sexuality. Think, for instance, of the negative effect high prolactin and low testosterone levels during breastfeeding can have on sexual desire and sexual arousability. Or think of the negative impact genito-pelvic pain caused by endometriosis can have on one's sexual experiences.

Still, it is important to note that the physical system does not have to be in pristine condition to enable people to have pleasurable sex. Many people continue enjoying sex despite e.g. being on anti-depressants, suffering from genital pathology, having a chronic disease, being blind, sitting in a wheelchair because of a spinal cord injury, etc.

One's sexual system does not have to be 100%, but it has to function sufficiently to allow people to experience what they want to experience.

3.1.3 Good Sexual Stimuli

Every system has its start-up requirements. Our sexual system is no different. It needs the input of sexual stimuli to get going and keep going. These stimuli can be internal (like memories, thoughts or fantasies) and external (like sound, touch, scents or just seeing someone you find attractive, hot or sexy). Both can do the job equally well. Most people have a general idea of which stimuli are the most valuable for themselves [4].

For most people in a stable relationship, the partner is an important source of various sexual stimuli. Partners can evoke erotic thoughts or fantasies, look really sexy when dressed in the right way (or not at all) or be the one who lights those lovely scented candles.

Stimuli are abundantly available. However, even when exposed to a potentially good stimulus, you still have to *experience it in a sexual way*. One's brain has to give sexual meaning and thus sexually validate a stimulus. In other words: allow oneself to interpret it sexually.

Whether or not this will occur will largely depend on one's personal background and frame of reference regarding sexuality. So the way people think about sex, their ideas and conceptions about sex, what is sexy, what is fun and so on, will largely determine if potential sexual stimuli will effectively become sexual stimuli for that person. So, the better you know your own and your partner's 'sexual frame of reference' (also called 'lovemap'), the easier it will be to find the proper stimuli to jumpstart your sexual system or your partner's.

The bottom line is that we need stimuli to get our sexual system going, but we have to experience' them as sexual stimuli to have the desired effect.

3.1.4   A Comfortable Context

Even after fulfilling the first two conditions, one still needs the proper context for the situation to develop in the desired sexual way.

When people feel their physical sexual system is starting up, and desire and arousal are building, time and place have to be suitable for that person to actually do something with those feelings. And again, independent of whether time and place is in reality fit for sex, it has to feel right. Both the physical context, your surroundings, and one's internal context, in other words one's mindset need to be good enough to allow our brain to see stimuli as sexual. When your mind is elsewhere, occupied with non-sexual thoughts, or when your previous (negative) experiences or beliefs come into the mix, even potentially stimulating surroundings to act upon your desire could be transformed into 'not-comfortable-enough' to proceed to a satisfying sexual experience.

3.1.5   The '3-Conditions Framework' as a Communication Tool

For many midwives and other HCPs, sexuality is not an easy topic to address. Midwives might feel personal barriers and think it is inappropriate to ask actively about sexual wellbeing or fear invading the intimacy of the couple's relationship. Still, research shows that women and men expect the HCP to start a conversation about sexual health, as they too feel the challenge of addressing such a taboo-laden topic [5]. Chapter 26 will offer the midwife/HCP a step-by-step plan, the 'one-to-one method', for starting a conversation with the woman (or couple) on sexuality-related topics. The second step in that model is: *'Let her tell her own story'*. The woman can, for instance, be invited talk about sexuality by asking about her current situation's biological, psychological and social aspects or exploring her ideas, concerns and expectations relating to her sexual life. Here we can also use the '3-conditions framework' to enable the client to explain her current situation fully. By actively asking the client about her physical health in relation to sexuality, the presence of sexual stimuli and by exploring how their experiencing the context, the client and her partner start to already paint a broader picture of their sexual life at that moment in time.

3.1.6   The '3-Conditions Framework' as a Diagnostic Tool in Case of Sexual Problems

The midwife does not always have the skills and knowledge to diagnose the sexual problems of her client accurately. On the other hand, this is far from always necessary.

We can trace most sexual problems to a disturbance of one or more of the three conditions for pleasurable sex. Either the physical sexual system is impaired (e.g. hormonal changes during breastfeeding), or the stimuli are insufficient to trigger desire and arousal (e.g. perception of a partner as less attractive due to excess weight gain) or the context is not comfortable enough (e.g. fear that the baby will start crying).

By actively exploring the three conditions for pleasurable sex, the midwife can gain a rudimentary idea of what might be causing the sexual difficulties, which will help her decide on the strategy, provide the necessary psychoeducation or other interventions to help the couple tackle their problem or refer to another HCP for specialised treatment.

3.1.7   The '3-Conditions Framework' as a Psycho-Education Tool

The couples that remain sexually satisfied during pregnancy tend to have greater sexual and relational wellbeing during the challenging post-partum period. This is a solid argument for pro-actively addressing sexuality in pregnant couples and counselling on how to keep their sex life satisfactory, which is not an easy challenge in a changing relationship, with a changing body, etc. [6] (see also Chap. 6).

One way to do so is by already actively discussing the three conditions for satisfying sex with the couple early in pregnancy. That can make them aware of how various changes can affect their sexual relationship.

With enough stimuli available and regularly a context allowing them to act upon their sexual desire, the sexual response will probably follow. Helping couples in this way to actively think about their sex life can enhance mutual understanding, which e.g. can facilitate acceptance of differences in desire. Understanding why each partner behaves in a certain way can help the couple deal with tense and tricky situations and prevent developing frustrations. The midwife can lay the foundation for prolonged sexual and relationship happiness by enabling this, resulting in greater overall health and wellbeing during pregnancy and post-partum (and probably during later parenthood).

It is, however, essential to recognise that people's experiences might differ when their physical sexual system is not functioning optimally or when e.g. physical stimulation occurs in the 'wrong context', for instance a non-sexual, or even negative context.

3.2   When Sex Is Not Working

The '3-conditions framework', as described above, can help understand why people are experiencing sexual difficulties. Decades of research delineated various conditions making sex difficult or even impossible to enjoy. These so-called sexual dysfunctions have been officially adopted as clinical diagnoses in the DSM V and the ICD11, internationally used systems for diagnostic descriptions. The DSM V describes them as follows:

> *Sexual dysfunctions are a heterogeneous group of disorders that are typically characterised by a clinically significant disturbance in a person's ability to respond sexually or to experience sexual pleasure.*

For calling something a sexual problem, it should cause distress to the person and/or their partner.

The rest of this chapter will give an overview of known sexual dysfunctions, starting with problems of sexual desire, moving on to problems with sexual arousal, orgasm problems, sexual pain problems and finish with some sexual problems that deserve special attention. Each of the sexual problems will be linked to the '3-conditions model', explaining how the model could show the cause of that problem. We will also address the sexual problem's relevance to midwifery practice.

Clinical practice indicates that people sometimes have problems in their physical, sexual functioning but are still perfectly sexually satisfied. Labelling something as 'problematic' instead of 'dysfunctional' induces a mindset with the client that makes treatment more manageable, given that 'when one has a problem, we just have to find a solution', whereas labelling something as 'dysfunctional' gives the impression that something is 'malfunctioning' or even 'broken', which is often not the case when women or couples present with sexual distress. Hence we favour the term 'sexual problem' above the clinical term 'sexual dysfunction'.[1]

3.2.1 Problems with Sexual Desire

Problems with sexual desire can arise when people experience not enough or too much sexual desire. The logical question becomes: what is not enough or too much? At this point, the interpersonal distress aspect comes in. It will become a problem when a woman or her partner experiences distress because of a low level or even no sexual desire. In the same way, a high level of sexual desire can become a problem when it causes distress in the relationship. Culturally and clinically, too low desire levels are typically associated with women and too high desire levels with men. Still, it is essential to note that gender is not an absolute defining factor in sexual desire. Women can experience distress because of high levels of sexual desire too, just as men can experience problems because of low levels or no sexual desire. In a partner relationship, the discrepancy between the levels of sexual desire can cause problems if the difference is experienced as too large. Such problems with differences in sexual desire can occur at all points in life, including during pregnancy and post-partum. It is also worth noting that differences in sexual desire can also be about the nature of sexual desire.

Viewed through the lens of the '3-conditions framework' sexual desire problems can e.g. arise from lack or abundance of suitable sexual stimuli, from the idea that there is seldom a proper context, or that almost any context is seen as fit for a sexual experiences.

---

[1] Be aware: sexual and relational problems can coincide and be related but they do not have to be. Couples with a very good relationship can have very poor sex. And very exciting, satisfying sex happens also in people who barely have a relationship.

3.2.2 Problems with Sexual Arousal

Problems with sexual arousal can arise when the body has difficulties generating enough physical arousal. The cardiovascular system, numerous muscles and neurotransmitters have to cooperate to create general and genital arousal. Also, without sufficient subjective arousal, in other words enough feelings of arousal, lubrication or erection will fail.

In midwifery, think of the role sexual arousal plays in boosting one's chances of conception. Good vaginal lubrication is needed for proper movement and viability of the sperm cells, and a good erection is required for intra-vaginal ejaculation (see also Chap. 5).

A common mistake is to focus on the most visible symptom women experience when arousal is not always running smoothly. Lack of arousal often translates into a lack of vaginal lubrication and pain. So, when a woman presents with pain during intercourse, we have to address both feelings of arousal and physical arousal.

Erections can fail in several ways: no erections, erections disappearing too soon or not getting hard enough for penetration. This will only become a problem when causing (inter-)personal distress. A prerequisite for the body to start generating physical arousal is the presence of enough effective sexual stimuli, eliciting a sufficient level of 'feeling aroused' to get the physical sexual system to start up (see above).

Viewed through the lens of the '3-conditions framework' sexual arousal problems can be caused by each condition, separately or simultaneously. Be aware to distinguish between low female arousability caused by low testosterone levels during breastfeeding and so-called 'psychogenic arousal problems', often caused by a lack of proper stimuli or comfortable context. In the first case, it's transient.

Different causes will require different treatment approaches. The '3-conditions framework' can help the midwife discriminate the aetiology of the sexual arousal problem, leading to more targeted interventions or referrals.

3.2.3 Problems with Orgasm

Problems with orgasm can take many different forms. Men and women can climax too slow, sooner then desired or not at all.

What is the relevance of problems with orgasm in midwifery? Conceiving will become rather difficult if the man cannot ejaculate or always ejaculates before vaginal penetration. Besides, many men and women view the ability to orgasm as an essential aspect of their sexual wellbeing. Research repeatedly reports on the link between high sexual wellbeing, general psychosocial wellbeing and partner attachment during pregnancy and post-partum. For more information, see Chap. 4 on The Health Benefits of Sexual Expression.

Viewed through the lens of the '3-conditions framework', orgasm problems can be caused by all three conditions. Good in-depth anamnesis will be paramount to tailor treatment successfully.

3.2.4   Sexual Pain Problems

Women (and also men) can experience pain when having sex. In nearly all cases of sexual pain, there will be a physical factor that is (co)causing the pain. For women, the physical origins of sexual pain can vary widely from pathologies like endometriosis or vulvodynia to anatomical issues, birth trauma (see Chap. 13) or a hypertonic pelvic floor (see Chaps. 10 and 16). Apart from the possible physical cause of sexual pain, women often find themselves in a vicious circle where they have had several painful sexual experiences, leading them to expect pain beforehand the next time. The expectation of pain causes 'bracing' for the pain and unwillingly tightening her pelvic floor muscles, making penetration more difficult and painful. So the anticipation of pain is confirmed. In addition, fearing pain will distract from sexual stimuli, making good arousal and lubrication more difficult, which is another possible cause of pain. Breaking this cycle requires, among other things, good psychoeducation. Still just insight into what is happening is sometimes not enough. Good inter-disciplinary cooperation with a clinical sexologist and pelvic floor therapist is often needed.

Detailed anamnesis is a necessary precondition before proceeding to treatment. A clear picture of the type and location of the sexual pain can aid in diagnosing potential underlying pathologies (e.g. pain when entering the vaginal canal is more associated with e.g. birth trauma, whereas pain experienced deeper in the vaginal canal could indicate e.g. endometriosis).

The importance of awareness of sexual pain problems in midwifery practice seems evident. In the childwish-phase, sexual intercourse without pain is an important condition to continue to have pleasurable sexual experiences when trying to concieve. The post-partum period is also a well-known risk phase for developing sexual pain.

Viewed through the lens of the '3-conditions framework', sexual pain can be caused by all three conditions, in other words, by problems with the physical sexual system, a lack of good stimuli or lack of a comfortable context. In sexual pain problems, there will almost always be an impairment of the physical sexual system. The HCP should be aware that the initial physical cause of the pain might be gone when the client consults about her pain problem.

3.3   The Midwife's Job When It Comes to Sexual Problems

People experiencing sexual problems deserve good care and guidance. Not all professionals are qualified to deliver intensive sexual therapy. But, happily enough, only a few people need that.

In 1974, Jack Annon developed a model used for the assessment and management of sexual problems, coined the PLISSIT model [7].

This PLISSIT model (Fig. 3.1) shows that people with different sexual problems can have different needs. It is a stepped model in the form of a pyramid, consisting of four distinct levels.

Fig. 3.1 The Plissit model.
(Adapted from Annon)

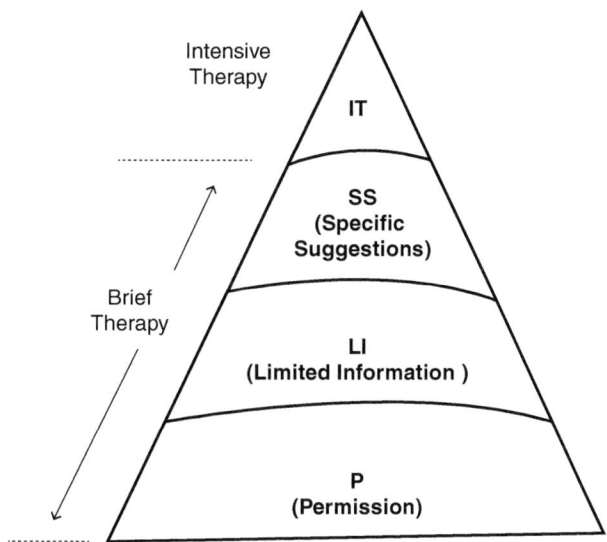

The first level of the model, 'P', stands for *'permission giving'*. At the large base of the pyramid, the first client group represents all potential clients. All people can benefit from knowing that their HCP is open to discussing any issue about sexuality that they might be experiencing. So all HCPs—midwives, gynae-cologists, sexologists, psychologists, physical therapists, nurses, etc.—should (be able to) create an environment where the client feels they can freely bring up sexual questions and worries. In addition to this, every woman and couple will benefit from a positive framing of sexuality. Being made aware by their HCP that it is okay to have sexual feelings, behave sexually and be sexual in a way that is not harmful to others can be an additional benefit that HCPs can create for their clients. In practice this translates to HCPs actively telling their clients 'if you ever have questions, concerns or problems with regards to sexuality, I'm always willing to listen'.

The second model level, 'LI', stands for *'limited information'*. Not all clients need information on sexual health, but a reasonably large group of people could benefit from such info. Think, for instance, of the midwife informing the client about the sexual side effects of hormonal contraception or explaining that it is per-fectly safe to have penetrative sex during a physiological pregnancy. As the group of clients in need of this intervention become smaller, the group of HCPs which we expect to be able to deliver limited information on sexual health become smaller also. Aplied to midwifery practice one could argue that midwives should be able to deliver limited information with regards to sexuality during an active child wish phase, pregnancy and young parenthood.

The third model level, 'SS', stands for *'specific suggestions'*. A smaller group of clients are actually experiencing sexual problems and will need some professional guidance to overcome these issues. Specific suggestions on how to handle the challenges they face can help them boost or regain their sexual wellbeing.[2]

Moving further through the levels the number of clients in need of this intervention becomes smaller. Also, fewer professionals will have the skills to provide such specific suggestions. Most healthcare curricula do not provide HCPs with the skills and knowledge they need to give this form of care. Often some additional training about sexual health is required. Such specialisation in sexuality or sexology is available for midwives in several countries. In some countries, the primary focus is on sexual health during the period of childwish, pregnancy and young parenthood. In other countries, midwives deal with the broader area of women's sexual health.

The final level of the model, 'IT', stands for *intensive therapy'*. The group of clients who effectively need in-depth sexual therapy is tiny compared to those who need the previously described interventions. It follows that only a small group of highly trained and specialised professionals such as clinical sexologists or physicians, psychologists and psychiatrists with additional training in sexual therapy are capable of providing such care. Even a very experienced sexologist cannot correctly deal with all sexual problems. Therefore sexology has developed into various sub-specialisations, 'reproduction sexology' being one of them.

The advantages of the PLISSIT model are that it allows professionals to position themselves in this model, thus deciding how far they can go in providing sexual health care for their clients. For midwives and gynaecologists, giving permission to talk about sexual concerns and providing clients with limited information on sexual health and wellbeing is a prerequisite. Those midwives and gynaecologists who find themselves working with client groups who often have real sexual concerns could seek some additional training to also become able to provide specific suggestions on sexual health and practice when needed. Still, if the HCP feels he is not the best person for addressing the client's questions and concerns on sexuality, it is important to stress that a good referral to a more specialised colleague is an equally good or sometimes better form of care than handling all issues by oneself.

In 2006, Taylor and Davis proposed a more nuanced version of this model, recreating it as the Ex-PLISSIT model [10]. Their additions updated the model with the healthcare norms and values of the new millennium. In the 1970s, health care had just started on the path to leaving paternalism behind. Autonomy as a value became much more central to health care, leading to client participation and a right to self-determination in matters of one's own health(care) becoming the new norm in healthcare. Today it is widely accepted that any therapeutic process has to be a process of co-creation, an interplay between HCP and client. We can see this value shift in the Ex-PLISSIT model, emphasising the importance of permission-giving

---

[2] Many exercises have been devised to help partners get to know just what works for their partner sexually (see, e.g. [8]). When selecting exercises that might help your clients to explore each other's sexual preferences, it is important to choose an exercise that is concise (not too time-consuming) and positively oriented (focussing on what works and previous good experiences, rather analysing what caused bad experiences). This way couples can learn 'what works and to do more of that' [9].

as the central element for any level of intervention, from permission-giving up to intensive therapy. The HCP should regularly check the client's current goals and, consequently, ask the client's permission to proceed in such a way that both HCP and client feel what is the best course of action to make their desire for change become a reality. Such a process of constantly focussing on the women/couple's desired outcome is essential in sexual health care. After all, cultural myths and taboos that exist in society about sexuality can easily cause the HCP to fill in what the client has not explicitly said because asking for detail would be 'uncomfortable' for both or 'too invading towards the client's intimate life'. By integrating permission-giving and a constant process of reflection, as elements of the model, it aims to keep the clients as co-pilots in the process, recognising them as the experts of both their own lives and their own problems, but also their own desired futures and the strengths they possess that can help get them to reach the goal.[3]

3.4 Conclusion

Sexuality, meant as a pleasurable and fulfilling form of human expression and bonding, can be a major source of physical, mental and social wellbeing. From trying to conceive till after childbirth, women and couples can, and many will, have sexual concerns and sexual problems. Thus, midwives and other HCPs should be aware of the necessary conditions to make sexuality a satisfying experience and thus a positive aspect of the couple's life. With the '3-conditions framework' of system, stimuli and context, this chapter offered an easy to use model to find out, together with the woman or couple, what might be causing the sexual problem and how to achieve a desired sexual future.

Providing good care also requires knowing one's strengths and limitations as an HCP. All midwives should be able to create a climate in which the woman and the couple feel safe to talk about sexuality and their sexual concerns or problems. We believe that every midwife should be able to give limited information on the effect of pregnancy, birth-related trauma, contraception, etc. on sexuality. Some midwives might even feel that they can proceed, with the tools presented in this chapter and this book, to take it one step further and give their clients specific suggestions on how to change their situations in their desired direction. Putting the client's needs and goals first will be the guiding principle towards helping women and couples 'making their sex work'.

Note: There will be books or blogs in most countries and languages to improve sexual communication and contact. We recommend the reader to look for good books or blogs in their own country/language area and integrate them into their midwifery and obstetric care.

---

[3] More practical guidelines for midwifes and other HCPs on how to ask questions and have a conversation with clients' as experts, focussing on their desired outcomes and strengths can be found in Geuens et al. [11].

References

1. Rosen RC, Barsky JL. Normal sexual response in women. Obstet Gynecol Clin North Am. 2006;33:515–26.
2. Bancroft J. Human sexuality and its problems. Amsterdam: Elsevier Limited; 2009.
3. Maister L, Fotopoulou A, Turnbull O, et al. The erogenous mirror: intersubjective and multi-sensory maps of sexual arousal in men and women. Arch Sex Behav. 2020;49:2919–33.
4. Lehmiller JJ. Tell me what you want: the science of sexual desire and how it can help you improve your sex life. Boston, MA: Da Capo; 2018.
5. Verhoeven V, Colliers A, Verster A. Collecting data for sexually transmitted infections (STI) surveillance: what do patients prefer in Flanders. BMC Health Serv Res. 2007;7:149.
6. Johnson C. Sexual health during pregnancy and the postpartum. J Sex Med. 2011;8:1267–84.
7. Annon JS. The PLISSIT model: a proposed conceptual scheme for the behavioral treatment of sexual problems. J Sex Educ Ther. 1976;2:1–15.
8. McCarthy B, Ross LW. Maintaining sexual desire and satisfaction in securely bonded couples. Fam J. 2018;26:217–22.
9. Burns K. Focus on solutions, a health professionals guide. Solution Books; 2016.
10. Taylor B, Davis S. Using the extended PLISSIT model to address sexual healthcare needs. Nurs Stand. 2006;21:35–40.
11. Geuens S, Dams H, Jones M, Lefevere G. Back to basics: a solution focused take on using and teaching basic communication skills for health care professionals. J Solution Focused Pract. 2020;4(2):70–80.

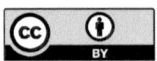

The Health Benefits of Sexual Expression

4

Woet L. Gianotten (ORCID)

4.1 Introduction

For a long time, medical professionals considered sexuality dangerous, based on undesired pregnancies, sexually transmitted infections, sexual abuse, masturbation or what was supposed to be 'hypersexuality'. Only in the last decades has the medical profession begun to acknowledge and accept that sexual expression has various benefits for relationships, bodies and minds.

The obstetric area showed a comparable shift in attention. In 1999, Kirsten von Sydow reviewed all English and German language articles of half a century [1]. She discovered that early research questions on sexual health were primarily negatively oriented (*'Can sex harm the baby?'*), then gradually action-oriented (*'Who has intercourse during pregnancy and post-partum?'*), finally going to longitudinal studies in which both partners were researched (*'How does the marital and sexual relationship develop when partners become parents?'*). Cultural changes have gradually prepared the medical community to accept that sexuality can be healthy for mothers and pregnancies.

Today we are moving towards a consensus that sexual expression has multiple inherent health benefits. This chapter will look into those health benefits.

It will start with some of the general benefits. Although not directly related to pregnancy, those benefits could favour the pregnant couple. And, of course, also the private life and health of midwives, other HCPs and partners.

The second part will focus on various fertility-related benefits of sexual expression and include some relevant explanations.

W. L. Gianotten (✉)
Department of Gynaecology and Obstetrics, Erasmus University Medical Center, Rotterdam, The Netherlands

© The Author(s) 2023
S. Geuens et al. (eds.), *Midwifery and Sexuality*,
https://doi.org/10.1007/978-3-031-18432-1_4

'Sexual expression' comprises all sorts of intimate and sexual behaviour (including erotic massage, arousal, orgasm, kissing, masturbation, intercourse, etc.). Perhaps (un)necessary to mention, this chapter will only deal with the consequences of sexuality without coercion, pain or other forms of personal distress directly related to sexual activity.

The range of health benefits is comprehensive, with some benefits very short-term and directly related to the sexual act. An example is the increased pain threshold for a short period after female genital stimulation [2]. Other benefits are real long-term. For instance, the greater longevity ('growing older') for women who, over the years, enjoyed sexuality more and for men who, over the years, ejaculated more frequently [3].

There are many explanations for why good sex promotes good health. It is partly because good sex is an essential part of our general wellbeing, one of the prerequisites for good general health. But there are more explanations. Sexual behaviour is for a reasonable amount also physical activity, and physical activity is healthy and delays the development of atherosclerosis, various chronic diseases, cancer and cognitive decline. For young couples, they found the energy expenditure during sexual activity to be approximately 85 kcal (or 3.6 kcal/min), and on average, sexual activity is performed at a moderate intensity [4]. Even without muscular activity, sexual arousal itself activates the circulation.

Various aspects of sexual action directly influence the homeostasis of the neurotransmitters and the neuroendocrine system. Cuddling and other sexual activities increase the testosterone level; orgasm changes the prolactin level; partnered sexual activity influences the person's immunity and stimulation of the female genitals increases the endorphin level. Oxytocin has a significant role in the reproductive triad of sexuality, birth and lactation. Caressing and massage (both touching and being touched), breast stimulation, arousal and orgasm increase the oxytocin levels. Oxytocin also has sedating and anxiolytic effects, and it can increase interpersonal trust [5]. Such influence of oxytocin is probably the reason why some men, after orgasm, fall asleep, and some others start talking.

The reader can find an extensive overview of the various benefits in a 'White Paper' of the PPFA [6] or more recent [7].

4.2 Sexuality-Related General Health Benefits

4.2.1 Cardiovascular Health and Longevity

In a 10-year follow-up, middle-aged men with 2 or more acts of intercourse per week had a 50% lower risk of dying than men who had intercourse once a month or less, with clear benefits in cerebrovascular and especially cardiovascular health [8]. It is probably not the act of intercourse itself but the thorough flushing of the cardiovascular and cerebrovascular system that accompanies arousal and orgasm. So, most likely other ways of reaching orgasm (including solo masturbation) are supposed to have the same benefits. A comparable explanation for the slower development of dementia is found in people with more frequent sexual activity [9].

4.2.2   Pain Reduction

Pain tends to be a killjoy for sexuality. However, one can also use sex as a way to reduce pain. An orgasm, for instance, diminishes migraine headaches in many female (and some male) patients. It is not yet exactly clear how that works.

Pleasurable sex can reduce pain through distraction, comparable with a romantic movie or an exciting sports match. That goes both for women and for men. For women, there is an additional sexual pathway to less pain. Pressure stimulation of the anterior vaginal wall and physical stimulation of the clitoris have an analgesic effect, with maximum impact when an orgasm is reached [2]. This increase in the pain threshold is the result of endorphins. But oxytocin seems to play a role as well. Women with higher oxytocin levels had a higher pain threshold [10]. The oxytocin increase caused by massage has anti-nociceptive effects, apparently via endogenous pain controlling systems [11].

4.2.3   Sexuality, Work and Marital Relationship

Employees engaging in sex at home reported increased positive effects at work the following day, both in terms of job satisfaction and job engagement [12].

4.2.4   Self-Esteem, Mood and Depression

Women have a higher chance of depression. Even in countries with close-to-perfect gender equality, the prevalence of depression in women is 50–100% higher than in males. It is supposed that, at least partly, this correlates with different levels of testosterone (T) and its mood-enhancing and depression-reducing action. Sexual activity itself increases the T-level both in men and women. In women (who are not on hormonal contraception), sexual thoughts also increase the T-level [13].

More sexual activity seems to be strongly connected to more happiness [14].

Self-esteem increases from positive sexual experiences with a partner and from accepting and embracing one's own sexuality and sexual desires. More self-esteem was also found to correlate to more masturbation. Women who masturbate have a more positive body image and less sexual anxiety [15].

In 2002, American research found that women who had intercourse without a condom were less depressed [16]. Under the title 'Does semen have anti-depressant properties?', the article received many adverse reactions, especially concerning STI risk. Semen contains many different substances that are easily absorbed by the vaginal wall. Testosterone, DHEA and zinc are all known to have anti-depressant properties [7].

4.3   Sexuality-Related Reproductive and Obstetric Health Benefits

From an evolutionary perspective, one may expect that sexuality has reproductive health benefits.

4.3.1   Menstrual Cycle

The monthly cycles appear to become more regular in women with more frequent sexual intercourse (and in women with more frequent same-sex sexual activities) [17].

Menstrual or pre-menstrual cramps can be relieved by orgasm, apparently by opening the cervical canal. Some women use masturbation to achieve this pain-relieving effect. When they combine it with intercourse and intra-vaginal ejaculation, there is the additional benefit of the semen's prostaglandins that assist in softening and opening the cervix.

With more frequent sex, women appear to have the intermediate-term benefit of postponing natural menopause (and the following hypoestrogenism) [18]. Ongoing sexual activity correlates with better vaginal health, especially in post-menopausal women. With frequent masturbation and coitus, there is less vaginal atrophy [19].

4.3.2   Fertility

'Good sex' is a relevant factor in conception and in maintaining a relaxed approach towards trying to conceive when success does not occur. However, professionals who counsell to couples who try to conceive, frequently tend to forget this.

A higher intercourse frequency, better arousal for the man, better arousal for the woman and proper timing of the various elements of the sexual play will together contribute to an increased conception chance. Chapter 5 will give a detailed explanation.

Recent research indicates that hormones influence menstrual-cycle-related changes in the immune response and, in that way, could influence implantation. Relevant differences in immune function have been found between sexually active women and sexually abstinent women [20].

4.3.3   Obstetric Advantages of Pre-conception Sexuality

The pregnant woman houses a system in which half of the tissues and antigens are paternal (from the father) and, therefore, 'a foreign body'. Since the placenta does not keep the woman's and the fetus' tissues wholly separated, a limited amount of fetal cells and fluid enters the woman's circulation (sometimes called microchimerism). After an organ transplant, we know that the human body tries to reject that foreign tissue. Gradually we are learning that some pregnancy disturbances (recurrent miscarriage and pre-eclampsia) could in some way be comparable to such 'transplantation reaction'. That seems to depend on the amount of immunological intolerance to the tissues of the baby (in fact, to the baby's paternal antigens). Sufficient maternal tolerance to the allogeneic fetal tissues can be developed by prior and prolonged exposure to paternal antigens in the seminal fluid, in that way protecting the fetus from rejection and facilitating successful implantation and placentation. That is where sexuality comes into the picture. For extra clarity: not semen per se, but semen of the father of the pregnancy.

In the first article on this topic, the researchers found less pre-eclampsia in women who had more experience with intra-oral ejaculation.

Women exposed to the paternal seminal fluid via absorption through the vaginal mucosa also have a lower risk for pre-eclampsia [21]. Accordingly, an increased risk for pre-eclampsia will be found (and is found) after vaginismus, after donor insemination, after a short relationship or a one-night-stand pregnancy, after being raped by a stranger and after consequent condom use (as in HIV couples).

On the other hand, women who had regular intercourse with ejaculation and without condoms will have a decreased risk. A condomless sexual intercourse period of 6 months is associated with less pre-eclampsia and less abnormal uterine activity (situations that can result in small-for-gestational-age babies [22]). It appears wise to consider such 'sexual pre-conception recommendations', although up to now, very few professionals discuss this with the women or the couple.

Although not researched, one may suppose that a relatively high 'uptake' of seminal fluid will occur after intra-rectal ejaculation, partly because of the highly vascular rectal mucosa and because an anal deposit of semen will stay relatively long in the rectum.

More recent is a study suggesting that oral sex (oral ejaculation and even more swallowing of semen) had, in a proportion of the cases, a possible protective role in the occurrence of recurrent miscarriage [23].

4.3.4 Sex During Pregnancy

The typical forms of sexual behaviour do not pose a risk to the pregnancy or the baby as long as the pregnancy is healthy.

Pregnant women with $\geq 1\times$ weekly intercourse at 23–26 weeks had a significantly reduced risk of pre-term birth [24]. Couples who, during late pregnancy, continue intercourse have a reduced risk of pre-term birth [25]. The same goes for women who have orgasms without intercourse [26].

Still, it is important to note that pre-term birth was found more in women with trichomonas vaginalis or mycoplasma hominis when at 23–26 weeks having 'frequent' intercourse (≥ 1/week), but not when having infrequent intercourse [24]. In women with vaginal infections in late pregnancy, the male-superior position is associated with more pre-term pre-mature rupture of the membranes and more premature birth [27].

When both heterosexual partners enjoyed sexual activity during pregnancy, the relationship was (4 months after the birth) evaluated as more positive in terms of tenderness and communication.

Researchers also looked at the relationship of couples 3 years after the birth. Those with mutual sexual joy before and during pregnancy had a more stable connection and were less negatively affected by the pregnancy than the couples without such mutual joy [28].

4.3.5   Sex and Parturition

Various elements of sexuality could contribute to the start of labour; oxytocin (via massage, breast/nipple stimulation and orgasm); prostaglandin (via semen and pounding the cervix by the penis) and uterine contractions (by orgasm). Whereas intercourse before the expected birth date did not seem to induce labour, reported sexual intercourse at term was associated with the onset of labour and reduced the need for labour induction at 41 weeks [29].

After the start of labour, the elements mentioned above of sexuality (except penetration) can keep the process going. Additional benefits are relaxation because of the pleasurable intimate contact and the increased pain threshold through elevated endorphin levels caused by genital/clitoral stimulation [2].

4.3.6   Long-Term Benefits

Sexuality is a significant bonding element for many couples at the start of their relationship. Then, during pregnancy, the importance of sexuality can enormously diminish for various physical, cultural and other reasons. In the first year after the birth, many women are more focussed on motherhood and the baby than on their partner, whereas many men prefer to return to their pre-pregnancy sexual pattern. Combined with the hassles of young parenthood, this can create much relationship tension, with 5% of couples divorcing after the first baby [30]. On the one hand, much of the sexual decline in post-natal relationships started during pregnancy. On the other hand, couples who continued during the pregnancy with satisfactory sex do far better after the birth [28].

4.4   Practical Implications

What could this list of potential health benefits teach about the role of the midwife or HCP in obstetric care?

In addition to the responsibility for a healthy mother, a healthy pregnancy and a healthy baby, we believe that good care should incorporate responsibility for healthy parenthood and healthy couplehood.

The conclusions will be evident with the parents' dyad at risk (especially after the first pregnancy) and knowing that sexuality can be an essential disrupting factor.

1. Address the importance of keeping the sexual and intimate life as good as possible. An exception is when one of the partners in the couple is clearly and explicitly not interested in sexuality.
2. Make it clear that investing in the sexual life will help maintain or regain intimacy, sexuality and the sexual relationship after the birth.
3. Make it also clear that sexual activity can help to reduce stress.
4. Regularly explain that there are no contraindications regarding sexual expression as long as the pregnancy is without complications. In case of real disturbances, explain very explicitly what is not allowed, but also what is allowed [see Chap. 12].
5. When relevant, explain the potential benefits of sexual expression for pain relief, stress reduction and easier sleep.

To say it in a very simplified way: sexuality and intimacy are relevant elements of care.

References

1. von Sydow K. Sexuality during pregnancy and after childbirth: a metacontent analysis of 59 studies. J Psychosom Res. 1999;47:27–49.
2. Whipple B, Komisaruk BR. Elevation of pain threshold by vaginal stimulation in women. Pain. 1985;21:357–67.
3. Palmore E. Predictors of the longevity difference: a twenty-five year follow-up. Gerontologist. 1982;22:513–8.
4. Frappier J, Toupin I, Levy JJ, et al. Energy expenditure during sexual activity in young healthy couples. PLoS One. 2013;8:e79342.
5. Kosfeld M, Heinrichs M, Zak PJ, et al. Oxytocin increases trust in humans. Nature. 2005;435(7042):673–6.
6. https://www.plannedparenthood.org/files/3413/9611/7801/Benefits_Sex_07_07.pdf.
7. Gianotten WL, Alley JC, Diamond LM. The health benefits of sexual expression. Int J Sex Health. 2021;33:478–93.
8. Davey Smith G, Frankel S, Yarnell J. Sex and death: are they related? Findings from the Caerphilly Cohort Study. BMJ. 1997;315(7123):1641–4.
9. Wright H, Jenks RA, Demeyere N. Frequent sexual activity predicts specific cognitive abilities in older adults. J Gerontol B Psychol Sci Soc Sci. 2019;74:47–51.
10. Grewen KM, Light KC, Mechlin B, Girdler SS. Ethnicity is associated with alterations in oxytocin relationships to pain sensitivity in women. Ethn Health. 2008;13:219–41.
11. Lund I, Ge Y, Yu LC, et al. Repeated massage-like stimulation induces long-term effects on nociception: contribution of oxytocinergic mechanisms. Eur J Neurosci. 2002;16:330–8.
12. Leavitt K, Barnes CM, Watkins T, Wagner DT. From the bedroom to the office: workplace spillover effects of sexual activity at home. J Manag. 2017;45(3):014920631769802.
13. Goldey KL, van Anders SM. Sexy thoughts: effects of sexual cognitions on testosterone, cortisol, and arousal in women. Horm Behav. 2011;59:754–64.
14. Blanchflower DG, Oswald AJ. Money, sex and happiness: an empirical study. Scand J Econ. 2004;106:393–415.

15. Hurlbert DF, Whittaker KE. The role of masturbation in marital and sexual satisfaction: a comparative study of female masturbators and nonmasturbators. J Sex Educ Ther. 1991;17:272–82.
16. Gallup GG Jr, Burch RL, Platek SM. Does semen have antidepressant properties? Arch Sex Behav. 2002;31:289–93.
17. Cutler WB. Love cycles: the science of intimacy. New York: Villard Books; 1991.
18. Arnot M, Mace R. Sexual frequency is associated with age of natural menopause: results from the Study of Women's Health Across the Nation. R Soc Open Sci. 2020;2020:7191020.
19. Leiblum S, Bachmann G, Kemmann E, et al. Vaginal atrophy in the postmenopausal woman; the importance of sexual activity and hormones. JAMA. 1983;249:2195–8.
20. Lorenz TK, Heiman JR, Demas GE. Interactions among sexual activity, menstrual cycle phase, and immune function in healthy women. J Sex Res. 2018;55:1087–95.
21. Saftlas AF, Rubenstein L, Prater K, et al. Cumulative exposure to paternal seminal fluid prior to conception and subsequent risk of preeclampsia. J Reprod Immunol. 2014;101–102:104–10.
22. Kho EM, McCowan LM, North RA, et al. Duration of sexual relationship and its effect on preeclampsia and small for gestational age perinatal outcome. J Reprod Immunol. 2009;82:66–73.
23. Meuleman T, Baden N, Haasnoot GW, et al. Oral sex is associated with reduced incidence of recurrent miscarriage. J Reprod Immunol. 2019;133:1–6.
24. Read JS, Klebanoff MA. Sexual intercourse during pregnancy and preterm delivery: effects of vaginal microorganisms. The Vaginal Infections and Prematurity Study Group. Am J Obstet Gynecol. 1993;168:514–9.
25. Reamy K, White SE, Daniell WC, Le Vine ES. Sexuality and pregnancy. A prospective study. J Reprod Med. 1982;27:321–7.
26. Sayle AE, Savitz DA, Thorp JM Jr, et al. Sexual activity during late pregnancy and risk of preterm delivery. Obstet Gynecol. 2001;97:283–9.
27. Ekwo EE, Gosselink CA, Woolson R, et al. Coitus late in pregnancy: risk of preterm rupture of amniotic sac membranes. Am J Obstet Gynecol. 1993;168:22–31.
28. Heinig L, Engfer A. Schwangerschaft und Partnerschaft [pregnancy & partnership]. Rep Psychol. 1988;13:56–9.
29. Tan PC, Andi A, Azmi N, et al. Effect of coitus at term on length of gestation, induction of labor, and mode of delivery. Obstet Gynecol. 2006;108:134–40.
30. Swaminathan S, Alexander GR, Boulet S. Delivering a very low birth weight infant and the subsequent risk of divorce or separation. Matern Child Health J. 2006;10:473–9.

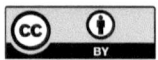

Part II

Introduction to Module 2: 'Nature Taking Its Course'

Woet L. Gianotten, Ana Polona Mivšek, and Sam Geuens

Module 1 focused on sexuality in general. It addressed how we define sexuality ('What is sex?'), it paid attention to the anatomy, physiology, and psychology; it showed in some way how sex works and how it doesn't work, and the last chapter dealt with the health benefits of various aspects of having sex.

Module 2 and Module 3 both focus on the day-to-day practice of the midwife, both addressing the sexual and intimacy consequences of the various stages from conception to young parenthood.

For the structure of this book, we have made two crucial subdivisions. We base the first subdivision on the various stages of the process, including active child wish, conception, pregnancy, labour and birth, the postpartum phase (combined with the first year of young parenthood), and breastfeeding. In addition, there is a chapter on the pelvic floor.

The second division deals with the difference between healthy/natural development, characterized within midwifery as 'physiology' and, on the other hand, those situations coloured by troubles, pathology, and high risk. We are aware that this is an artificial division since there is a gradual transition between what is healthy and what is problematic.

With sexuality being the essential perspective, in both modules, the chapters are named 'Sexual aspects of ….' Module 2, called 'Nature taking its course', will deal with physiological processes. Module 3, named 'Nature losing its way', will deal with sexuality in the same series of topics as in Module 2, but now when the situation has become problematic, pathological, or very high risk.

Apart from these divisions, we recommend readers, in particular midwifery students who use this book as a textbook, to start with Chap. 26, dealing with 'talking sex', which is an essential skill.

Chapter 5: Sexual Aspects of Getting Pregnant (Conception and Preconception)

Up till very recently, sex was needed to get pregnant. Especially the start of that period tends to be pleasurable for many couples. There are several reasons to lose that pleasure easily. One of the explanations is the higher age at which women decide to become pregnant when the chance of conception is already decreasing. Another explanation is the idea of the malleability of life, which gradually developed in many high-income societies. Then, 'still not being pregnant' can be a real blow to a couple's identity.

This chapter will describe the gradual move from pleasurable sex towards 'conception inefficiency', which happens in part of healthy couples who try to conceive. That is different from where fertility is disturbed due to sexual dysfunctions or infertility.

The chapter will also cover the relevant elements of 'good conception sex' to help people understand how they can positively influence the chance to get pregnant (and proceed to successful nidation).

Finally, the chapter will give ample information on sexual aspects of preconception care, a fairly new approach.

Chapter 6: Sexual Aspects of Pregnancy

Especially during the first pregnancy, many changes occur in the woman, the relationship, and her partner. This chapter will describe the wide range of elements influencing sexuality and intimacy. It will start with the physical changes. Both pregnancy and sexual arousal are characterized by hypercongestion of the internal and external genital organs (and the breasts). On the one hand, being pregnant can facilitate sexual arousal, with more sexual dreams and easier orgasms. The accumulating effect of much sexual arousal and the existing hypercongestion due to pregnancy itself can however, on the other hand, cause pain in the breasts and the vulvar area. In the last trimester of pregnancy, the quality of orgasm can change from clonic to tonic (and painful). Sexual desire can change in different directions and is influenced by physical factors, but also by fear of miscarriage or premature birth; and by changing appearance and sense of self. Some women feel better and others less attractive than ever. Some partners love their pregnant partner's appearance, and others have issues with that. In this period, existential changes in the relationship occur, with parenthood bringing on new responsibilities and a substantial decrease in the previous freedom.

Chapter 7: Sexual Aspects of Labour and Birth

Whereas some women experience the natural birth as very painful and devastating, for some others, it can be an overwhelming sensual or nearly erotic experience that resembles an orgasm. Birth, orgasm, and breastfeeding are similar processes, all strongly associated with oxytocin. That makes oxytocin one of the potential factors when couples look for a way to influence labour proactively. This chapter will pay attention to various aspects of physical/sexual stimuli that could affect the start of labour and its continuation. It will also describe several ways of dealing with pain.

The birth (especially first one) is not only a physical process but also a significant life event, influencing the bonding between the partners towards parenthood. So, the chapter will also look into the partner's role and how to optimally navigate through this process.

Chapter 8: Sexuality of the Couple in Postpartum and Early Parenthood (1st Year)

The first birth is a major life event for all involved parties: woman, partner (and couple). And for the baby, who will get a complex role in the triangle of care and attention.

This chapter will address the relevant elements that together shape parenthood and couplehood.

That process is somewhat different for the average woman and the average man. Many men more or less tend to return to their pre-pregnancy level of sexual desire rather quickly. On the other hand, women need much more time before having consolidated in their new role as mothers, simultaneously reconsidering their role as sexual partners.

The woman's physical and sexual system has been worn out by the hormonal changes and maybe periods of low or no sexual activity. Especially when breastfeeding, her low oestrogen levels keep the vagina atrophic, and her low androgen levels keep arousability low. Together those factors create a substantial risk of developing dyspareunia. Besides these physical aspects, the woman and her partner undergo great psychological adaptations in the postpartum period.

This chapter will address how to optimally navigate through this phase of 'transition to parenthood' and new couplehood.

Chapter 9: Sexual Aspects of Breast and Lactation

Besides nutrition for the baby, the breasts are in many cultures in many ways connected to sexuality and intimacy. They have many sexual functions. An essential erogenic zone, a relevant factor for female identity causing insecurity or pride, a source for pain and a source for pleasure.

There are striking similarities between breastfeeding, birth, and orgasm. Oxytocin orchestrates all three of these processes, with all three also comparably influenced by the ability 'to relax' (sometimes called 'to let down').

During parturition, breast stimulation can influence the process of birth. Once lactation has started, it can affect sexuality both positively and negatively, which partly results from hormonal changes. Finally, when the lactating woman gets sexually excited or has an orgasm, milk can appear and be a source of confusion for some couples and a source of pleasure for others.

The chapter will include also the HCP's role in counselling on the advantages and disadvantages of breastfeeding. It is the best nutrition for the baby, a vital factor in the bond between child and mother, and it has long-term health benefits for both. On the other hand, breastfeeding can cause severe fatigue, lack of sex drive, dyspareunia, and the fear of disfigurement.

Chapter 10: Sexual Aspects of the Female Pelvic Floor

The last chapter of this module is devoted to the pelvic floor (PF). Whereas maternity care always considered the PF muscles an essential part of the birth and its disturbances, the pelvic floor gradually became also known as a vital element for both sexual pleasure and sexual problems.

This chapter will start by explaining its role in posture and sexuality. It will delineate differences between the normotonic, the hypotonic, and the hypertonic pelvic floor and their influences on sexuality.

The chapter gives some primary education on assessing pelvic floor function.

After explaining the PF concerning pregnancy and birth, the chapter will also address aspects of prevention and prehabilitation. In other words, this chapter will also deal with how to optimally prepare the pregnant woman for a relaxed birth with as low as possible negative consequences regarding vaginal laxity or pelvic floor prolapse.

Sexual Aspects of Getting Pregnant (Conception and Preconception)

5

Woet L. Gianotten ⓘ

5.1 Introduction

This chapter will address various conception-related aspects of sexuality. It will offer relevant information for the midwife, though, in many countries, midwives only become involved after conception has taken place. On the one hand, such information is essential because understanding sexual troubles that develop in the 'trying to conceive'-phase can have (and probably will have) consequences for sexuality during pregnancy and post-partum. But also because in some countries, the midwife is involved in the broader area of reproductive health. That includes pre-conception care, an area supported by the WHO [1]. This chapter will integrate sexuality in pre-conception care, although almost nowhere mentioned in the literature.

That approach is a logical consequence of 'chain care', where the awareness of the ultimate intended outcome upgrades multi-disciplinarity among all professionals.

> We use the term 'chain care' here. Medical care today exists in an era of superspecialisation. In our field, a couple can come in contact with fertility expertise, obstetric expertise, childbirth expertise, neonatal expertise, sexology expertise and family & relationship expertise. Each profession will focus on its own specific area and influence the couple with relevant recommendations. In that fragmented way, however, both the professional and the couple easily forget the ultimate intended outcome: happy family life and happy couplehood.

W. L. Gianotten (✉)
Department of Gynaecology and Obstetrics, Erasmus University Medical Center, Rotterdam, The Netherlands
e-mail: woetgia@ziggo.nl

© The Author(s) 2023
S. Geuens et al. (eds.), *Midwifery and Sexuality*,
https://doi.org/10.1007/978-3-031-18432-1_5

> In 'chain care', the various professions not only cooperate (multi-disciplinarity) but are also aware of the ultimate intended outcome and integrate that awareness into their approach.

'Good sex' is a relevant factor in conception. This chapter will deal with such 'good conception sex' and explain how factors like intercourse frequency, quality of male arousal, quality of female arousal and proper timing can contribute to the chance to conceive.

That may seem rather unromantic. It is also true that many pregnancies just happen without planning. However, especially in the Western World, many pregnancies are deliberately planned. Such a 'planned approach' is part of the lifestyle of many modern couples, who want to design their own life and future. For them, when conception does not happen soon enough, it is not uncommon to get confused. As a result, couples fairly quickly look for medical assistance to keep the parenthood part of their life plan on track. Unfortunately, many professionals then turn to diagnostics and treatment, forgetting (and denying) that sex is the common way to get pregnant.

When conception does not happen in due time, many couples end up in a vicious circle where 'no-conception-yet' creates poor sex and where 'poor sex' diminishes the chance to conceive and eventually can threaten the quality of the intimate relationship [2].

This chapter intends to provide some clarity in such processes and will successively address:

- How sexual pleasure can get lost in healthy, 'trying to conceive' couples
- Sexual aspects of pre-conception care
- The sexual physiology of conception.

The chapter will not deal with disturbed fertility resulting from sexual dysfunction or the sexual aspects of infertility. We will approach those areas in Chap. 11.

5.2   'Conception Inefficiency' - Losing Sexual Pleasure Along the Way

If fertility is not disturbed, many couples will get pregnant without needing great (conception) sex. That does not really matter as long as conceiving is not, or not yet, important. However, for many contemporary couples, the reality is somewhat different. In the affluent Western World, many couples wait for an extended period before they feel ready to step into parenthood. Then, after discontinuing contraception, they tend to believe that conception will take place within 2 or 3 months.

Some couples will be lucky, and many then experience a boost in self-esteem because of getting pregnant. Others will be less lucky with the risk of disappointment lying in wait. Not succeeding in this area (which usually means not-yet succeeding) can really diminish the couple's self-esteem. That alone can already considerably decrease sexual desire. Wanting so badly to conceive can quickly influence also the couple's spontaneity and sexual timing schedule, resulting in stress, less intimacy and intercourse without genuine arousal. A vicious circle can develop between 'poor sex' and lower conception chance. That does not mean sub-fertility, rather 'conception inefficiency'.

In older fertile women, additional stress can develop when the fear of 'being too late' starts interfering.

Such a period of poor sex (because of 'no-pregnancy-yet') can spill over into the pregnancy and then into the post-partum phase, finally having negative influences on the relationship quality and happy parenthood.

5.3 Sexual Aspects of Pre-conception Care

According to the WHO, the ultimate aim of pre-conception care is to improve maternal and child health in the short-term and long-term [1]. From a sexual health point of view, we prefer to broaden that WHO intention and explicitly include the couple's health, which for an important part means the couple's sexual health.

Based on that perspective, we will focus on four phases that should belong to pre-conception care:

1. The phase before conception ('sex for adapting to paternal antigens')
2. The phase of conception ('what to do and not to do when wanting to conceive')
3. The period of pregnancy ('how to invest in future sexual wellbeing')
4. The post-partum period ('how to restart one's sexual life').

We will give this information to the woman/couple in a narrative way (including some do's and don'ts) and add some explanation for the HCP.

We will give the explanatory narratives for the woman/couple in italics.

5.3.1 The Phase Before Conception

A fascinating new line of obstetric knowledge deals with immunology. Some pregnancy disturbances appear to happen less when the mother has had ample exposure to paternal semen (the ejaculate of the father of this pregnancy). Regularly having condomless sex for 6 months is associated with less pre-eclampsia and less abnormal uterine activity (resulting in small-for-gestational-age babies) [3]. There are also indications that paternal semen exposure can prevent part of recurrent abortions. For a more extensive explanation, see Chap. 4.

For practice, you have to know if the couple regularly had sex in a way that the woman was exposed (vaginally, orally or anally) to the paternal semen. In other words: you have to ask the clients.

If the answer is negative, you can use the following narrative:

> When a woman is pregnant, half of the baby is foreign material (antigens from the father). That foreign material can cause trouble for the pregnancy. It increases the risk for high blood pressure problems and abnormal womb activity, resulting in too small babies. Besides, it seems that it can be an underlying reason for miscarriages.
> We are learning that the woman can get adapted to the antigens of this specific father. Research shows that regular exposure to his semen diminishes those risks. So, we recommend considering postponing conception for half a year and regularly having sex with exposure to semen and without condoms. That could also have an extra benefit, since semen is partly absorbed, with anti-depressant influence [4].

That should be followed by some practical explanation, depending on why there was no yet exposure to paternal semen. Sometimes that information will ask for a balancing act with exposure in the non-fertile days of the cycle.

5.3.2   The Phase of Conception

> 'You'll be in the process of trying to get pregnant.
> Some couples will be lucky because they just conceive effortlessly. Congratulations to them!
> In other couples, however, it'll take more time. The focus then quickly moves away from sexual pleasure towards 'We have to get pregnant', sometimes resulting in vicious circles of disappointment, stress and sexual timing that is not only not productive but also not based on sexual pleasure and desire.
> Let's be clear. That doesn't work!
> On the one hand, pleasure and intimacy are relevant elements towards conception. Higher levels of sexual arousal in women and men increase the conception chance.
> The same goes for more frequent sexual intercourse and a relaxed approach.
> There is also another reason to pay attention to good sex and sexual pleasure. The way you will have and enjoy sex during this period of conception will influence the quality of your sexual life during the pregnancy, which subsequently will affect how your sexual relationship will take shape after birth'.

For the couple, sex after pregnancy might seem far away. It can be very beneficial to make couples aware that keeping a good sexual life during this conception phase will spill over into a good sexual life during pregnancy and post-partum. That will finally benefit all parties, with better bonds between the partners and between parents and baby.

Recommendations for Couples

Do:
- *Invest in sexual pleasure and sexual desire.*
- *Try as much as possible to be at the same time parents-to-be and lovers. Giving priority to sexuality and intimacy (above career, social media, friends and relatives) is a long-term investment in a sound future as partners and lovers.*
- *When using ovulation as an indicator moment, be aware that the chance to conceive is highest with intercourse on day 2 before ovulation.*
- *Continue ejaculating regularly. Too long intervals between ejaculations will diminish the quality of the sperm. Once ejaculation every 1–3 days appears the good frequency for conceiving. So, masturbation can sometimes be helpful to keep the sperm quality optimal.*

Don't:
- *Don't continue sexual intercourse when it hurts. The pain usually means that you are not (or not yet) sufficiently aroused.*
- *Don't stop intercourse because the day of ovulation is over. Semen appears to facilitate proper ingrowth (nestling) in the womb.*

5.3.3   The Period of Pregnancy

'*When you are pregnant, there is a real possibility that changes will occur in your intimate and sexual life. Sexual desire can increase or decrease. In some couples, the changes will go in the same direction for both partners, but frequently it turns out to be different.*

Moreover, these things change throughout pregnancy because of physical adaptations in the woman and emotional anticipation of your future role as parents.

So we emphasise that the quality of your sexual life during the pregnancy will affect your sexual life after childbirth.

Once the baby is born, many couples struggle to get their sex life back on track.

In the first year after the baby is born, sexuality is an important reason for the tension in the relationship.

We also know that couples who successfully keep an active and satisfying sex life during pregnancy will have less (sexual) tension afterwards.
In other words: investing in a healthy and satisfying relationship and sexual life throughout pregnancy is a long-term investment in good couplehood and good parenthood.

Recommendations for Couples
Do:
- *Pay extra attention to sexual pleasure and sexual desire.*
- *If you are not (yet) used to it, try already at the beginning of the pregnancy to learn to enjoy sex without penetration. Next to being fun, it will provide an extra leeway towards the end of pregnancy, when penetration may no longer be possible or pleasurable.*

Don't:
- *Don't continue sexual intercourse when it hurts. That usually happens because of a lack of arousal.*
- *In the second half of the pregnancy, refrain from having intercourse in the male-superior position. Not only because the big belly makes that position unpleasant for many women, but also because it can be a risk factor for more prematurity and premature rupture of the membranes.*

The HCP has several roles concerning sexuality and intimacy during pregnancy.

On the one hand, create a sexuality-friendly open atmosphere and clarify that whenever the woman or her partner has worries or questions, they should bring them up.

On the other hand, proactively educate couples on possible sexual alterations due to a shifting relationship and changes in the woman's body and function. This way, we invest in the sexual future after birth and the transition to parenthood.

5.3.4 The Post-partum Phase

When dealing with couples in the period around conception, it might seem strange to talk about the post-partum phase already. However, good chain care requires anticipation of the subsequent phases. After all, most couples finally strive for a healthy family with a healthy child living under the wings of a healthy couple. Given that many couples face relationship tension in the post-partum year, with sexuality problems upfront, we believe that discussing common peri-partum and post-partum realities should be an integral part of pre-conception care [2].

In the first post-partum months, the mindset of the majority of young mothers is primarily focussed on the baby and not on the partner. Regularly, her hormones and her vagina are not yet ready for intercourse, especially not when she is also breastfeeding or when she has experienced any form of birth trauma.

On the other hand, many young fathers want to return to their previous sexual pattern, with testosterone levels far higher than the mother has, which usually means more sexual desire. At the same time, men can get seriously confused by their new roles as fathers and the sudden change from a dyad to a threesome. Sexuality is a common male 'method' for stress relief. That combination of factors can cause confusing or severe complications in the couple's sexual life. Such disappointment and alienation after childbirth can easily have negative repercussions for the sexual future of the couple [2].

> It might seem strange to address sexuality for the period around and after birth. However, during that phase, your sexual life can get entirely disrupted.
>
> There is nothing wrong with the sexual routine you have developed together. That sexual routine, however, is most probably not very useful in the later stages of pregnancy and the first months after birth. Certainly not when you intend to breastfeed the baby.
>
> Since those sexual disturbances can have long-lasting effects on the relationship and negatively influence parenthood, it seems wise to anticipate and be prepared.
>
> So the challenge here is: How to keep sexuality rewarding and connecting during this period?
>
> We'll address the two most important topics: 'Sexually keeping up with each other' and 'The automatism to end a sexual encounter with penetration and orgasm'.
>
> Regarding sexually keeping up: in all couples, the partners differ in their level of sexual desire. That doesn't need to be a problem. However, dealing with those differences can be difficult and might become a problem. Couples who learn how to deal with those differences tend to have a happier and more satisfying sex life. As the pregnancy proceeds and after birth, that becomes very relevant.
>
> Regarding penetration (with or without orgasm) as end-of-sex: Many couples develop a routine to end a sexual encounter by penetration and intravaginal (male) orgasm. There is nothing wrong with that, however, such automatism precludes relaxed intimacy when the vagina is sore. In the last pregnancy months and after birth, it is common that the woman is not ready for penetration.

*Then, when 'real sex' means penetration, a sexual encounter inevitably will
end in pain for her, resulting in distress and disappointment for both.*

*Many couples avoid that trap by 'intimate masturbation': cuddle until the
woman's need for intimacy is satisfied and the partner can proceed to
extra-vaginal stimulation and orgasm while lying in her arms.*

*When negotiated and agreed upon by the couple, such sexual routine adapta-
tions resulted in many couples in sexual encounters with less tension, less
pain, fewer feelings of guilt and more intimacy.*

*We honestly believe that no couple should get pregnant before they feel suffi-
ciently at ease with sex and orgasm without the need to vaginal
penetration.*

5.4   Recommendations for the Professional

Let us assume that the reader believes in the benefits of such sexual anticipation as
a form of sexual health prevention. It will not be easy for many HCPs to integrate
this into pre-conception care. Here are some arguments in support:

- Couples who have learned to cope with differences in sexual desire and who can
  cope with sex without penetration will benefit throughout the rest of their
  relationship.
- Honest, open information about sexuality generally improves the relationship of
  trust between the woman, the couple and the HCP.

Do:
- Prepare a leaflet with the required sexual information in your patients'
  language(s).[1]
- If this sexual anticipation talk is new, try to practise with your partner or colleague a few times. Talking out loud about sex is different from just saying it in
  your mind.
- The next step could be to practise with a friendly couple a few times. Discussing
  sex with a male partner present is different anyway.
- Adapt (within your comfort zone) your narrative to the language of the couple.
- Ask the couple how they, with the provided information, could develop changes
  in anticipation of the future. That sometimes causes a confidence boost when a
  couple succeeds in 'helping themselves' with their own ideas.

Don't:
- Be careful not to let your own sexual frame of reference prevail.

---

[1] The website www.zanzu.be gives relevant reproductive health information in 15 different
languages.

- Don't let the leaflet replace your own verbal connection when using flyers. It is better to hand out a leaflet at the end of your conversation, and next time ask if that raised any questions.
- Sometimes it is tempting to recommend couples: 'Do this or do that!' directly. That is not wise in terms of the professional relationship with the couple. When a couple obediently follows your 'direct sexual advice', you run the risk of virtually becoming a part of their 'sex scene', which can be very tricky. It is better to recommend indirectly via experiences of other couples: *'I know that some couples in the same situation did such and so. For many, that helped rather well. So, maybe that is something for you to consider!'*.

5.5   The Sexual Physiology of Conception [5]

In healthy couples who do not use contraception, the average time required for conception is 5.3 months, and 25% of couples have conceived after 1 month of unprotected intercourse [6]. Since, for some other healthy couples, it can take more than 1½ years, it feels a bit like a lottery.

As long as a couple is fertile, they can get pregnant, even when their sex is clumsy. However, it will be evident that the chance of conception is far higher with good procreative sex.

In this part, we will first address the various aspects of 'optimal sexual logistics' (timing, choreography, etc.), and we then will close with some recommendations on how to improve sexual desire when that threatens to get lost.

5.5.1   Frequency of Intercourse

Frequently engaging in coitus enhances the chance of conception considerably. With intercourse 4×/week, the chance of conception is 4–5× greater than with intercourse occurring ≤1/week. With a regular menstrual cycle, intercourse 2–3×/week appears okay.

5.5.2   Timing of Intercourse

For conception, one needs spermatozoa and a fresh ovum. Healthy spermatozoa can survive up to 6 days in the woman's body. The ovum survives 12–24 h after ovulation (although some unintended conceptions seem to happen 48 h after ovulation). For conception, intercourse should take place in the 'fertile window'. That is the period from 6 days before till 12 h after ovulation. The optimal time within the fertile window is when the cervical mucus is abundant, whitish and slippery as egg white. Another reliable (but much more expensive) method is an ovulation test. The best time for intercourse is 2 days before ovulation [7].

Between ejaculation and fertilisation, spermatozoa undergo capacitation, which takes 1–4 h before they are ready for their job. Capacitation is a chemical process in the cervical mucus and cervical crypts, enabling the sperm cell to impregnate the ovum. From the ejaculated pool, continuously new capacitated spermatozoa start their journey. Remember that an ejaculate contains some 50 million spermatozoa.

The conception chance is highest when sufficient viable spermatozoa are already available at the ovulation site. That supports the advice to regularly have intercourse during the fertile window (and the 2 days before ovulation). So, couples who wait for intercourse till the ovulation test indicates actual ovulation will miss the optimal opportunities for conception.

After having conceived, the embryo has to implant successfully in the nidation window (day 6–12 after ovulation). Proper nidation (usually at day 9) appears to be positively influenced by regular intercourse. Probably acting via humoral immunity by which the emerging embryo is accepted by a woman's body, despite being a 'foreign invader' [8].

5.5.3 Frequency of Ejaculation

It is not wise to ejaculate very frequently (several times per day) when trying to conceive because that will diminish the sperm quality. On the other hand, 'saving' (prolonged period of abstinence till ovulation) also decreases sperm quality. Abstinence of 5 days gives the optimal quality and amount of sperm, relevant for male partners with limited opportunities for sexual contact. For couples living together, the optimal frequency is probably once every 1–2 days, because of the above mentioned benefits of repeated intra-vaginal ejaculation.

5.5.4 Female Sexual Arousal

Whereas the vaginal surface is typically just moist, sexual arousal creates lubrication, a fluid with several functions. Lubrication has fertility functions next to pleasure and preventing mechanical irritation (which causes pain). With a high O_2 content and the proper pH, the lubrication fluid facilitates metabolism, mobility and lifespan of the spermatozoa [5].

The vagina of the sexually not-aroused woman has an acid pH (between 3.8 and 5.0) in which yeasts and other pathogens cannot grow. Spermatozoa, however, are immobilised at a pH <6.3. That is why lubrication fluid has a neutral pH of around 7.0.

Besides, good lubrication will make the penis slide better, prevent dyspareunia and increase sexual pleasure. That is another relevant argument for good arousal since it will increase the chance of repeated sex and thus the chances of conception. Artificial lubricants were supposed to harm spermatozoa. However, recent research corrected this idea [9]. Lubricant use gave a slight increase in the conception rate.

At high arousal, the cervix and uterus move away from the posterior vaginal wall (the 'tenting effect'), preventing the bulk of sperm from entering the cervix before capacitation has started to take place [2].

5.5.5 Male Sexual Arousal

With a high level of male sexual arousal, the sperm quality gets better [10]. There is also a timing element. With a more extended pre-ejaculatory arousal period, the sperm concentration will improve [11].

Good arousal will also increase the chance of repeated sex with a higher chance of conception.

5.5.6 Female Orgasm

Orgasm's impact on conception chances is still not fully clear [12]. Immediately after ejaculation, the sperm coagulates and then (after approximately 10 min) deco-agulates. Since the spermatozoa first need some hours before being capacitated and viable to start the journey to the ovum, an orgasm most probably will not favour conception with the ejaculate of this sexual encounter.

That could be different from the ejaculated sperm of last evening. Around the ovulation period, subendometrial smooth muscles send peristaltic waves from the cervix to the Fallopian tube at the side of the ovulation. Oxytocin, peaking during orgasm, facilitates those myometrial waves. From that perspective, orgasm could bring the sperm of last evening to the site of ovulation. But maybe more important here again, a satisfactory orgasm can be a good reason to repeat the sexual encounter and by the higher frequency enhances the conception chance.

Recommendations (for narratives or folders) for the couple to improve their sexual life when sexual pleasure is dwindling

When you dearly want to get pregnant, but don't have success, you can easily lose your sexual desire. The pressure to sexually perform well will not increase sexual pleasure. And neither 'having sex at fixed times' nor 'enjoying sex on command' is easy. After all, one cannot be forced to have fun. From such situations, we have learned some strategies to improve your sex life. Many of those recommendations aim to create conditions for intimacy since intimacy is an important condition for sexual desire and enjoyable sex.

- *Make sure you will not be disturbed. Keep social media out of the bedroom (just turn off that smartphone, TV and doorbell).*
- *Create time for intimacy. Doing things together with nobody else around can reestablish your bond. Doing household chores or craftwork together can work as foreplay. Some couples benefit from physical activities like working out, dancing, sporting or enjoying wellness treatment together.*
- *Create intimacy. A cold, non-cosy bedroom with an iron board in the corner is not very erotic.*
- *Take joint responsibility to strengthen your sexual relationship. Instead of repeatedly reminding the other what is not working, you better indicate what could bring you in a more sexual mood. Many couples enjoy thinking back to the exciting moments when they fell in love or had good sex.*
- *Accept being different. Usually, women are more sensitive to undivided attention, romance and intimacy, and men are more sensitive to variety, visual cues (from lingerie to nudity) and explicitly shown excitement.*
- *There tends to be a lot of arousal at the edge of your comfort zone. Depending on the limits of your comfort zone, you could try to spice things up. Examples are incense, massage oil, sauna, romantic movies, X-rated movies, toys, etc.*
- *Some alcohol can create extra relaxation, looseness and sexual ease for some couples. That is not dangerous for the baby before nidation (usually at day 9 after ovulation) as the fetus is still wholly separated from and not influenced by the mother's circulation.*

References

1. WHO on preconception. https://www.who.int/maternal_child_adolescent/documents/preconception_care_policy_brief.pdf.
2. von Sydow K. Sexuality during pregnancy and after childbirth: a metacontent analysis of 59 studies. J Psychosom Res. 1999;47:27–49.
3. Kho EM, McCowan LM, North RA, et al. Duration of sexual relationship and its effect on pre-eclampsia and small for gestational age perinatal outcome. J Reprod Immunol. 2009;82:66–73.
4. Gianotten WL, Alley JC, Diamond LM. The health benefits of sexual expression. Int J Sex Health. 2021;33:478–93.
5. Levin RJ. Recreation and procreation: a critical view of sex in the human female. Clin Anat. 2015;28:339–54.
6. Bancroft J. Sexual aspects of fertility, fertility control and infertility. In: Bancroft J, editor. Human sexuality and its problems. 3rd ed. London: Churchill Livingstone; 2009. p. 439–63.
7. Dunson DB, Colombo B, Baird DD. Changes with age in the level and duration of fertility in the menstrual cycle. Hum Reprod. 2002;17:1399–403.
8. Lorenz TK, Demas GE, Heiman JR. Partnered sexual activity moderates menstrual cycle-related changes in inflammation markers in healthy women: an exploratory observational study. Fertil Steril. 2017;107:763–73.e3.

9. McInerney KA, Hahn KA, Hatch EE, et al. Lubricant use during intercourse and time to pregnancy: a prospective cohort study. BJOG. 2018;125:1541–8.
10. Yamamoto Y, Sofikitis N, Mio Y, et al. Influence of sexual stimulation on sperm parameters in semen samples collected via masturbation from normozoospermic men or cryptozoospermic men participating in an assisted reproduction programme. Andrologia. 2000;32:131–8.
11. Pound N, Javed MH, Ruberto C, et al. Duration of sexual arousal predicts semen parameters for masturbatory ejaculates. Physiol Behav. 2002;76:685–9.
12. Levin RJ. Can the controversy about the putative role of the human female orgasm in sperm transport be settled with our current physiological knowledge of coitus? J Sex Med. 2011;8:1566–78.

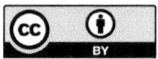

Sexual Aspects of Pregnancy

6

Ana Polona Mivšek ⓘ and Xuan-Hong Tomai ⓘ

6.1 Introduction

This chapter is the first of two dealing with sexuality during pregnancy. Whereas Chap. 12 will address sexuality in complicated pregnancies, this chapter will focus on the uncomplicated, physiological pregnancy. It will start by briefly summarising the physiological and psychological changes in pregnancy that impact a woman's sexuality with attention to changing body awareness and changing social roles. Sexuality is also influenced by the partner, the society and culture of the couple. Those elements, however, will get limited attention. Chapter 22 will give details on the sexuality of the male partner in the phase of pregnancy and young parenthood, and Chap. 23 will delineate cultural aspects. Healthcare professionals (HCPs), usually midwives, who have the expertise to guide women through pregnancies, need to address this vital area of sexuality with all its changes for women and couples.

6.2 Pregnancy: A Unique But Challenging Time

All couples enter partnership and pregnancy with their shared experiences, behaviours, dreams [1]. A woman's thoughts and feelings about pregnancy, her acceptance of it and consequently her attitude towards sexuality in pregnancy are very

---

The original version of the chapter has been revised. A correction to this chapter can be found at https://doi.org/10.1007/978-3-031-18432-1_31

A. Polona Mivšek (✉)
Faculty of Health Studies, University of Ljubljana, Ljubljana, Slovenia
e-mail: polona.mivsek@zf.uni-lj.si

X.-H. Tomai
Department of Obstetrics and Gynecology, University of Medicine and Pharmacy,
Ho Chi Minh City, Vietnam

much influenced by how the couple decided to become pregnant. Some women experience pregnancy as a loss of identity and perceive their bodies as no longer their own, while others thoroughly enjoy this period. A planned pregnancy that both partners desire can increase the enjoyment of pregnancy and, consequently, sexuality during this time [1].

Many other factors influence a woman's attitude towards pregnancy and sexuality also: her current life situation, sense of security, relationships with others, self-acceptance, reaction to the hormonal changes of pregnancy and last but not least, her expectations of motherhood.

The partner's support and attention can strongly impact the woman's feelings about pregnancy [2]. However even if the pregnancy was planned and desired by both, it is normal to have ambivalent feelings. Nowadays, most women have the opportunity to build a career, have a baby and step a while out of the career path. Then, dedicating one's life to a dependent child can be perceived as losing one's professional identity, freedom, etc. In this context, confronting these significant lifestyle changes can lead to grief and a sense of loss. Despite mutual consent with the partner for a child, these women's feelings of sacrifice can affect their (sexual) relationship.

Pregnancy also challenges the partner. Some will experience insecurities about career and parenting abilities. Besides, the pregnant woman gradually changes from a lover to a mother, which can affect the climate of the relationship. Therefore, it is important to talk about feelings during pregnancy and address insecurities so that they do not become a problem for the couple. If such emotional challenges are left unresolved, they can easily affect the couple's relationship and sexual wellbeing over time.

Despite the individual differences in the way women experience (each and every) pregnancy and even the different stages of the same pregnancy, there are some general physiological and psychological changes that pregnancy brings to each woman and her partner, which already can change sexuality during this time.

6.3   Physical and Psychological Changes in Pregnancy Which Might Influence Sexuality

As indicated above, during pregnancy, the woman experiences changes in all areas of her life—physical, emotional and social. We will discuss only those most likely affecting her intimacy and sexuality.

6.3.1   Physiological Body Changes

In the first trimester of pregnancy, specific physiological changes (such as the absence of menstruation) can positively impact a woman's sexuality. Other changes, such as nausea and fatigue, are normal, but not pleasant and can negatively affect sexual desire and arousability.

In the second trimester of pregnancy, the volume of the breasts increases, which some women find uncomfortable or even painful, affecting sexual intimacy. Some women might feel more feminine because of the increased breast size and some might not. The increased blood flow to the genitals strengthens the sensitivity of this area, which can facilitate the achievement of orgasm and increase sexual desire. Nausea usually disappears during this time, and most women begin to enjoy the pregnancy, which can also affect their levels of sexual desire and willingness to have sex.

In the third trimester, women may experience heaviness and shortness of breath as the uterus grows. Fatigue becomes again more familiar. Women often report insomnia because even at night, they have to urinate frequently. The enlarged uterus can cause feelings of clumsiness and affect self-confidence. And the awareness that the baby will soon be a reality can trigger a change in social roles (with the focus shifting from partner, employee, etc., almost exclusively to motherhood). All of these situations can be reasons why interest in sexuality can wane.

The above-mentioned physical symptoms are not pathological, but they are not always pleasant and interfere with a woman's daily activities. It is relevant to remember that nowadays, many women postpone their pregnancies. Pregnancies at an older age of the mother and father however increase the risk of complications and these are addressed in the next chapters.

6.3.2 Psychological Changes

Reva Rubin, a maternity nursing specialist, described that a woman goes through three stages of psychological acceptance during pregnancy, usually corresponding to the trimesters [3]. These psychological considerations and focusses also play an important role in the context of a woman's interest in sex.

In the first trimester woman's interests are directed towards how being pregnant will change her life. She largely will focus on herself and her physical changes. This self-centred view is necessary for woman and her transition to motherhood, but it can lower sexual desire because her mind is pre-occupied with the changes she is going through.

In the second trimester, attention turns to the baby; it is usually closely associated with awareness of the first movements of the fetus. Protective feelings towards the unborn child come to the forefront, and the child's benefits are the focus of the woman's attention, so it is common and logical that fear of harming the baby during sexual intercourse arises. Some researchers say that fear of the harmful effects of sex on the baby is a main reason for low sexual activity in pregnancy [4]. However, as Gianotten [1] writes, these fears are often culturally based. Couples might also have more sex during pregnancy than before. For instance, one tribe in Africa frequently practises intercourse during pregnancy because the act is crucial to 'finish' the baby (intercourse has to create all body parts). Southeastern Nigerians also practise sex during pregnancy because they believe it dilates the vagina and facilitates childbirth [5].

The third trimester is often marked by the woman becoming aware of the upcoming birth. That realisation can cause anxiety due to worries about the safety of herself and the baby. Common issues also include awareness of the changed body image or disturbing physical changes caused by pregnancy.

6.3.3   Social Changes

How woman accepts this period is also affected by how her culture views the pregnancy. How is pregnancy portrayed in the media? And how is it taken by the relevant intimates-especially her partner. Because of her physical changes, the idea of the baby (and impending parenthood) is more tangible to the pregnant woman than to her partner. Realising and accepting the imminent fact that their roles will change dramatically will arise later in her partner. Since this can create tension in the relationship, addressing and explaining this 'time gap' in accepting future parenthood can be beneficial. An unsatisfactory relationship and disturbed intimacy usually will impair sexuality and vice versa. As said, the pregnant woman's male partner usually does not feel the physiological changes of pregnancy, however some do - psychosomatic symptoms are called 'couvade syndrome' and reflect the woman's fatigue, exhaustion and nausea. Some claim that couvade syndrome is more common in men facing unplanned pregnancies, suggesting that it is often related to unresolved issues of paternity acceptance [6]. Couvade symptoms have also been linked to possible hormonal changes in the male partner, such as a drop in cortisol and testosterone levels. That can also decrease sexual desire as a side effect [7]. Couvade symptoms are more common during first pregnancy, especially in the first trimester and around birth [1]. However, even without experiencing any physical changes, pregnancy significantly impacts the man's emotions, which requires psychological adjustment and recognition by his partner and their HCPs. Just as in pregnant women, ambivalent feelings about pregnancy and the baby are common and not abnormal among expectant fathers. Joy and anxiety about the future may be intermingled.

In some cases, men have concerns about future financial responsibilities. And some can feel excluded from the dyad formed between the expectant mother and the coming baby. Common concerns are also fears about the birth process. Childbirth is felt as dangerous for his wife and the baby and not in his control. All these feelings affect the dynamics of the partners and can therefore also affect their sexual life.

These changes are relevant for understanding pregnancy's changes to a couple's relationship.

The following sections will provide information about the woman's sexuality and include details on every trimester. Chapter 22 will pay extra attention to the male partner, and Chap. 21 to the lesbian couple's pregnancy. Although a bit old, we derived much information from an extensive meta-analysis on sexual behaviour in pregnancy by Kirsten Von Sydow [5], and we will draw some parallels with more recent research.

6.4   Sexuality in Pregnancy: Diversity of Normalcy

As explained above, both partners' physical and psychological factors may influence their sexual desire and response. In an uncomplicated pregnancy, the couple may continue with sexual activity until the end of the pregnancy [8], but the couple's desire may vary as the pregnancy progresses. Some researchers report less sexual activity by couples during these 9 months [9]. On the other hand, rare studies have found that some couples regularly continue having sex until childbirth [10]. More commonly, a decline is reported, estimated to be as high as 50% [11]. Some couples stop having sex as soon as they know they are pregnant [5]. In general, a slight decrease in the frequency of coital activity is observed in the first trimester, followed by a slight increase in the second trimester and a sharp drop in desire and coital activity at the end of pregnancy. Studies that examined sexual desire, arousal and frequency of orgasm report a reduction in all of these parametres of sexual function [12]. In interpreting information from different research articles, the midwife/HCP must be aware of often interfering cultural biases plaguing sexuality research from both the respondents' and the researcher's sides.

Sexual desire and ability to become aroused and achieve orgasm in pregnancy is very individual; it varies from woman to woman, pregnancy to pregnancy and even trimester to trimester. It is also very much related to the quality and satisfaction of the partnership [13]. The quality of sexuality before the pregnancy has a significant impact on sexual satisfaction post-partum and during young parenthood [1]. Therefore, in terms of prevention, it is vital to regularly address and eventually educate on sexuality and intimacy in pre-natal check-ups to prevent developing problems or resolve them promptly.

6.4.1   First Trimester

The commonly accepted view is that women in the first trimester are less interested in sexual activity due to fatigue, nausea or morning sickness. Women prefer non-genital stimulation to penetration [5]. However, this may also be the result of uncomfortable or even painful sensations. In nulligravid and primigravid women, breast volume can increase by 25% during sexual arousal. When the hypercongestion of arousal augments the pregnancy-related physiological enlargement of the breasts, the breasts can cause discomfort or even pain (and eventually avert women from sex) [1].

Experts report differences in sexual desire among couples, with the male desire usually being higher. That difference can cause tension in the relationship through feelings of rejection from the partner with greater desire and guilt from the partner with lower desire [6]. Therefore, good health care should address sexuality individually, starting from the perception of this couple's sexuality during pregnancy. HCPs should avoid assuming fixed norms and average behaviours not to provoke feelings of inadequacy. They should start from a frame of reference in which any changes in women's sexuality as a direct result of pregnancy are normal. We think that providing all couples with appropriate education about sexuality is neccessary. Some midwifery researchers caution that only quantitative measures of changes in sexual components, usually estimated with validated instruments (the FSFI as most commonly used), cannot explain the broader context of changes in the couple's sexuality and partnership and are not explanatory enough, because they do not capture individual aetiology of individuals' issues [14]. Therefore starting by assessing this couple's ideas about sexuality and their common sexual practice can help avoid misconceptions and miscommunication.[1]

6.4.2   Second Trimester

In the second trimester, increased vasocongestion of the vagina and vulva may improve sexual arousal and sexual desire in some women so that they have similar or even higher levels of sexual desire and arousal than before pregnancy. Another advantage of the pregnancy is perceiving the moist vagina as sexual lubrication and this acts as a potential trigger for greater arousal. Hypercongestion can also contribute to more intense orgasms, and some women may experience multiple orgasms. For about 50% of women, their ability to orgasm improves during this time (some even experience reaching orgasm faster). However, these physical changes can also have disadvantages. Pregnancy-induced hypercongestion combined with sexual arousal can lead to vulvar numbness or hypersensitivity and even pain during penetration. As a result, about 30% of women are unable to or have difficulty reaching orgasm.

Male hormone levels also alter when the man is expecting a baby. They have low testosterone and cortisol levels, while oestrogen levels are higher. During pregnancy, also their prolactin levels increase [7]. Low testosterone may be the reason why sexual desire decreases in some of the expectant fathers. Therefore, the sexual desire of women in the second trimester is sometimes higher than that of their male partners [1].

All women can usually feel fetal movements by the end of the 20th week of pregnancy. According to Reva Rubin [3], this is a trigger for women to perceive the unborn baby as a separate individual, no longer a part of their body, but an entity in its own right. However, feeling the baby's movements after coitus can be psychologically unsettling for some women; they may fear that the baby is uncomfortable or even in pain, or they may lack a sense of privacy—they can have the feeling that they are not alone with their partner during intercourse. Therefore, it is helpful to explain to expectant mothers and fathers that baby movements after orgasm are normal and that intercourse and orgasm cannot hurt her. The baby is secured by amniotic fluid in the amniotic sac, within the uterus.

6.4.3   Third Trimester

Similar to the functional changes, sexual behaviour also changes as pregnancy progresses. In the third trimester, the decrease in sexual activity is common again. Reasons may include an enlarged uterus, overly sensitive nipples and enlarged

---

[1] Practical tools on how to effectively 'Talk sexuality' with women and couples can be found in Chap. 26.

breasts that cause physical discomfort [15]. During this period, women experience a prolonged period of arousal, which often leads to a different orgasmic experience. The normal, rhythmic, clonic contractions can be replaced by one prolonged, tonic spasm, which can be experienced as painful [5]. After intra-vaginal (or anal) ejaculation, the semen's prostaglandins may intensify the orgasm contraction. Complete resolution can become impossible due to the constant state of hypercongestion in the vaginal and vulvar areas [1].

During pregnancy, the body changes dramatically, leaving some women feeling unattractive in the last trimester [15]. Acceptance of the changed body image is not only related to weight gain but also to many other changes in the pregnant body (larger breasts, stretch marks, hyperpigmentation of the skin, oedema of the ankles, etc.) and also to physical functioning (some feel clumsy, slow, some report stress incontinence, etc.). Nonetheless, some women feel more attractive during pregnancy; the hormones and congestion make them glow and shine, sometimes leading to a greater sense of femininity. The perception of the attractiveness of the pregnant body increases a woman's sexual desire and enjoyment of sex. Results from Pascoal et al.'s [16] study suggest that body dissatisfaction is strongly associated with sexual distress, which is associated with lower sexual and relationship satisfaction [13]. This confirms older findings reported by Von Sydow [5]. Male partners also have various perceptions. Some men are attracted to pregnant bodies, while others are not. There is much debate about the public image of pregnant women, particularly concerning the influence of the media and pregnant celebrities [6].

The most common fears of couples who engage in penetrative sex during pregnancy are injury to the unborn child, induction of pre-mature birth, rupturing of the membranes or causing infection [11]. Therefore, one of the main tasks for midwives and other HCPs accompanying the couple through the pregnancy is to answer the expressed (and also the not-asked) questions, clearly explaining the physiological changes during pregnancy and the associated potential risks to sexuality and reassure where needed. For example, logical and straightforward advice such as that the onset of labour is a complicated process and that in normal pregnancies, labour cannot be induced by sexual intercourse until the baby is at term.

6.5 Counselling Sexuality to Pregnant Couples: Overcoming the Taboo

Many HCPs avoid talking to women and their partners about sex in pregnancy, often arguing that they do not want to invade the couple's privacy. On the other side, couples expect them to open up this conversation and hope that they will not have to bring up the subject themselves [15]. The topic of sexuality in pregnancy is sometimes hidden or made misty by using the term intimacy when meaning sex. Another miscommunication occurs when HCPs or couples say sex when meaning penetration. Buehler [6] writes that it is essential to address sexuality directly. Our readers will find more detailed information on *'how to do'* this in Chap. 26. At the same time, we need to be aware that talking about sexuality might bring to light other things that, at first glance, have nothing to do with sexuality but underpin the climate in the relationship and can have a profound impact on the couple's relationship and therefore also on sexuality. That is why it is crucial to take enough time when starting the conversation about sexuality in pregnancy. Ideally, the first conversation should occur already when planning a pregnancy or at the beginning of the pregnancy. We should include both partners in that conversation about sexuality (if needed, followed by individual talks). In many countries, men are actively involved in their partners' pregnancies, attending pre-natal checks and ultrasound examinations, providing birth support, and caring for the baby, so they are also more emotionally affected by pregnancy. In general, gender roles are changing and these changes are even more profound when it comes to the active involvement of fathers-to-be in the perinatal period. HCPs should use their presence at antenatal visits, antenatal classes and counselling sessions to open up the topic of sexuality and intimacy as well. Investing in feelings of mutual support and emotional empathy and maintaining a connection through shared intimate and/or sexual experiences before and during pregnancy are necessary to maintain a solid relationship foundation to survive the challenges of the post-partum period and early years of raising children. Therefore, facilitating an open conversation about sexuality during pregnancy should become a part of routine holistic care for pregnant couples.

There are sexual issues that can be quickly resolved. For example, with counselling about different sexual positions, we can resolve the challenge of abdominal pressure in late pregnancy. Usually, women prefer woman-on-top positions, side positions or posterior positions [5], which are more suitable due to the enlarged uterus. Psychoeducation regarding the baby's safety during intercourse can also relieve some of the stress in the couple. It is also beneficial to discuss with the couple sexual activities that are different from coital activity, which are acceptable to them. In such a way, the HCP can help reconnect them when they suffer from desire differences. Some couples need advice regarding relief from the tension caused by 'pent-up sexual energy'. Non-penetrative forms of sexuality can become very relevant, especially in the third trimester and early post-partum period (the sexual restart phase). Exploring sensual pleasure and intimacy as outercourse[2] options and developing new sexual scripts will be very new for many couples but can help resolve sexual frustrations successfully. We call this process 'renegotiating intimacy'. For example, masturbation or mutual masturbation may help to keep the couple's sexual relationship healthy during pregnancy [1] and might be acceptable to some clients. However, attitudes towards masturbation are also shaped by cultural acceptance and expected male/female roles in the society. Cultural norms and prejudices can have a massive impact on sexual behaviour of the individual, and for pregnancy, in particular, every culture has unwritten rules. Women can feel confused when their feelings and desires differ from society's norms. Therefore, in counselling, HCPs should emphasise the individual variability of sexual response in

---

[2] Outercourse is usually the term for all kinds of extended sex without penetration.

pregnancy, reassuring the couple. Women receive a lot of misleading advice, so HCPs need to start the conversation about sexuality to debunk myths and traditional beliefs and try to reduce unfounded fears and anxieties. We should conduct such conversations with sensitivity and respect.

6.6 Conclusion

Sexual behaviour in pregnancy is influenced by various hormonal, emotional and social factors, reflecting the biopsychosocial nature of sexuality. This mixture of influences 'gives birth' to a very different sexual life during pregnancy. The woman may have less or more sexual desire than her partner. She may have trouble accepting her pregnant body image, or her partner may have a problem accepting his lover becoming a mother. Both may have barriers to sexuality at this time, stemming from cultural misbeliefs. The woman may have concerns about becoming a mother. The partner may also have ambivalent feelings about pregnancy, even with strong child-wish. Partners may feel left out of the process, as the pregnant woman is the radiant centre of everyone's attention. Situations are complex, so there is no prescribed guide on what to advise all pregnant women and their partners regarding sexuality during pregnancy except that maintaining their sexual wellbeing is an essential factor in their general health and wellbeing. It is essential to talk in-depth about sexuality, listen actively and without prejudice, create an intimate atmosphere and maintain professional standards while building a trusting relationship in which couples feel safe to share their thoughts, problems and desires.

References

1. Gianotten WL. Pregnancy and sexuality. In: Tepper MS, Owens AF, editors. Sexual health. Vol 2. Sex, love and psychology. Westport: Praeger; 2007. p. 167–96.
2. Crooks RL, Baur K. Conceiving children. In: Our sexuality. 13th ed. Boston: Cencage Learning; 2015. p. 332–68.
3. Rubin R. Maternal identity and the maternal experience. New York, NY: Springer; 1984. Google Scholar.
4. Mazuchova L, Kelčikova S, Duricekova B, Malinovska N. Perceived changes and concerns of women related to sexuality in pregnancy in the context of the importance of being informed. Kontakt. 2018;20:e244–9.
5. Von Sydow K. Sexuality during pregnancy and after childbirth: a metacontent analysis of 59 studies. J Psychosom Res. 1999;47:27–49.
6. Buehler S. Counselling couples before, during and after pregnancy: sexuality and intimacy issues. New York: Springer; 2018. p. 93–111.
7. Berg SJ, Wynne-Edwards KE. Changes in testosterone, cortisol and estradiol levels in men becoming fathers. Mayo Clin Proc. 2001;76:582–92.
8. Jones C, Chan C, Farine D. Sex in pregnancy. Can Med Assoc J. 2011;183:815–8.
9. Gałązka I, Drosdzol-Cop A, Naworska B, et al. Changes in the sexual functioning during pregnancy. J Sex Med. 2015;12:445–54.
10. Pauleta JR, Pereira NM, Graça LM. Sexuality during pregnancy. J Sex Med. 2010;7:136–42.
11. Corbacioglu Esmer A, Akca A, Akbayir O, et al. Female sexual function and associated factors during pregnancy. J Obstet Gynaecol Res. 2013;39:1165–72.

12. Banaei M, Azizi M, Moridi A, et al. Sexual dysfunction and related factors in pregnancy and postpartum: a systematic review and meta-analysis protocol. Syst Rev. 2019;8:161.
13. Vannier SA, Rosen NO. Sexual distress and sexual problems during pregnancy: associations with sexual and relationship satisfaction. J Sex Med. 2017;4:387–95.
14. Bender SS, Sveinsdottir E, Fridfinnsdottir H. "You stop thinking about yourself as a woman". An interpretive phenomenological study of the meaning of sexuality for Icelandic women during pregnancy and after birth. Midwifery. 2018;62:14–9.
15. Güleroğlu F, Beşer N. Evaluation of sexual functions of the pregnant woman. J Sex Med. 2014;11:146–52.
16. Pascoal PM, Rosa PJ, Coelho S. Does pregnancy play a role? Associaton of body dissatisfaction, body appearance, cognitive distraction and sexual distress. J Sex Med. 2019;16:551–8.

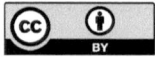

Sexual Aspects of Labour and Birth

Woet L. Gianotten (ORCID)

7.1 Introduction

Giving birth and becoming parents encompasses many challenges, both physical, emotional and social, with changes influencing sexuality, intimacy and the relationship between the woman and her partner. This chapter will focus on the 'sexual aspects' of those challenges and changes.

Maybe even more than in other chapters of this book, the language used here can confuse. For some HCPs, using the word sexual in the context of delivering a baby puts them too far out of their comfort zone. Therefore terms 'nipple stimulation' or 'genital touching' appear more appropriate. For others, the 'neutral' use of medical or anatomical terms will create distance and debunk the intimate value of what happens.

This chapter aims to provide helpful information for optimal midwifery care during labour and birth. It will start by addressing some of the variety in 'sexual aspects of birth' that exists among cultures and subcultures. After that, the relation between the various elements of sexuality/intimacy and the start of labour will get attention, followed by how those elements could influence a smooth continuation of labour. We will give ample attention to the connections between sexuality/intimacy and pain relief methods used during birth.

The last part of this chapter will approach other aspects of sexuality/intimacy and relationship. The birth of a baby is a major life event for all parties involved, especially the first birth being the tipping point from woman to mother, from man to father and from couplehood to parenthood.

W. L. Gianotten (✉)
Department of Gynaecology and Obstetrics, Erasmus University Medical Center, Rotterdam, The Netherlands

© The Author(s) 2023
S. Geuens et al. (eds.), *Midwifery and Sexuality*,
https://doi.org/10.1007/978-3-031-18432-1_7

7.2   Cultural Aspects of Sexuality in Relation to Childbirth

When one mentions (during teaching HCPs) that some women undergo labour 'nearly as a sexual experience', part of the female students tend to react with a mixture of disapproval and denial.

On the one hand, one can consider such a reaction as a not very constructive frame of reference for good intrapartum practice. The reality is that while giving birth, some women have an orgasm (sometimes called birthgasm). For part of those women, that happens without conscious stimulation, whereas some other women deliberately stimulate themselves to orgasm to relieve labour pain. On the other hand, a reaction of 'impossible' apparently represents the mental scripts and communications currently dominant in their society and in 'the medicalized culture'.

In an extensive review, Mayberry and Daniel looked at the explanations behind the apparent disconnection between sexuality and birth [1]. Among them are, for instance, deeply held negative cultural beliefs about sexuality and the gradual change from the intimacy of home birth to the more impersonal and sterile hospital settings. As a result, the current medicalised obstetric care does not favour or use the potential benefits of 'sexual stimulation'. This reality becomes most evident in the area of pain-relief practices. Nowadays, labour and childbirth are predominantly perceived as physically painful events in various cultures. When a culture has developed the belief that that process is meant to be unbearable and traumatic, it becomes difficult for pregnant women (and HCPs) to accept the information of women who do not primarily experience the birth process as painful. Reports from anthropology made clear that in various traditional cultures, 'sexuoerotic stimulation' was applied by the pregnant woman, the husband or the midwife, creating a fluent birth process [2].

In the second half of the twentieth century, the Western world gradually developed a more open attitude towards sexuality and increased female autonomy. That also happened in pregnancy, childbirth and breastfeeding, with leading roles for three professionals mentioned here. Niles Newton was an English research psychologist (1923–1993) who reintroduced the value and pleasure of breastfeeding. Sheila Kitzinger was an English anthropologist (1923–2015) and became an advocate for home birth, breastfeeding and the pregnant woman's autonomy. Michel Odent is a French obstetrician (1930–) who became an advocate for birth without medical intervention, as long as not needed, use the doula, 'natural oxytocin' and (immediately after birth) skin to skin contact between mother and baby. Their approach clarified that the processes of 'sexual' arousal, orgasm, childbirth and lactation have much in common, all being (partially) orchestrated by oxytocin release. They made clear that each of those processes can easily be disturbed by distraction and that the woman should be able to let herself go to succeed. Those developments allowed more intimacy and acceptance of sexual/erotic aspects.

Over the last decades of the twentieth century, other developments gradually counterbalanced this process. There was an increase in the medicalisation of pregnancy and birth, with more hospital births, continuous monitoring and more medicinal interventions for pain relief (nitrous oxide, epidural anaesthesia, etc.), diminishing the women's chances of experiencing an autonomous labouring process. These developments created the current situation in some countries, where more than half of all deliveries end in a caesarean section.

7.3 Sexuality and the Timely Start of Labour

In many eras and cultures, professionals and couples have been afraid that intercourse or orgasm could increase the risk of pre-term birth. In healthy pregnancies, both intercourse and recent female orgasm during late pregnancy (till 36 weeks) appeared to reduce the risk for pre-term birth [3].

This chapter deals with the consequences of sexual activity in term pregnancy.

To prevent post-term birth, unprotected intercourse is recommended as one of the strategies to initiate labour. Responsible for this effect is the exposure to prostaglandins, partly exogenous from the semen and partly endogenous from the cervical manipulation (similarly as in stripping the membranes) [4].

7.4 Sexual Aspects of the Induction of Labour

Internet shows numerous 'natural ways to induce labour' with sex mentioned frequently. Although being an important topic, very little research has been done in that area [5]. One can explain that as a taboo, but also because research in this period is complex for ethical and practical reasons. Articles on 'sex to induce labour' tend to limit themselves to only a part of the potential. Here we will elaborate on all the known possibilities and their accompanying explanation. The starting point of this explanation and advice is a healthy term pregnancy

7.4.1 Breasts and Nipples

In the early 1980s, they developed a nipple stimulation contraction test to assess fetal wellbeing, based on the finding that stimulation of the nipple(s) frequently resulted in uterine contractions in late pregnancy. In that protocol, the pregnant woman stimulated her breasts (*through her clothes*) for 2 min, followed by 5-min rest. When there were no adequate uterine contractions, the next cycle of 2-min stimulation and 5-min rest was started, etc. One 2-min cycle or less stimulation was enough for 43% of the women, 39% needed two cycles and 15% required three cycles to induce contractions [6]. In a meta-analysis comparing breast stimulation versus no intervention, 37% versus 6% were in labour at 72 hrs [7]. In two of the breast-stimulation trials, they found an additional benefit in an 84% reduction in post-partum haemorrhage.

Of course, the mediator here is oxytocin. Around the onset of labour, uterine sensitivity to oxytocin markedly increases [8]. Implementation for the non-research practice: forget the 'not through the clothes', do not stop just because of a 2-min restriction, and (when feasible) let the loving partner deliver this stimulation;

Stimulation will have a more intense effect when performed by the partner due to the intimate connection and (hopefully) the partner's knowledge and experience on how to stimulate her nipples optimally.

7.4.2 Touch

Caressing and massage increase the level of oxytocin. Among its many effects are nurturing and sedating and anti-stress and anxiolytic effects.

7.4.3 Intercourse/Penetration

As long as the membranes are not ruptured, both intercourse (penetration) and ejaculation can have a function in labour induction. HCPs know that the direct internal touching/pressure of vaginal examination can cause a surge in oxytocin (the Ferguson reflex). The same happens with other forms of vaginal penetration. Such touching of the cervix also releases (endogenous) prostaglandin. Ejaculation can add a labour-inducing effect since seminal plasma contains (exogenous) prostaglandin (PGE2 and PGF) in higher concentrations than in the common cervical ripening agents.

Anal penetration also causes the oxytocin release of the Ferguson reflex and the endogenous prostaglandin due to touching the cervix. The (exogenous) prostaglandins deposited in the anus will not reach the cervix but indirectly via the circulation after easy absorption through the anal wall.

7.4.4 Arousal and Orgasm

Sexual arousal and orgasm both cause an increase in oxytocin levels. The increase is most clearly seen at orgasm, with, at 5 minutes after orgasm, still a high level [9]. Orgasms typically have clonic contractions, but the contraction pattern can change into one tonic contraction in the last 6-8 weeks of pregnancy. Such a strong contraction can cause rupturing of the membranes.

Some 25–30% of women experience the so-called cervico-uterine orgasm, accompanied by strong uterine contractions. That orgasm needs the stimulation of the cervical area and is orchestrated at the T12-L2 centre in the spinal cord.

Hypothesis: As long as the membranes are not ruptured, stimulating the cervix and 'G-spot area' with a penis, finger, dildo or vibrator could be a valuable opportunity for physiologically furthering labour.

7.4.5 Implementation

The limited research in this area tends to deal with only one of the above-mentioned elements. However, in daily practice, combining those various elements is expected to have an added value. The midwife appears the right professional to address those possibilities.

7.5   Sexual Aspects of 'Keeping the Process Going'

After labour has started, several of the above-mentioned elements could be benefi-cial to keep the process going. In trying to explain the cause-effect relationship, it is difficult to distinguish between the direct influence on the progress of labour and the indirect effects by influencing the degree of experienced pain.

7.5.1   Touch

Well-received caressing and massage will increase the level of oxytocin, influencing both uterine contractions and relaxation. Massage also increases dopamine and serotonin levels and decreases the cortisol level [10]. With the progress of labour, an increase in plasma cortisol level is needed to maintain maternal/foetal wellbeing and facilitate the regular labour progress. Well-applied (and well-received) non-erotic or erotic skin contact may prevent cortisol levels from going too high.

7.5.2   Breasts and Nipples

Stimulation of breasts and nipples (especially when playful and intimate) will increase the oxytocin level and, as such, have a direct effect on uterine contractions and an indirect effect (via sedation) of less pain. The added value is bonding with the partner.

7.5.3   Sexual Arousal and Orgasm

An increase in oxytocin levels accompanies both sexual arousal and orgasm.

Orgasm will give strong uterine contractions and a temporary altered state of consciousness. Well-received stimulation of the genital-clitoral area has extra ben-efits since it significantly increases the pain threshold through endorphin release. Outside pregnancy, the effect of self-applied vaginal stimulation on pain thresholds was studied. When such stimulation produced orgasm, the pain detection threshold increased significantly by 107% and the pain tolerance threshold by 75% [11].

7.6   Labour Pain and Sexual Aspects

The amount of pain that people experience and remember is influenced by factors like context, cause and what the pain means to the person. For instance, chronic pain and pain related to surgery tend to be overestimated, whereas pain induced by intense sports tends to be underestimated [12]. Nearly every runner has experience with pain, and that amount is acceptable because of having control over it. There appears to be a wide variety of responses regarding recalling the pain of childbirth. Researchers compared the neurophysiology of pain at childbirth and the pain of running a marathon. Both are not only physically exhausting but also emotionally intense experiences. Oxytocin (mediating uterine contractions in childbirth and maintaining the fluid balance in running) has analgesic properties and also plays an essential role in memory formation and recall [12]. When women interpret the pain as productive and purposeful, it is associated with positive cognitions and emotions. That appears to be at least one of the context factors that create the above-mentioned variety in childbirth pain recall. A culture telling that childbirth is meant to be a painful and traumatic event neither creates positive expectations nor an atmosphere where intimacy and trust can easily develop [1].

Intimacy and trust are essential for several reasons. Trust is needed to let the process happen smoothly. Intimacy is relevant to allow the woman and her partner to feel at ease for massage, breast stimulation and other 'pseudosexual stimulation' by which the oxytocin and endorphin levels can increase and, in that way, keep the process going and the pain acceptable. In the choreography of 'sexual labour pain relief', orgasm appears the most valuable and practical element.

Besides, intimacy is a critical element of the bonding between the partners during this major life event.

7.7 The Relational Aspects and Sexual Implications of Childbirth

Especially the first birth is a pivotal moment in partnership. It is a major life event where the woman and her partner experience extreme fatigue and hormonal changes that strongly influence emotions. How that will affect their future relationship will depend on many different factors. There are areas on the globe where pregnancy and birth predominantly belong to the woman's realm and where the vast majority of her social contacts are with other females. Then the male partner's role and his reactions are relatively less critical. In other parts of the world, the connection between the woman and her partner can be rather different. Having less family around and being emotionally far more dependent on each other, their interaction during childbirth will strongly influence their bond as a couple and, subsequently, their joint parenthood. After all, the first birth is also the transition from a dyad to a triad, influencing their (sexual) relationship.

During the birth, some husbands get lost or become a nuisance. Others turn into valuable supporters by which the birth can become a moment of mutual personal growth.

A key element in that process is how the partner deals with the labour pain. Most people have no experience with the pain of someone else. When the midwife can co-create an intimate context; when the woman is open to her husband's presence and support and when the husband can caress, massage and generate 'intimate, physical labour pain relief', their sexual relationship will get a boost instead of the adverse effects commonly referred to as 'the uncoupling of birth'.

References

1. Mayberry L, Daniel J. 'Birthgasm': a literary review of orgasm as an alternative mode of pain relief in childbirth. J Holist Nurs. 2016;34:331–42.
2. Pranzarone GF. Sexuoerotic stimulation and orgasmic response in the induction and management of parturition – clinical possibilities. In: Kothari P, Parel R, editors. Proceedings of the first international conference on orgasm. New Delhi: Bombay VRP Publishers; 1991. p. 105–19. Available https://www.researchgate.net/publication/280495439.
3. Sayle AE, Savitz DA, Thorp JM Jr, et al. Sexual activity during late pregnancy and risk of preterm delivery. Obstet Gynecol. 2001;97:283–9.
4. Caughey AB, Snegovskikh VV, Norwitz ER. Post-term pregnancy: how can we improve outcomes? Obstet Gynecol Surv. 2008;63:715–24.
5. Kavanagh J, Kelly AJ, Thomas J. Sexual intercourse for cervical ripening and induction of labour. Cochrane Database Syst Rev. 2001;2001:CD003093.
6. Huddleston JF, Sutliff G, Robinson D. Contraction stress test by intermittent nipple stimulation. Obstet Gynecol. 1984;63:669–73.
7. Kavanagh J, Kelly AJ, Thomas J. Breast stimulation for cervical ripening and induction of labour. Cochrane Database Syst Rev. 2005;3:CD003392.
8. Gimpl G, Fahrenholz F. The oxytocin receptor system: structure, function, and regulation. Physiol Rev. 2001;81:629–83.
9. Carmichael MS, Humbert R, Dixen J, et al. Plasma oxytocin increases in the human sexual response. J Clin Endocrinol Metab. 1987;64:27–31.
10. Field T, Diego MA, Hernandez-Reif M, et al. Massage therapy effects on depressed pregnant women. J Psychosom Obstet Gynecol. 2004;25:115–22.
11. Whipple B, Komisaruk BR. Elevation of pain threshold by vaginal stimulation in women. Pain. 1985;21:357–67.
12. Farley D, Piszczek Ł, Bąbel P. Why is running a marathon like giving birth? The possible role of oxytocin in the underestimation of the memory of pain induced by labour and intense exercise. Med Hypotheses. 2019;128:86–90.

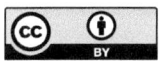

Sexuality of the Couple in Postpartum and Early Parenthood (1st Year)

8

Deirdre O'Malley ⓘ, Agnes Higgins ⓘ, and Valerie Smith ⓘ

8.1 Introduction

The birth of a baby is, for many, a joyous occasion; however, during the months that follow, significant changes often occur within couples' relationships. For many couples, during the first 12 months after birth, their intimate relationship transforms, in particular, aspects of their sexual relationship. Couples have reported that extreme tiredness, adapting to new parenting roles, baby care and concern over baby's well-being have impacted their relationship priorities, with their sexual relationship often moving down their list of priorities. While many relationship changes are normative and may be transitory, parents must be advised of the possibility of changes to their intimate and sexual relationships so they are aware and prepared for these should they occur. It is also important that couples are provided with evidence-based, practical information, research-based when possible, on sexual health post-partum, including strategies to maintain a satisfying intimate relationship with their partner during the first year post-partum. This chapter will explore and discuss this multi-dimensional view of sexual health in post-partum and early parenthood (up to 1 year).

D. O'Malley (✉)
Department of Nursing, Midwifery and Early Years, Dundalk Institute of Technology, Dundalk, Co Louth, Ireland
e-mail: deirdre.omalley@dkit.ie

A. Higgins · V. Smith
School of Nursing and Midwifery, University of Dublin, Trinity College, Dublin, Ireland

© The Author(s) 2023
S. Geuens et al. (eds.), *Midwifery and Sexuality*,
https://doi.org/10.1007/978-3-031-18432-1_8

8.2   Post-Partum Sexual Health

This textbook views sexuality and post-partum sexual health as multi-faceted concepts utilising a biopsychosocial approach. Facets include physical dimensions (vaginal lubrication, orgasm and dyspareunia), social dimensions (adapting to parenthood, changed roles), psychological (perception of body image, sexual desire, fear, worry and anxiety) and relational (intimacy, emotional and practical support, perception of sexual desire in the partner and changed roles) dimensions. Yet, an examination of the literature from the last 20 years highlights a predominant focus on the physical facets of post-partum sexual health. Many of the published studies appear to focus on the objective measurement of aspects of sexual health such as sexual desire, dyspareunia, vaginal lubrication, orgasm and timing of resumption of first sexual intercourse after birth and do so through the use of measurement tools, scales and questionnaires. These study reports often use the language of sexual dysfunction and sexual problems when, for example, women indicate that they have not had an orgasm in the preceding 4 weeks or that their sexual desire has lessened since the birth of their baby. This adverse labelling, however, does not take account of the transitional nuances or natural changes that women, and their partners, may experience after childbirth and as they adapt to being parents of a new baby. In more recent years, there is a growing body of evidence, predominately from qualitative enquiry, that has identified and given credence to the multi-dimensional aspects of post-partum sexual health. For example, O'Malley and colleagues emphasise the importance of communication within the couple dyad, communication about tiredness, stress associated with adapting to parenthood, sexual desire or lack of sexual desire as a means of maintaining sexual wellbeing post-birth [1]. How women perceive their body image (and changed body image after birth) has been shown to impact the couple's sexual wellbeing after birth [2].

8.3   Intimacy

Intimacy and sexual wellbeing may, for some, be closely aligned, although not necessarily so. In considering sexual wellbeing for couples post-partum, it would be remiss, however, not to consider the concept of intimacy and the role it may play. It is generally recognised that there are four types of intimacy: physical intimacy (e.g. hugs, kisses and sexual activity), emotional intimacy (e.g. closeness, trust and love), cognitive intimacy (e.g. sharing ideas and thoughts) and spiritual intimacy (e.g. bonding over spirituality). Post-partum women have described intimacy as closeness with their partner, a closeness not shared with any other person. Women have described non-sexual touch, such as back rubs, holding hands, cuddles and hugs, as intimacy. They have talked about the importance of sleeping in the same bed, sitting on the same couch, watching a television show together and good morning kisses as aspects of intimacy with their partner. Women have been clear in their narratives that maintaining these non-sexual aspects of intimacy is essential to their sexuality and sexual wellbeing during the first year after birth [1].

Features of satisfying relationships are varied, but commonalities in how couple's relationships evolve after the first child's birth have been reported. In a longitudinal study carried out over 8 years with 820 first-time parents, for example, reported factors affecting the quality of the intimate relationship 6 months after the birth of the baby were: coping by adjusting to parental role, mutual support as new parents, the couple's intimacy (i.e. togetherness and love) and coping by communication (i.e. verbal and non-verbal confirmation) [3], thus supporting the notion that sexual health after birth is multi-dimensional. Furthermore, features associated with long-term relationship satisfaction in couples with children included cohesiveness within the couple, effective communication and maintaining sensuality and sexuality [3, 4]. Sharing parental and household responsibilities, good communication and emotional, physical and sexual intimacy have also been identified as features of a satisfying intimate relationship after the first baby's birth [5].

The following sections will examine some of the common post-partum sexual health issues women and healthcare professionals have identified as important.

8.4   Resuming Sexual Activity After Birth

Sexual activity is the many ways in which humans express their sexuality, sometimes solo, often together. We also do it through writing, art, music and how we communicate with each other. Common sexual activities include masturbation, vaginal sex, anal sex, oral sex, sex toys, role play (acting out sexual fantasies), deep kissing, intimate massage, etc. Sexual activities enable a vulnerability and deeper level of intimacy that has been shown to lead to greater relationship satisfaction. After birth, a frequent concern for couples is the resumption of any form of sexual activity, particularly when penis-in-vagina penetration may be started. For healthcare professionals (HCPs), this is also a question that does not lend itself to a definitive answer, with many HCPs advising women to resume sexual activity '*when you feel ready*'. Yet, post-partum couples appear to need specific information. For example, many want to know when other couples resume sexual activity or if they 'have to wait' until their six-week or final post-partum assessment. As a HCP, being asked these questions can be challenging because each couple is different, and what might be appropriate advice for some couples might not be appropriate for others. Many women report that they wait until they feel physically recovered from the birth, that is, when perineal or abdominal wounds have healed or when lochia has ceased [1]. Some women may wait until uterine afterpains and wound pain have resolved. Regardless of each individualistic scenario, women collectively appear to experience varying levels of fear when they talk about resuming sexual intercourse after birth. They frequently describe a fear of pain (further addressed in Sect. 8.5.1) and a fear of how sexual intercourse will feel. Many wonder if they will experience sexual satisfaction and the feeling of closeness with their partner in the same way as they previously did. Partners also worry about pain, that is, causing their partner pain and when the 'right' time is.

Much of the discussion on the timing of resumption of sexual activity after birth is focussed exclusively on vaginal/penile penetration. Reported rates of vaginal/penile penetration resumption range from 41% at 6 weeks [6], 51–65% at 8 weeks [6, 7] and 78% ($n = 1020$) at 12 weeks after birth [6], although much lower rates have also been reported; for example, 30% ($n = 146$) in one study at 12 weeks post-partum [8]. Women, however, did tend to resume some form of sexual activity, other than penetrative vaginal sex, earlier in the weeks and months after birth (approximately 10–12% of women), although the exact detail on what types of sexual activities were resumed is generally lacking from studies. Crucially, we are not aware of any studies that have specifically examined sexual health post-partum in women who are in same-sex relationships. Occasionally, a tiny number of women in same-sex relationships have been identified in larger samples of women in opposite-sex relationships with no comparisons made to determine if their experience of their post-partum sexual health differs from opposite-sex couples.

In our own research, involving 21 women in opposite-sex relationships in Ireland up to 2 years post-partum, we explored women's experience of their sexual health after the birth of their first baby through in-depth one-to-one interviews. Women described how they planned when they would resume vaginal sex. They mentioned the baby being in a different room, being away from the baby and home or the baby having an overnight with immediate family [1]. Women explained that they planned to resume sex after a night out with their partner, for example, going for dinner and drinks. Some women planned to start sexual intercourse as soon as they could post-birth, for example, 4 weeks post-partum. They wanted emotional and physical closeness with their partner. They wanted to feel attractive, feel sexually desired and experience sexual satisfaction. Nonetheless, many other women explained that sexual intercourse was something that took many months to resume. For these women, baby care, infant feeding, adapting to motherhood and the desire for sleep were more important during the first 3 or 4 months after birth. When preparing to resume sexual activity and vaginal penetration, women describe additional considerations: the mode of delivery and the presence of perineal wounds. Some women preferred to wait until they had their final post-partum assessment, traditionally 6 weeks after birth, particularly those who had a caesarean section or operative vaginal birth. Women with perineal stitches also described waiting at least 6 weeks until they received reassurance from their medical practitioner that their wounds had healed, which did not necessarily mean that they resumed sexual activity immediately after 6 weeks. It was rather another factor that women considered when planning to resume sexual activity.

Little is published regarding the partner's views on resuming sexual intercourse after birth. Nonetheless, many women in their narratives have described him waiting for their lead on timing or coming to an agreement as a couple that sexual intercourse will be less of a priority for the first few months as they focus on adapting to their new roles. Of course, while sex may be postponed in the short-term, the conversation about sex and sexual desire needs to take place for each member of the couple to remain sexually satisfied in their intimate relationship. Complacency can set in, with sex becoming a sporadic event. On the other hand, many women feel pressure from their partners to engage in sexual intercourse after birth. In particular in couples with a limited sexual repertoire.

An example is when sexual activity and orgasm are strongly associated with penetrative sex. Some men and couples may have a 'penetration imperative' not having learned how to masturbate to reach orgasm. Men can solo masturbate, but mutual or intimate masturbation can also provide sexual pleasure in these circumstances. Each individual and couple must explore their own and each other's bodies to find ways to experience sexual pleasure and climax if that is their ultimate goal.

> Pregnant and post-partum women can be directed to get information on resumption of sex after birth from reputable websites. Examples might include www.babycenter.uk and www.tcd.ie/mammi/. The MAMMI study has developed a suite of videos for women and healthcare professional on sexual wellbeing after birth. They have been translated into Spanish, Dutch, Lithuanian and Romanian.

When to give information on the resumption of sexual activity after birth is fundamental and ought to be individualised to the woman, her literacy skills and preferred language. Frequently, women are discharged from maternity services 24 h after a normal birth and 72 h after a caesarean section, although this may vary from country to country. In some instances, depending on the model of maternity care, women might receive a home visit or two from a community midwife with a final post-natal assessment undertaken by a general practitioner or obstetrician approximately 6 weeks after the birth. Post-partum discharge advice often relies on a 'tickbox' approach, a list of wide-ranging issues that need to be discussed with a woman before discharge from maternity services. The list may include but is not limited to: post-natal depression, registering the birth of the baby, prevention of Sudden Infant Death Syndrome (SIDS), audiology screening, screening for metabolic disorders and contraception. This is the only window of opportunity to discuss with women when to resume sexual activity after birth in many countries. Yet, for many women, it may be an inappropriate time to bring up the topic of restarting penetrative sexual activity. It could be a time of extreme tiredness, physical discomfort, getting to know their new baby, establishing feeding and a desire to leave the maternity service and go home. This raises the question of 'When might be the appropriate or 'right' time?' to start the discussion.

One solution that could be considered is to discuss the issue of sexual health post-partum during antenatal parenthood education classes. This topic may be appropriate in antenatal discussions on adapting to parenthood after birth. However, as many women do not attend antenatal parenthood education classes, a large population of women may not receive information on sexual health after birth. Therefore, post-partum home visits, if included in the model of care or the six-week post-natal assessment, may be a more appropriate time. This final post-natal assessment has been criticised for its 'check-list' approach and being baby-centric, with little time devoted to maternal health and wellbeing. Frequently, contraception is belatedly addressed during this assessment, but the actual issue of resuming sexual activity is often ignored. Thus, midwives may find no alternative opportune time to address the resumption of sexual activity after birth other than as part of discharge planning. In these less-than-ideal circumstances, midwifery students and registered midwives could advise women that they can resume sexual activity when they feel physically and emotionally ready to do so while also acknowledging that this will vary from woman to woman and that it is usually planned by the woman rather than spontaneous. Women who have their birth complicated by perineal tears, sutures and/or instrumental births may be advised to avoid penetrative sex for 4–6 weeks until wounds have healed.

Women concerned about pain and discomfort during penetrative sex could also consider exploring oral sex as a means of sexual satisfaction. This may be oral stimulation of the vulva or clitoris (cunnilingus) or oral stimulation of the penis and testicles (a 'blow job' or fellatio). Couples might also consider solo or mutual masturbation. However, be sensitive to women's views and norms. For example, the notion of oral sex may be offensive depending on their cultural beliefs and sexual norms. A gradual build-up to sex and artificial lubricants can also be advised. Lastly, as maternity HCPs, you should equip yourselves to comfortably, and knowledgeable provide direction for women on where to source additional evidence-based information on post-partum sexual health. This may be in web addresses, links to learning packages or support services in your area, such as sexual health midwife or nurse, psychosexual therapist or a women's health physiotherapist or pelvic floor therapist.

8.5   Sexual Health After Birth: What Is Normal?

An abundance of research reports a high prevalence of sexual health issues after birth, particularly so in first-time mothers. However, wide prevalence rates vary, ranging from 18–61% 3 months after birth [9] to 9–40% at 12 months post-partum [10]. Research is generally consistent in the reported types of issues: dyspareunia (pain during penetration), vaginal lubrication, sexual desire, sexual arousal and orgasm. Many commonly used measurement tools are based on Masters and Johnson's Sexual Response Cycle [11], suggesting that human sexual response follows a linear model progressing through four phases: excitement, plateau, orgasm and resolution. This model is often criticised as being dated and male-orientated, without attention to female sexual motivation, emotional intimacy and relational dynamics. The following section examines what women, couples and healthcare professionals should consider as normative changes to sexual health after birth.

8.5.1   Is Dyspareunia Normal After Birth?

Genito-pelvic pain disorder is commonly referred to as sexual pain disorder or dyspareunia and often encompasses pain during sexual intercourse, pain during penetration and rarely pain at orgasm. The potential for dyspareunia during first and

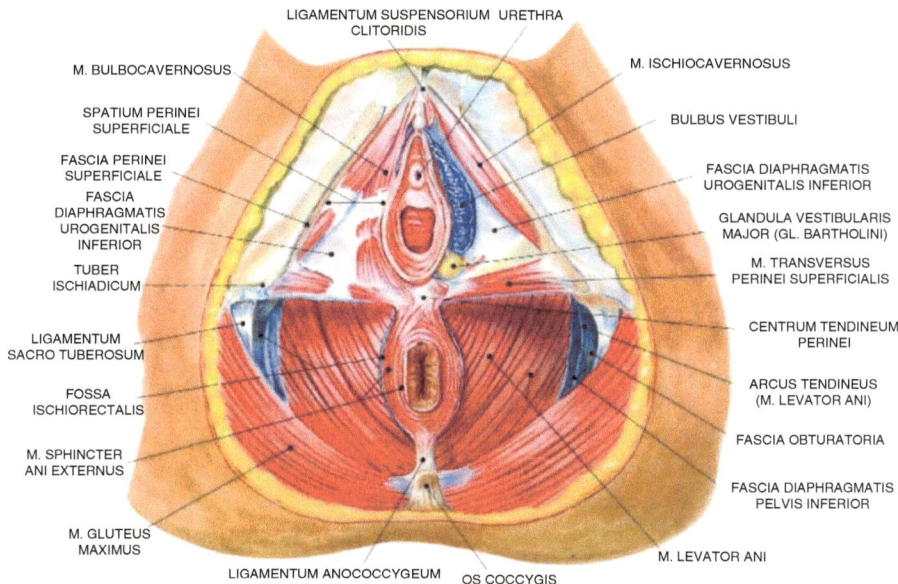

LIGAMENTUM SUSPENSORIUM URETHRA
CLITORIDIS

M. BULBOCAVERNOSUS

M. ISCHIOCAVERNOSUS

SPATIUM PERINEI
SUPERFICIALE

BULBUS VESTIBULI

FASCIA PERINEI
SUPERFICIALE

FASCIA DIAPHRAGMATIS
UROGENITALIS INFERIOR

FASCIA
DIAPHRAGMATIS
UROGENITALIS
INFERIOR

GLANDULA VESTIBULARIS
MAJOR (GL. BARTHOLINI)

TUBER
ISCHIADICUM

M. TRANSVERSUS
PERINEI SUPERFICIALIS

LIGAMENTUM
SACRO TUBEROSUM

CENTRUM TENDINEUM
PERINEI

FOSSA
ISCHIORECTALIS

ARCUS TENDINEUS
(M. LEVATOR ANI)

M. SPHINCTER
ANI EXTERNUS

FASCIA OBTURATORIA

M. GLUTEUS
MAXIMUS

FASCIA DIAPHRAGMATIS
PELVIS INFERIOR

LIGAMENTUM ANOCOCCYGEUM   OS COCCYGIS

M. LEVATOR ANI

Fig. 8.1 The female pelvic floor

subsequent vaginal penetrative sexual intercourse after childbirth is possible. During the second stage of labour, the pudendal nerve can get damaged by compression from the fetal head, or stretch injury may develop from prolonged pushing. The levator ani muscles, stretched during birth, shrink post-birth. Women sometimes report a sensation of tightness that was not experienced before birth (See the pelvic floor in Fig. 8.1). Combined with frequently reported vaginal dryness post-birth, this can result in pain and discomfort during sex.

During the first 3 months post-partum, dyspareunia is common, with prevalence rates ranging from 45% to 62% [10, 12]. For many women, this is transitional. The prevalence decreases as the months pass. In a meta-synthesis of 22 studies ($N =$ 11,457), the estimated prevalence of dyspareunia was 42% at 2 months, 43% at 2–6 months and 22% at 6–12 months [12], although remaining high enough to warrant attention. It is relevant to consider and explore the extent of dyspareunia. Is the pain mild or excruciating, constant or passing, experienced upon vaginal entry or deep penetration? Table 8.1 provides some insight into the experience of pain during the first intercourse after birth based on a study involving 1,507 first-time mothers in Australia [13]. The distressing experience of severe and persistent dyspareunia will be addressed in Chap. 14.

While it is important to inform and discuss the frequency of dyspareunia after birth with women, these prevalence rates provide limited insight into how dyspareunia impacts women and their sexual health and how they eventually resolve the pain. Consequently, the midwife's task is to offer possible strategies and solutions for women and their partners to resolve dyspareunia and experience satisfying sexual encounters. Discuss the cycle of pain with the woman and her partner and clarify that pain results in reduced sexual arousal and lubrication. Penetration without or

Table 8.1 Intensity of pain during first vaginal intercourse occurred at any stage in the first 12 months post-partum [13]

	N = 1122	
	N	%
No pain	161	14.3
Mild pain	357	31.8
Discomforting pain	380	33.9
Distressing pain	150	13.4
Horrible pain	56	5.0
Excruciating pain	18	1.6

with minimal lubrication will cause pain. A high pelvic floor tone adds to the pain and the persisting cycle. Evidence based on women's narratives highlights that women are active participants in seeking strategies and solutions to manage and overcome dyspareunia and that these are diverse [1]. In the first instance, midwives can support women to open the conversation with their partners about their experience of pain, encouraging women to identify where she feels the pain, what exacerbates it and what eases it. The HCP can advise women to use a slow build-up to penetration ('slow foreplay'). Women have described engaging in self and mutual masturbation or oral sex as means of foreplay and becoming sexually aroused [1]. The midwife could suggest trying different sexual positions in which the woman has more control over penetration, such as the woman being on-top, side-lying/spooning or holding and leading the penis into the vagina. Advice should be adapted to where the woman feels pain. For instance, pain felt in the posterior vagina indicates trying the doggy position. Although women in same-sex relationships are not visible in the literature on post-partum sexual health, the principles of open communication, expressing sexual needs and trial and error concerning sexual activities that are pain-free and provide sexual satisfaction most likely are universal. Nonetheless, there is an urgent need to research this discreet population of women about their post-partum sexual wellbeing needs.

8.5.2 Do All Post-Partum Women Experience a Lack of Vaginal Lubrication After Birth?

Changes to vaginal lubrication are commonly self-reported by women in the immediate months after birth. For example, 57% of women experienced a lack of vaginal lubrication 3 months post-partum, reducing to 30% 12 months after birth [12]. The experience of a lack of vaginal lubrication results from fluctuating levels of circulating oestrogen post-partum. There is an immediate drop in oestrogen and progesterone after the birth of baby and placenta, with varying estimates of 6 weeks to 6 months on when levels return to their pre-pregnancy concentrations. Low oestrogen levels affect the epithelial lining of vaginal mucosa resulting in a thinning of the mucosa and a diminished lubrication capacity. Increased circulating cortisol levels can occur when new parents experience stress as they adapt to their new roles as parents, caring for a new baby. When cortisol levels rise, there is a corresponding reduction in testosterone levels. This can result in diminished sexual desire and a lack of vaginal secretions. Furthermore, decreased levels of melatonin associated with a lack of sleep are thought to hinder oestrogen secretion. For women who are breastfeeding, oestrogen levels are suppressed longer. Prolactin (necessary for lactation) is known to impact testosterone, which, coupled with tiredness and a low mood, may negatively influence sexual desire and sexual arousal.

Notwithstanding the endocrine reasons for post-partum vaginal dryness, another potential cause is not engaging in ample foreplay before penetration and thus not being sufficiently lubricated. Without proper foreplay and feelings of desire, lack of vaginal lubrication lurks. Added to that some women describe that their motivation for engaging in sexual activity was not to satisfy their own sexual desire but that of their partners. The midwife should counsel women on the frequency with which women experience a lack of vaginal lubrication post-partum and encourage women to communicate their sexual needs, desire for sexual activity or a lack of desire with their partner. A solution to manage the lack of vaginal lubrication is using a water-based lubricant during sexual activity when she really wants to engage in penetrative sex. Artificial lubricants should not be used to replace sexual stimulation and arousal completely. Midwives can recommend a good quality organic, water-based lubricant irrespective of feeding choice. Perfumed and flavoured lubricants and lubricants with superfluous additives often contain glycerine that can irritate the vagina and increase discomfort or pain. Condoms and silicon-based sex toys respond well to water-based lubricants. Silicon-based lubricants last longer than water-based lubricants (no reapplication). However, they are difficult to wash off, and they are not suitable for silicon-based sex toys or sex aids.

8.5.3 Do All Women Experience a Lack of Sexual Desire After Birth?

The desire for sleep and alone time can be stronger than the desire for sexual activity for many new parents during the first 12 months after birth. However, the desire for intimacy usually remains. As discussed in the introduction to this chapter, the desire for emotional and physical intimacy remains an important feature of the couple's relationship and is a source of relationship satisfaction. Many studies report a high prevalence of a lack of interest in sex or no sexual desire ranging from 61% at 3 months post-partum to 40–51% 12 months after birth by first-time mothers [10, 13]. It is important to discuss these prevalence rates and their meanings for women and their partners. For many, the change in sexual desire experienced after birth is a normative adaptation to parenthood, particularly in the first few months. Once communicated to and understood by the couple, this often alleviates or prevents associated distress. Nonetheless, most first-time mothers were insufficiently prepared for the experience of reduced sexual desire [1]. Women who discussed their feelings on adapting to motherhood, stress associated with baby care and a lack of interest in sexual activity with their partner tended to manage the change in sexual desire with greater ease than their counterparts who had difficulty conveying their needs to their partners. When changed sexual desire is communicated honestly within the couple dyad, it becomes less problematic. Some couples give themselves time to prioritise the baby and new routines, for example, 6 months, expecting that they then can plan time-away or alone time as a couple. In the first instance, we suggest that couples prepare themselves for changes in sexual desire after birth and that they discuss the kind of pleasurable sexual activities that are not penetration-focussed. Secondly, we suggest that maternity HCPs give tips to couples on opening the dialogue on sex, that is, allocating time to discuss a sexual activity and writing down feelings and sexual desires.

In our post-partum interviews, some women described distress at their lack of sexual desire. They felt utterly unprepared for that and described their sexual relationship as 'broken'. Many women mentioned a discordance between their own and their partner's sexual desire. Most commonly, the male partner's desire for sexual activity was greater than that of the female partner. The distress often materialised due to not talking to their partner about their feelings of stress in adapting to motherhood, tiredness, concern over the baby's wellbeing, loss of sexual desire and the need to have alone time. Throughout all the literature on sexual health after birth, the consensus is that effective communication within the couple dyad on the social, relational, psychological and physical dimensions of post-partum sexual health is fundamental for post-partum sexually and emotionally satisfying intimate relationships. Maternity HCPs can suggest that couples can 'start from the beginning'. In other words, if not used to talking about sex and sexual pleasure, they can start now. They can forget everything that has come before and outline their expectations for the next year or two regarding their intimate and sexual relationship. It is important that intimacy and affection are discussed, that each person identifies what makes them happy and feel special and that sex and sexual pleasure become part of their conversation. We suggest that couples set time aside in a neutral environment to discuss these issues. Each person should use 'I', owning their feelings, desires and fears and not be afraid to state what one does and does not want or enjoy. We argue that both partners take responsibility for their own pleasure. We emphasise the importance of listening to each other and asking questions.

8.6 Conclusions and Key Points

Post-partum sexual health is multi-dimensional. It is individual to the woman, her partner, her culture and her personal expectations. The lack of visibility of women in same-sex relationships in the literature is noteworthy and problematic. This group of women is not represented and therefore unlikely to receive post-partum sexual health information and advice relevant to their needs.

8.7 Key Points of Note from the Chapter

- Post-partum sexual health is multi-dimensional, encompassing physical, social, psychological and relational dimensions.

- Emotional intimacy and non-sexual touch are important to women and help maintain satisfying relationships. Holding hands, kissing, sleeping in the same bed, cuddling and spending alone time with her partner are valued by women and a significant part of their intimate relationships.
- Women want specific, timely information about resuming sexual activity after birth. When can they resume sexual activity after birth? Approximately 80% of nulliparous women had resumed vaginal/penetrative sexual intercourse 3 months after birth.
- Resuming sexual activity after birth was not spontaneous. Women and their partners planned it. Women considered their physical and emotional recovery from birth, their mode of birth and the presence of perineal trauma and abdominal wounds. They also considered being away from home and away from the baby having time to enjoy their partner's company.
- About 85% of nulliparous women experience discomfort during first vaginal penetration. The midwife can provide possible strategies to resolve experienced pain:
  - Slow build-up to penetration
  - Other forms of sexual activity before penetration or as a source of sexual satisfaction. For example, masturbation, oral sex, use of sex toys and sexual role play
  - Use of different sexual positions that enable the woman to control penetration, such as the woman on-top or side-lying. In the doggy position, changing the direction of the penis may provide relief depending on where she feels the pain.
  - Use of good quality, plain water-based lubricants.
- One-fifth of women continue to experience dyspareunia 1 year after birth.
- Women did resume other forms of sexual activity, e.g. masturbation and oral sex before vaginal penetration.
- Approx. 57% of women experience a lack of vaginal lubrication in the immediate months post-partum. There are several endocrine reasons why post-partum women experience a lack of vaginal lubrication. We recommend that all women, irrespective of feeding choice, should be advised on the benefit of using a good quality water-based lubricant for first and subsequent sexual intercourse. Additive-free water-based lubricants will not irritate the vaginal wall mucosa and can be used with condoms and silicone sex toys. Artificial lubricants should not be used to replace sexual stimulation and arousal completely.
- Maternity healthcare providers should open the conversation about post-partum sexual health antenatally and encourage women to think about and discuss their sexual preferences and needs with their partners. Couples should be advised to anticipate changes in their sexual relationship and consider strategies to manage this.
- In couples with a 'penetration imperative', solo and mutual masturbation should be recommended to achieve sexual pleasure and orgasm.

- Maternity HCPs need to be sensitive to women's cultural and personal expectations regarding sex and intimacy since some women may be embarrassed to discuss that topic.
- Many couples experience a change in their feelings of sexual desire as adapting to parenthood, tiredness and baby-care take priority. Discussing these feelings within the couple dyad is relevant in adapting sexual health after birth.
- Some couples experience a discordance in feelings of sexual desire. If that is not communicated within the couple, it can cause conflict.
- Good communication within the couple dyad is essential in maintaining good post-partum sexual health.
- Advise women that if sexual health issues persist and cause them distress, they should speak to a healthcare professional with expertise in sexuality and intimacy.

8.8   Case Study

Leila, a 38-year-old first-time mother. Four months ago, she had a vacuum birth of her son Sam and acquired a second-degree tear that was sutured. Her perineum has healed well, and she has been post-natally well. She is exclusively breastfeeding Sam. Leila has a seven-year relationship with Raul, Sam's father. They had regular, satisfying sexual encounters pre-pregnancy, at least once a week. This pattern continued during pregnancy. Since Sam's birth, Leila and Raul tried vaginal intercourse on two occasions, 8 weeks and 12 weeks post-partum. Leila found penetration quite painful on both occasions, and she did not experience sexual satisfaction. She felt her vaginal lubrication lacking, and her vagina felt 'tight'. Leila has told Raul of her discomfort, and he felt bad for causing her pain. Leila is aware that Raul has more feelings of sexual desire, and she feels bad because she has no desire for sex. Leila discussed these issues with her community nurse-midwife when Sam had his vaccinations.

The community nurse-midwife initially carried out an assessment. The nurse confirmed Leila's mode of birth and if her perineum had been sutured. The nurse-midwife inspected her perineum and questioned the presence of pain or discomfort in the perineum. She asked about Leila's recovery from birth, her feeding choice and how she and Raul were settling into parenthood. She inquired about Leila's relationship and if they are good communicators? Do they talk about sex and sexual desire? Do they discuss adapting to parenthood and any challenges they may be experiencing? The nurse-midwife asked about their sexual relationship before pregnancy and after the birth. She asked about their preferred sexual activities and sexual satisfaction.

The nurse-midwife urged Leila to open the conversation with Raul, he was feeling bad about her discomfort during sexual intercourse, and she was feeling bad about his feelings of sexual desire. Rather than each feeling bad, it would be more beneficial to explain their feelings and make a plan.

The nurse-midwife suggested that they agree on a day and time when they can be sexually intimate, for example, a Friday or Saturday night when the baby is sleeping and when they may not have to worry about work the following day. At the weekend, they may have an opportunity to together have dinner, watch a television show or share a beer or wine. They might begin slowly engaging in some of the sexual activities they enjoyed before pregnancy and birth. The nurse-midwife suggested using a good quality water-based lubricant with no additives to assist vaginal lubrication, which may have contributed to the discomfort felt. Leila and Raul might consider mutual masturbation to lengthen foreplay and heighten Leila's feelings of sexual desire and arousal. The nurse-midwife and Leila discussed that a sexual encounter need not end up in vaginal penetration but that each sexual encounter should provide sexual pleasure. In case they attempt penetration, the nurse-midwife suggested trying different positions, for example, Leila being on-top. This way, she can control the penetration.

Leila and the nurse-midwife talked about the statistics on the prevalence of sexual health issues after birth and how sexual desire changes for many women. Adapting to parenthood, baby care, tiredness and alone time are often higher up the priority list for women in the immediate months after birth. The nurse-midwife suggested that Raul is likely tired, is also adapting to parenthood and likely concerned about baby care, too and that his feelings of sexual desire are not known to Leila unless they discuss these feelings.

The nurse-midwife advised Leila to return to her if there was no improvement within the next 4–6 weeks to make a new plan.

References

1. O'Malley D, Smith V, Higgins A. Women's solutioning and strategising in relation to their postpartum sexual health: a qualitative study. Midwifery. 2019;77:53–9.
2. Bender SS, Sveinsdóttir E, Fridfinnsdóttir H. "You stop thinking about yourself as a woman". An interpretive phenomenological study of the meaning of sexuality for Icelandic women during pregnancy and after birth. Midwifery. 2018;62:14–9.
3. Ahlborg T, Strandmark M. Factors influencing the quality of intimate relationships six months after delivery–first-time parents' own views and coping strategies. J Psychosom Obstet Gynaecol. 2006;27:163–72.
4. Hansson M, Ahlborg T. Quality of the intimate and sexual relationship in first-time parents - a longitudinal study. Sex Reprod Healthc. 2012;3:21–9.
5. Pardell-Dominguez L, Palmieri PA, Dominguez-Cancino KA, et al. The meaning of postpartum sexual health for women living in Spain: a phenomenological inquiry. BMC Pregnancy Childbirth. 2021;21:1–13.
6. McDonald EA, Brown SJ. Does method of birth make a difference to when women resume sex after childbirth? BJOG. 2013;120:823–30.
7. Faisal-Cury A, Menezes PR, Quayle J, et al. The relationship between mode of delivery and sexual health outcomes after childbirth. J Sex Med. 2015;12:1212–20.
8. Zhuang C, Li T, Li L. Resumption of sexual intercourse post partum and the utilisation of contraceptive methods in China: a cross-sectional study. BMJ Open. 2019;9:e026132.

9. McDonald E, Woolhouse H, Brown SJ. Consultation about sexual health issues in the year after childbirth: a cohort study. Birth. 2015;42:354–61.
10. O'Malley D, Higgins A, Begley C, et al. Prevalence of and risk factors associated with sexual health issues in primiparous women at 6 and 12 months postpartum; a longitudinal prospective cohort study (the MAMMI study). BMC Pregnancy Childbirth. 2018;18:196.
11. Masters W, Johnson V. Human sexual response. New York: Little Brown; 1966.
12. Banaei M, Kariman N, Ozgoli G, et al. Prevalence of postpartum dyspareunia: a systematic review and meta-analysis. Int J Gynaecol Obstet. 2021;153:14–24.
13. McDonald EA, Gartland D, Small R, Brown SJ. Frequency, severity and persistence of postnatal dyspareunia to 18 months post partum: a cohort study. Midwifery. 2016;34:15–20.

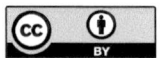

Sexual Aspects of Breast and Lactation

9

Z. Burcu Yurtsal ⓘ and Dilek Uslu ⓘ

9.1   Introduction

This chapter will address various aspects of sexuality that, in some way, are related to breastfeeding.

It will start with the relation between breast and sexuality, followed by the relation between breastfeeding and sexuality.

Both physiology, psychology and behaviour, and the relationship between the woman and her partner will get particular attention in either of those parts, with the remark that in real life, it is, of course, difficult to separate those factors since they tend to influence each other in a sometimes unpredictable choreography. As a sideline, we will share some ideas on the social aspect of breastfeeding. This chapter deals with the natural situation, whereas Chap. 15 will deal with disturbances of this process.

Midwives should be familiar with the whole range of possible responses to sexuality concerning breastfeeding. So that they can counsel women and couples appropriately and tackle the concerns and expectations, often entailing some psycho-education on what the woman can expect during this phase [1].

The original version of the chapter has been revised. A correction to this chapter can be found at https://doi.org/10.1007/978-3-031-18432-1_31

Z. B. Yurtsal (✉)
Midwifery Department, Faculty of Health Science, Sivas Cumhuriyet University, Sivas, Turkey
e-mail: zbozboga@cumhuriyet.edu.tr

D. Uslu
Doctor's Center Nisantasi, Istanbul, Turkey

9.2   The Breast and Sexuality

9.2.1   Physiology of Breast and Sexuality

In the breasts, the first sign of sexual arousal is the erection of the nipple (with left and right breast often not equally responding to sexual arousal). In full arousal, the increase of nipples is 0.5–1.0 cm. Such nipple erection can also occur during anxiety and non-sexual arousal. The second sign of arousal is increased venous flush, which shows a rash on the skin. Later in the arousal phase, the areola becomes swollen, by which the (visual) nipple erection seems to diminish. After orgasm, that areolar swelling quickly disappears, by which the nipple erection appears to return.

The breast volume can increase by 20–25% with full arousal. That happens both in the woman who never was pregnant and in the primigravid woman. Such volume increase during arousal is less after having breastfed one baby. After having nursed a second baby, there is no more volume increase during sexual arousal, probably because of the extensive development of the venous drainage system during those lactation periods.

In the primigravid woman, the increase in volume (due to arousal hypercongestion) is added to the pregnancy congestion. This combination can cause pain in the nipple and areola area, especially at the end of the first trimester. Later in pregnancy, that complaint usually disappears.

The tactile sensitivity of all areas of the female breast is (after puberty) more significant than in men, with maximal sensitivity at midcycle (in women without hormonal contraception) and during menses [2].

9.2.2   Psychology and Behaviour

At the start of puberty, breast development can create some pain in the breasts. Women can experience this period of change as positive (a sign of becoming a woman), but it also can be very unsettling. That variation depends on many factors like the age at which the breast development starts (somewhere between 'too early' and 'too late'); her mother's implicit breast-related attitude and explicit education regarding the breasts; cultural messages about decency or honour; and the threat of the 'male gaze'.

Gradually, the breasts play a role in the woman's female identity, which appears very culture-bound. Whereas in many African countries, the breast is predominantly a symbol of motherhood, in some other cultures, it is predominantly a symbol of femininity, accompanied by feminine pride in some women and insecurity in many women.

Gradually, the breasts can also play a role in a woman's lovemap.[1] For many women, the breasts become an erogenic zone. When women were asked about breast or nipple stimulation and sexual arousal, approximately 80% indicated that such

---

[1] Lovemap; this represents the person's (or couple's) highly individual set of erogenic zones, ways to become aroused, erotic scripts, et cetera.

stimulation caused or enhanced sexual arousal, whereas 7% indicated that such manipulation decreased arousal [3]. In Dutch research, 15% of women stated that they had experienced an orgasm purely due to breast stimulation [4]. The combination of 'breast and sexuality' is clearly an area with much variety and is greatly influenced by culture [1].

There is much sexual variety in how the breasts and nipples are stimulated and how they are part of the woman's or the couple's lovemap. Knowing about that lovemap is not relevant for the HCP, except when it causes confusion or interferes with breastfeeding or when it becomes relevant related to an apparent sexual problem.

9.2.3 Breasts and the Partner

The female breasts are also an important 'erogenic zone' for most partners, both for visual and for tactile pleasure. The same goes for the female partner in lesbian relationships.

The stimulation of breasts and nipples triggers the release of oxytocin in the woman's brain, which will focus her attention on the partner, strengthening her desire to bond with him (or her).

However, this represents the literature that originated almost entirely from the Western World. Anthropologists found in many cultures that the female breasts had no sexual meaning for men [1]. When men grow up with the idea that a woman is either a mother or a lover, her transition to breastfeeding apparently can make his sexual desire disappear.

9.2.4 Social Aspects

The female breasts have been a centre of attention from time immemorial. In the oldest human sculptures, they represented a symbol of fertility. Some cultures have tried to conceal them to varying degrees, whereas others implicitly or explicitly exposed the breasts. In some indigenous tribes of Southern and Eastern Africa, the women walk bare-breasted. In orthodox religious countries and the USA, a nipple will never be shown on television. At the same time, in nearly every American heterosexual porn story, the size of the female breasts is mentioned. Such cultural realities will undeniably influence how girls and women feel at ease (or not) with their breasts and body.

9.3 Breastfeeding

9.3.1 Benefits for Mother and Child

Breastfeeding has numerous benefits for both mother and child. In the mother, a period of breastfeeding reduces the future risk of endometrial cancer, ovarian cancer, breast cancer, and type 2 diabetes. Stimulation of the breasts is seen as having

Fig. 9.1 Motherhood

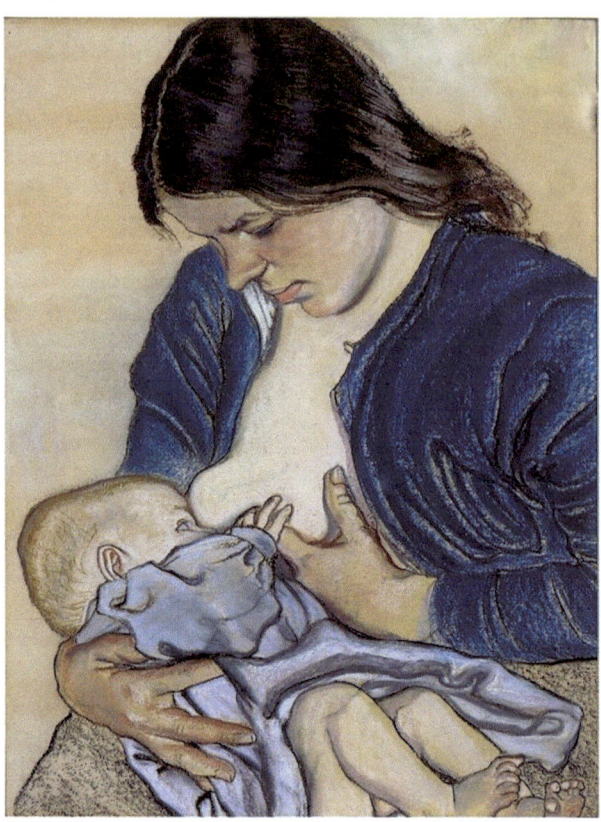

Painting by Stanislaw Wyspiański (1905)

health benefits. There is a hypothesis that breast cancer will occur less in women who experienced much sexual stimulation and suction of breasts and nipples [5]. Breastfeeding can assist women in birth spacing, and it can turn negative relationships between mother and baby into positive ones [6], and it can positively affect the mother's emotional well-being (Fig. 9.1).

In infants, it stimulates cognitive development and protects against gastrointestinal tract infections, necrotizing enteric colitis, allergic diseases, celiac disease, inflammatory bowel disease, SIDS, obesity, diabetes, and leukaemia.

The WHO recommends starting breastfeeding ('nursing') within one hour after the birth and suggests nursing exclusively for 6 months following birth unless medically contraindicated [7]. A high HIV viral load is one of the few contraindications.

9.3.2 Physiology of Breastfeeding

Before the first pregnancy, the breast consists mainly of adipose tissue with lactiferous lobes that drain into the lactiferous ducts, then drain into the lactiferous sinus, and then into the nipple–areolar complex. During the first trimester, the ductal system expands and branches out into the adipose tissue in response to the increase of oestrogen with ductal proliferation and elongation and a decrease in adipose tissue. The acinar cells proliferate into lactocytes. In pregnancy, each breast's volume increases by approximately 400 g. The increased oestrogen levels cause well-elevated prolactin levels. At 20 weeks, the mammary glands are sufficiently developed and start producing milk components ('colostrum') under the influence of prolactin (lactogenesis I). At this stage, the high levels of oestrogen and progesterone inhibit the production of 'mature milk'. Towards the end of pregnancy and especially immediately after birth, the levels of oestrogen and progesterone decrease, allowing milk production and eventual 'let-down' for breastfeeding. With the post-partum withdrawal of luteal and placental sex steroids and placental lactogen, the prolactin increase activates the alveolar cells to release milk into the alveoli and smaller ducts. Some 30–40 h after birth, the complete milk production is induced by prolactin (lactogenesis II), and the colostrum production alters into 'mature milk' production in this transitional phase. After that, milk production is further driven by milk removal (lactogenesis III). The combined storage capacity of the breasts is between 80 and 600 ml of milk (with L and R not always equal). In this stage, prolactin and oxytocin mechanisms balance the consumption and production of milk.

Oxytocin has a role in the milk-ejection reflex.

The high prolactin levels at childbirth and immediately post-partum fall within a week to half the childbirth level. In the breastfeeding woman, the prolactin levels go up and down, peaking some 45 min after the start of feeding. With frequent feeding (>8×/day), the levels stay high.

Without breastfeeding, the level will be back to pre-pregnancy within a week.

Whereas during pregnancy, the production of prolactin is suppressed by oestrogen and progesterone, the increased prolactin levels in lactating mothers cause a decrease in oestrogen and androgen. The low oestrogen level creates in the vagina an atrophic state (as in menopause). The low androgen causes decreased arousability and, in many women, decreased sexual desire, by which breastfeeding women tend to restart sexual life later.

The sensitivity of the breasts increases tremendously within 24 h after childbirth, which may be the key to activating the suckling-induced discharge of oxytocin and prolactin and inhibiting ovulation during lactation [5].

9.3.3 Social Aspects of Breastfeeding

Breastfeeding is a relevant element in the strong bonding between the mother and her child, generated by the baby's sucking reflex that triggers the release of oxytocin in the mother's brain. When anthropologists looked into various pre-industrial cultures, they found that cultures with long-continued breastfeeding showed less suicide and had less violence [8].

Despite knowing the benefits, health care does not succeed in having most women breastfeed for months.

Whereas in many African countries breastfeeding in public is the norm, it is frowned upon in many other countries. However, many of those countries have laws that allow women to breastfeed their babies in public. The reasons seem manifold. Under the pressure of cultural taboos, many young women see themselves as an object first and as a person second. When society implicitly associates the breast with sexuality, or when society associates the nude breast with indecency, it quickly can induce guilt and shame in nursing mothers, negatively affecting the nursing process. We believe that women should be encouraged to breastfeed and reclaim the naturalness of doing so in public worldwide. We should not forget that the first step to protecting babies is breastfeeding, which benefits the health and welfare of the baby, mother, family, and community [9].

9.4   Breastfeeding and Sexuality

We have to be aware of various factors that play a role when discussing the topic of 'breastfeeding and sexuality'. Successively we will address aspects of physiology, the influence of society, psychology and behaviour, the partner relationship, and the role of the midwife or other HCP. Finally, we will look at the essential troubles that can develop and potential ways to deal with them.

9.4.1   Physiology Aspects

Physiology has an essential link between breastfeeding and sexuality, with a significant role for oxytocin. Oxytocin causes the happy, contented feeling after breastfeeding, with stress reduction and the overall relaxation that breastfeeding conveys. Uterine contractions during breastfeeding are a well-known aspect of uterine involution, primarily known because they can be rather painful, even more so in multigravid women. However, uterine contractions can also have other ('more sexual') consequences. A group of 153 Dutch mothers was asked about sensations during breastfeeding. Of them, 71% had experienced pleasurable contractions in the womb area, and 34% had experienced a feeling of sexual arousal. Surprising was that 8% indicated having experienced an orgasm just by breastfeeding [4]. According to an extensive meta-content review of research articles, one-third to one-half of breastfeeding mothers described breastfeeding as erotic ('an intense physical lust') [10].

Such oxytocin connection goes as well the other way round. When getting sexually aroused (especially when having an orgasm), milk can leak or be sprayed outside forcefully. The breasts (and especially the nipples) are more sensitive in the months of breastfeeding.

During the months of breastfeeding, various hormonal and non-hormonal factors influence sexual desire. Prolactin is known to reduce sexual desire. Although diminishing from the very high levels around childbirth, prolactin stays high throughout the nursing period. The high prolactin levels also influence the gonadal hormones causing low oestrogen levels. Oestrogen should be low because oestrogen diminishes the milk flow. That, however, also causes an amount of vaginal atrophy (as if the woman is in her menopause). The androgen levels are also low, especially the testosterone level. That can cause both the absence of desire and low arousability. A complicating sideline among women is the big difference in their sensitivity to androgen levels. The low androgen levels are also causing lowered assertiveness and low energy or fatigue.

9.4.2 Society and Culture

Culture strongly influences the priorities in the woman's roles after childbirth. Saha reviewed the sexual advice literature in the United States over three decades [11]. When promoting breastfeeding, HCPs reflected the societal view that the husband owned the female breasts and that women must please their partners by timely returning to intercourse.

Research in the Philippines looked at the relationship between lactation, sexuality, and relationship commitment by comparing non-pregnant women, non-cycling breastfeeding women, and cycling breastfeeding women (i.e. without or with monthly bleeding). Cycling breastfeeding women have the highest sexual functioning and relationship commitment scores [12].

9.4.3 Psychology and Behaviour Aspects

Above we already addressed that some women experience sexual sensations during breastfeeding. When the woman with this experience has never heard of this as normal, she can get confused. In a research questionnaire, the question on 'erotic response during breastfeeding' had a high (37%) rate of non-response, indicating that this is a 'rather touchy area' [10]. A quarter of women had experienced feelings of guilt because of such sexual feelings, and some had stopped breastfeeding.

Leaking milk during lovemaking can confuse, depending on how well the woman can balance her roles as a mother and a lover. Whereas this is threatening for some women, other women thrive on it.

The higher sensitivity of breasts and nipples can be the start or intensification of breast sexuality in some couples. In other women, the former sexual ways of stimulating now can have lost their sexual, arousing effects. For some other women, all forms of sexual breast play can be too much in this period or have to be toned down.

Such vast differences can also be found in the reaction to the changed appearance of the breasts. For some women and their partners, this can be a feast of femininity; for others upsetting or nearly disgusting. All these areas need integration into health information.

Studies often measure breastfeeding sexuality in comparison with pre-pregnancy sexuality, but breastfeeding and the feelings involved may create new forms of sensuality and satisfaction. Usually, a relatively strong and sensual connection develops between the mother and the baby [13]. However, for mothers (and also for researchers), it does not seem easy to separate sensuality and sexuality.

9.4.4 Partner and Relationship Aspects

Just as in young mothers, partners show a wide range of reactions. These reactions can be negative, including jealousy because the baby gets so much attention. Perceived devotion to the child at the partner's expense and the intimacy between mother and child, fostered during breastfeeding, can elicit jealousy from new fathers [14]. The mother may also feel jealous when she is the breadwinner and her male partner takes the primary caregiving role and develops an extra close relationship with the child. Higher levels of attachment anxiety in both mothers and fathers are associated with greater jealousy of the partner–infant relationship. Attachment anxiety is characterized by mistrust in the relationship and preoccupation with the possibility of rejection or abandonment.

So, elevated attachment anxiety in oneself or one's partner may play a maladaptive role in adjustment to the transition to parenthood by sparking jealousy of the partner–infant relationship. Such feelings can contribute to a decline in romantic relationship adjustment during the early postpartum period. Given that the quality of a couple's romantic relationship sets the stage for establishing parent-child and co-parenting relationships, jealousy of the partner–infant relationship could have broader negative implications for the developing family system [14]. The attractive prenatal shape and firmness of the breasts, that maybe increased prenatal erotic desire and arousal, will change and perhaps influence desire [1]. Some partners will be turned off by the carnal aspects of breastfeeding, whereas others will get highly fascinated or even aroused by the voluptuousness of breastfeeding.

Such shifts in sexual sensations and experiences will rarely become troublesome, providing the partners have a more or less similar emotional reaction to these new experiences and feelings.

The leaking of milk during the woman's sexual arousal or orgasm can induce some couples to wish to drink from her breasts. There is no contraindication to that, as long as both wholeheartedly agree (and the baby keeps adequate nutrition).

9.4.5 Changed Sexual Function in the Breastfeeding Woman (and Couple)

We have already mentioned the strong influence of hormonal changes on breastfeeding women. High prolactin, low oestrogen, and low androgen levels tend to be accompanied by low sexual desire, low arousability, atrophic vaginal wall, low energy, and decreased assertiveness.

Added to that are the nightly feeding sessions causing a lack of sleep. Combined with an emotional focus on the baby, it is easily possible that the young mother is not in the mood for extensive sexual contact.

That can be different for the male partner. Most men have more sexual desire than their female partners, fitting with their higher testosterone levels. Besides, after the first childbirth, many men are in some way confused by their new role, which can cause stress. For many men, sexuality is one of their ways to deal with stress. Especially when a couple has developed the routine to finalize sex with penetration, there is a reasonable risk for dyspareunia. When dyspareunia happens once, that does not need to be so bad. However, repeated dyspareunia can become a vicious circle where pain, less sexual desire, and mutual tension and separation can have long-term adverse effects. This can create the following scenario:

> The male partner wants sex. He is neither very good at understanding that his wife is not yet ready for that, nor is he capable of picking up her non-verbal signals. The woman is tired but feels guilty when disappointing him. Her lack of arousal will prevent lubrication. Because their communication is inadequate for this situation, they will too quickly proceed to penetration. Penetration in the atrophic and not lubricated vagina will cause pain. So there will be no sexual pleasure for the woman, and maybe feelings of guilt in the man. Besides, her low testosterone level has reduced her assertiveness. Because of her 'learned social role', she will not stand firm and reject penetration. In the long run, the pain and the memory of pain can eventually become part of a vicious dyspareunia circle (pain → low desire → pain).

That is not good for the mother, not for the couple, and not for their joint partnership and parenting [15]. Much research data on post-partum sexuality show this lower sexual reality in lactating women [16, 17]. Sexual inactivity and dysfunctional problems are partly translated into lower partnership quality. This sexual scenario is regularly found in common sexological practice as a precursor of later sexual relationship problems.

Most literature shows that resumption of sexual activity is earlier in multiparous women and later in older women. Sexual functioning apparently is also influenced by the type of breastfeeding, with the partial breastfeeding women showing better vaginal lubrication [18].

9.5 Long-Term Breastfeeding

A small group of women continues for an extended period with breastfeeding. That can go up to several years, with some mothers 'tandem feeding' both a baby and a toddler. In Finnish research, both surrounding people and the women themselves had mixed reactions to that [19]. It brought these mothers much emotional pleasure, although some vehemently denied that there was any sexual pleasure in it [19].

9.6   Weaning

Weaning is the process of replacing breastmilk with other foods, the process by which the baby gradually gets used to eating family or adult foods and becomes less dependent on breastmilk. The process varies from culture to culture and is often tailored to the child's individual needs. Weaning is said to be on time when the child is 24 months old [20].

After complete weaning, it takes several menstrual cycles before the breasts have returned to their previous size.

Australian research looked into the changes at (complete) weaning of the first child [21]. After 2–3 weeks, there was less fatigue and better mood, and after 3–4 weeks, sexual activity and intercourse frequency increased. That indicates that breastfeeding keeps the testosterone levels low, by which sexual desire can be low and fatigue high.

In the phase between full breastfeeding and (complete) weaning, ovulation will return.

In the nonlactating woman, the first ovulation can occur 25 days after childbirth, although most women will not ovulate until six weeks post-partum.

In lactating women, a later return of ovulation is found with a higher frequency of breastfeeding sessions, with a longer duration of each feed and less supplementary feeding [22]. Exclusive breastfeeding reduces the ovulation risk by 98–99% up to 6 months post-partum, as long as there has been no menstruation, and by 94–97% after an anovular menstruation. These findings suggest that contraceptive use is indicated among women who resume menstruating before six post-partum months or continue breastfeeding beyond 6 months.

Since a new conception is not recommended within 18 months after birth, it will be evident that good post-partum care includes proactive attention to contraception. Chapter 20 will address that topic.

9.7   Clinical Implications for Midwives (and Other HCPs)

Breastfeeding or not? Midwives and HCPs have to find a proper balance in providing information. In good care, such information should be adequate and realistic, both on the benefits for the mother, the baby, and the mother–child relationship and potential consequences for sexuality. Despite all our good intentions, the woman and the couple have to decide to breastfeed without us creating feelings of guilt in them.

Prevention and Pre-lactation Counselling We recommend routinely including the combination of breastfeeding and sexuality in couple counselling and prenatal classes [16]. Those are the situations where one should not beat around the bush but be clear and explicit.

Below is an example of a way to already in advance give adequate information on potential sexual consequences:

'Be aware that breast-feeding probably will influence your sexual connections in many ways. Your desire can decline, but you can also get aroused by nursing. You could lose milk when you are aroused, and you can like that, or it can make you uncomfortable or even disgusted (and the same goes for your partner).

You can get so intimately connected with the baby that you forget your partner (which can make your partner jealous). Your partner can lose all sexual desire or, on the contrary, dearly wants sexual intimacy and orgasm.

Those are all perfectly normal reactions! Due to hormonal changes, it can take many weeks before your vagina is again ready for penetration. If you are not yet prepared and try penetrating, it will cause pain.

Be assured that pain can quickly turn into longstanding pain and a longstanding absence of desire. When orgasmic relief is needed, we recommend other stimulation or different ways to reach orgasm. Especially at this stage, they are a far better solution than penetration'.

Lactation Counselling As recommended by WHO and UNICEF, all relevant professionals should invest in counselling for early initiation and continuation of breastfeeding, and in that way, benefitting maternal and infant health. That should be done in the post-partum checks, home visits, Internet, phone, lactation apps, et cetera [23].

Lactation Problems Sexual problems related to disturbances in breastfeeding will be addressed in Chap. 15.

Dealing with Troublesome Sexuality In this phase, many couples experience sexual disturbances. Since most couples are too shy to address that to their HCP, the professional should pro-actively question sexual disturbances. At this point, the midwife has several advantages. Midwives understand the influence of hormones and the physical consequences of childbirth and maybe episiotomy. Above all, they benefit from the trust developed throughout the entire period of pregnancy and birth.

There is the confusion of changing roles and responsibilities, fatigue, drowsiness, and perineal soreness. Then, confusion and conflict can grow between the woman and her partner on resuming the prenatal or pre-pregnancy pattern of sexuality. Here, the empathetic midwife can guide the couple to renegotiate and rediscover sexuality and intimacy and assist in the foundation of happy couple life. Among the needed tools are a clear explanation of the underlying causes, respect for the difference between the partners, and indirectly providing solutions. For instance, in this way:

…That is what happens in many couples. The woman loves hugging and cuddling, but she is too tired, and her vagina is too sore for penetration. Continuing to penetration will not only give pain, but then her desire for hugging and cuddling will completely disappear. In that situation, some couples have learned to hug and play without continuing to penetration. When the man likes or feels the need to have an orgasm, he gives it himself with his wife in his other arm. Maybe that is something also for you to consider…?

References

1. Avery MD, Ducket L, Frantzich CR. The experience of sexuality during breast-feeding among primiparous women. J Midwifery Womens Health. 2000;45:227–37.
2. Robinson JE, Short RV. Changes in breast sensitivity at puberty, during the menstrual cycle, and at parturition. Br Med J. 1977;1(6070):1188–91.
3. Levin R, Meston C. Nipple/Breast stimulation and sexual arousal in young men and women. J Sex Med. 2006;3:450–4.
4. Gianotten WL. Zwangerschap en orgasme (Pregnancy & Orgasm). Tijdschr Verloskundigen. 1988;13:326–9.
5. Robinson VC. Support for the hypothesis that sexual breast stimulation is an ancestral practice and a key to understanding women's health. Med Hypotheses. 2015;85:976–85.
6. Else-Quest NM, Hyde JS, Clarck R. Breastfeeding, bonding, and the mother-infant relationship. Merrill-Palmer Q. 2003;49:495–517.
7. UNICEF WHO on breast-feeding. https://apps.who.int/iris/bitstream/handle/10665/326049/WHO-NMH-NHD-19.22-eng.pdf?ua=1.
8. Prescott JW. Phylogenetic and ontogenetic aspects of human affectional development. In: Gemme R, Wheeler CC, editors. Proceedings of the 1976 international congress of sexology. New York: Plenum Press; 1976.
9. Yurtsal ZB. The importance of breast-feeding in public places in Turkey. In: Ozdemir B, Shapekova NL, Bilal AK, et al., editors. Developments in health sciences. Sofija: St. Kliment Ohrodski University Press; 2017:347–52.
10. von Sydow K. Sexuality during pregnancy and after childbirth: a metacontent analysis of 59 studies. J Psychosom Res. 1999;47:27–49.
11. Saha P. Breastfeeding and sexuality: professional advice literature from the 1970s to the present. Health Educ Behav. 2002;29:61–72.
12. Escasa-Dorne MJ. Sexual functioning and commitment to their current relationship among breast-feeding and regularly cycling women in Manila, Philippines. Hum Nat. 2015;26:89–101.
13. Convery KM, Spatz DL. Sexuality & breast-feeding: what do you know? MCN Am J Matern Child Nurs. 2009;34:218–23.
14. Olsavsky AL, Mahambrey MS, Berrigan MN. Adult attachment and jealousy of the partner–infant relationship at the transition to parenthood. J Soc Pers Relat. 2020;37:1745–65.
15. Yurtsal ZB. The impact of lactation on the sexual life of Turkish couples. Int J Caring Sci. 2020;13:626–35.
16. Wallwiener S, Müller M, Doster A, et al. Sexual activity and sexual dysfunction of women in the perinatal period: a longitudinal study. Arch Gynecol Obstet. 2017;295:873–83.
17. Eaton MA. Maternal sexuality during lactation: the influence of breast-feeding recency and relationship quality. Dissertation. 2018. https://digitalrepository.unm.edu/psy_etds/272.
18. Holanda JBL, Richter S, Campos RB, et al. Relationship of the type of breast-feeding in the sexual function of women. Rev Lat Am Enfermagem. 2021;29:e3438.
19. Säilävaara J. Long-term breastfeeding: the embodied experiences of Finnish mothers. Nord J Fem Gend Res. 2020;28:43–55. https://doi.org/10.1080/08038740.2019.1694581.

20. La Leche League International. Anonymous. 2011. https://apps.who.int/iris/bit-stream/10665/39335/1/9241542373_eng.pdf.
21. Forster C, Abraham S, Taylor A, et al. Psychological and sexual changes after the cessation of breast-feeding. Obstet Gynecol. 1994;84:872–6.
22. Gray RH, Campbell OM, Apelo R, et al. Risk of ovulation during lactation. Lancet. 1990;335(8680):25–9.
23. Eroğlu V, Yurtsal ZB. Emzirme ve Cinsel Yaşam ('Breastfeeding and sexual life'). In: Yurtsal ZB, editor. Anne Sütü ve Emzirmede Kanıt Temelli Uygulamalar ('Breast-milk and breast-feeding; evidence-based practices'). New Delhi: Anadolu Nobel Medicine Bookstores; 2018:139–43.

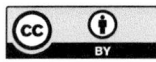

Sexual Aspects of the Female Pelvic Floor

10

Liesbeth Westerik-Verschuuren (ID),
Marjolijn Lutke Holzik-Mensink,
Marleen Wieffer-Platvoet, and Minke van der Velde (ID)

10.1 Introduction

Because of its essential functions in the choreography of sexuality and childbirth, two chapters of this book deal with the pelvic floor (PF). This chapter will start with addressing the PF and its role in sexuality. Next, we will address the PF during pregnancy, childbirth, and post-partum. Childbirth and the post-partum period are crucial moments with potential PF damage. So, this chapter will also look at aspects of preventing PF disturbances with extra attention to 'prehabilitation' (preparing the PF for optimal functioning during childbirth and post-partum). Since most people are not very aware of the functioning of their PF, they can easily and unnoticed get outside the optimal muscle tone (between too high and too low). There is a gradual transition from optimal to significant PF disturbances.

In some countries, PF physiotherapy developed into a highly specialized profession geared to treating PF disturbances. Some of those disturbances existed before getting pregnant, whereas others originated during pregnancy or childbirth. Chapter 16 will deal with the severe PF disturbances and their implications on sexuality and quality of life.

L. Westerik-Verschuuren (✉)
Bekkenfysiotherapie Twente, Center of Expertise for Pelvic Floor Physiotherapy,
Enschede, The Netherlands

SOMT University of Physiotherapy, Master Pelvic Physiotherapy,
Amersfoort, The Netherlands
e-mail: l.westerik-verschuuren@somt.nl

M. Lutke Holzik-Mensink · M. Wieffer-Platvoet
Bekkenfysiotherapie Twente, Center of Expertise for Pelvic Floor Physiotherapy,
Enschede, The Netherlands

M. van der Velde
Seksuologiepraktijk Twente, Center for Sexology, Enschede, The Netherlands

Men can have as well PF disturbances. This chapter will only address the PF disturbances that can impair conception.

10.2   What Is the Pelvic Floor?

The pelvic floor, literally the floor of the pelvis, is a layer of muscles and connective tissue that spans the bottom of the pelvis (see Fig. 10.1). They are striated, voluntary muscles that, although hidden from view, can be consciously contracted (squeezed) and relaxed. The PF consists of multiple muscles which stretch from the os coccygis (tailbone) to the pubic bone and from one tuber ischiadicum (sitting bone) to the other. In women, the PF muscles surround the hiatus genitalis, the space for the passage of the urethra, vagina, and anus. Together, these muscles support the pelvic organs (bowel, uterus, and bladder) and give conscious control of the bladder and bowel. They also contribute to core stability and motor control. Together with the musculus multifidus, the abdominal muscles, and the thoracic diaphragm, the PF muscles keep the structure of the spine and pelvis stable and maintain the posture of the trunk. In addition, the pelvic floor muscles have a role in sexual function.

The PF looks like a hammock or trampoline and can move up (contraction) and down (relaxation). They can also move ventrally (from the back to the front) and inward. So during contraction, the PF muscles make a lifting, closing, and ventral movement. Therefore, contraction of the pelvic floor muscles makes the pelvic organs lift, closes the urethra, vagina, and bowel, and pulls the urethra, vagina, and bowel forward (ventral ward). That is how one can support the pelvic organs and control or delay micturition and defecation until convenient.

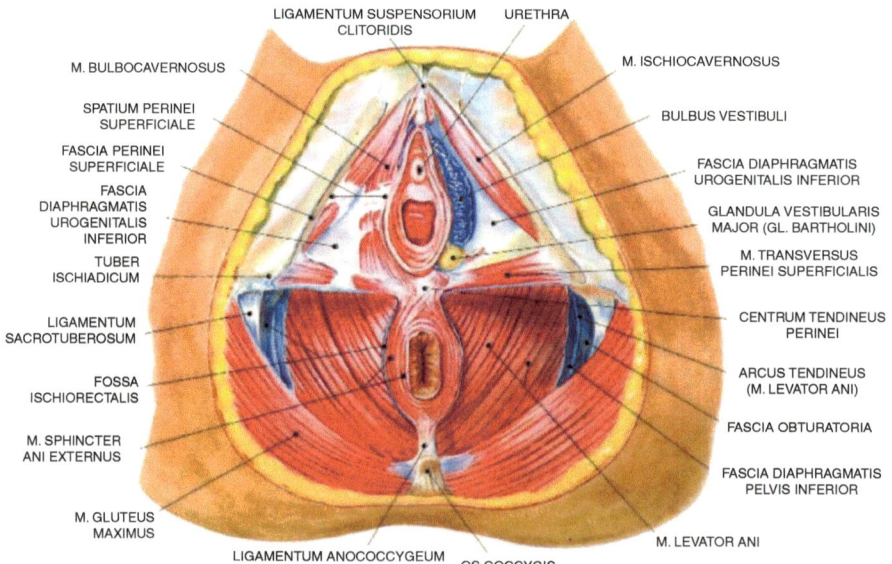

Fig. 10.1   The female pelvic floor

The PF muscles play a role in the sexuality of men and women. In men, they are important in getting and maintaining an erection and ejaculation. In women, voluntary contractions (squeezing) of the PF contribute to sexual sensation and arousal. The pelvic floor has a different role in each sexual response phase. In everyday life, the PF muscles are relaxed. When the woman becomes sexually aroused, the blood circulation increases and the erectile bodies of the clitoris get engorged, causing thickening of the vaginal wall and creating a cushion around the vaginal entrance to allow smooth penetration. At the same time, lubrication appears. When sexual stimulation continues, the muscle tension of the PF increases. In particular, the m. bulbospongiosus and m. ischiocavernosus contract and prevent the veins from emptying. In this plateau phase, alternating contracting and relaxing the pelvic floor leads to a more intense sensation, more friction between the vaginal wall and penis, and increased sexual arousal. During orgasm, the PF muscles involuntary and rhythmically contract, and, as a result, the hypercongestion of the veins will empty. The orgasm experience depends on the strength of the muscle contractions, so a well-trained pelvic floor contributes to a more intense sexual experience. In addition to the contraction of the pelvic floor muscles, the smooth muscles of the uterus might also contract rhythmically, thus intensifying the orgasm experience. In the resolution phase, the muscles relax, and all tissues recover to normal. About half of the women can have several orgasms in a row.

If the PF muscles are too tensed (hypertonicity) or too relaxed (hypotonicity), women's sexuality usually is disturbed.

A hypertonic pelvic floor can lead to painful intercourse. The sexual response cannot properly start up. The hypertonic muscles inhibit the extra blood circulation needed for the vaginal wall and the erectile tissues of the clitoris. The vaginal surface stays thin, and lubrication is insufficient, causing dyspareunia. The hypertonic PF muscles close and nod the vagina causing the feeling of a narrow and short vagina, an extra reason for pain at penetration. See Fig. 10.2.

Painful intercourse can have an overwhelming impact on women, affecting self-esteem and self-confidence. This condition can need counselling and maybe

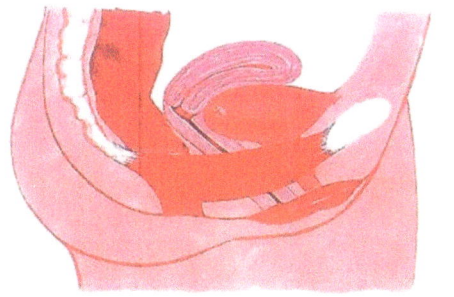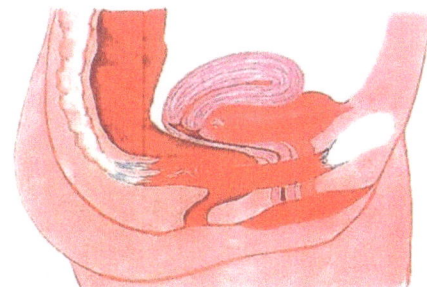

M. Levator ani (relaxed)   **M. Levator ani (contracted)**

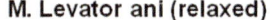

Fig. 10.2 The difference between relaxed and contracted levator ani muscle. On the left, the PF is relaxed, with the vagina straight and accessible. On the right, the PF muscles are squeezed. The vagina is curved and less accessible

coaching. If a woman does not understand why she feels pain during intercourse, she probably increasingly tenses her pelvic floor, reacting to the pain, and can develop a vicious cycle of '*(expected) pain* → *muscle tension* → *pain*'. Education is vital, as is re-education and relaxation of the pelvic floor. HCPs specialized in women's health like pelvic floor physiotherapists, nurses, or midwives can give such education.

A *hypotonic pelvic floor* causes other sexual problems or inconvenience. During the excitement phase, blood circulation can increase, and the erectile bodies can fill, but the veins will deflate, and the vaginal wall might stay unlubricated because the bulbospongiosus and ischiocavernosus muscles do not contract sufficiently. Besides, the weak levator ani muscle contractions do not close the genital hiatus well, and there will be not enough friction between the vagina and the penis. Both partners will feel less, which can decrease excitement.

Furthermore, a weak pelvic floor can cause vaginal noise or vaginal flatus. Because the vagina cannot be closed sufficiently, air will be sucked in or blown out, causing noises. Most women feel ashamed and embarrassed by this phenomenon.

Squeezing the PF muscles can increase the friction and thus improve the sensation and reduce the vaginal noise. Though this condition, also called 'vaginal laxity', does not hurt physically, it can need counselling. With an underactive pelvic floor, women will not experience pain, but they do not have a satisfying sexual life. Proper training will strengthen the PF muscles, increasing her ability to close the hiatus, increasing the friction during intercourse, and decreasing the risk of vaginal noise.

Unfortunately, there is still a taboo on talking about the pelvic floor or pelvic floor function, particularly sexual dysfunctions. Furthermore, the pelvic floor muscles have few sensors and have just a tiny area on the motor and sensory cortex. All this leads to a low level of awareness of the pelvic floor.

Being aware of the function and properly controlling the pelvic floor muscles will lead to good bladder and bowel control and to satisfying sex. Some authors call it the 'love muscle'. PF re-education is an essential part of the job of women's health caregivers, such as PF physiotherapists and midwives.

10.3   Prevention of Pelvic Floor Disorders

The risk factors have to be known to understand the prevention of pelvic floor disorders (*PFDs*). Many studies looked at the various risks. Overall risk factors after childbirth are delivery itself, instrumental delivery (forceps, vacuum), pelvic floor disorders before pregnancy, higher maternal age (>36 years), higher maternal BMI (>30), higher child weight (>4000 g), larger foetal head circumference (>35.5 cm), longer duration of the second stage of labour (>1 h), (median) episiotomy, lacerations, occiput posterior or forehead position, and shoulder dystocia. Some of these risks can be influenced, such as using forceps or vacuum or the duration of the second stage, others not.

Several authors developed flowcharts to prevent primary and secondary PFD or prediction models focusing on potential, expectable PFD.

For primiparous women, Jelovsek developed PFD-prediction models to discuss before birth the probability of developing those disorders and thus make an individual birth plan for every woman, facilitating decision-making in the prevention of incontinence [1].

'UR-CHOICE' is another prediction model for PFD. They fine-tuned the model with extensive long-term results [2]. See http://riskcalc.org/UR_CHOICE/.

To prevent primary disorders, one should carefully observe the function of the pelvic floor, avoid the use of forceps and routine episiotomy, and limit the duration of the second stage. Under these conditions, one can indicate vaginal birth.

However, with factors such as a foetal head circumference >35.5 cm, a maternal age >35, a maternal BMI >30/35, and a family history of pelvic floor disorders, one should consider Caesarean section.

All authors report the importance of good awareness and control of the PF muscles. During expulsion, the muscles have to be relaxed and optimally stretchable. With good (realistic) and honest education, pelvic floor muscle training (including relaxation exercises) and perineal massage, one can reach this. In some centres, the Epi-No® is used (see below). Women will benefit from being coached on adequately using their PF muscles.

10.4   How to Assess the PF Muscles

A woman with a well-functioning pelvic floor can consciously squeeze and relax her PF muscles. Unfortunately, correctly contracting the PF muscles is not easy. In Belgian research, 53% of post-partum women could not perform a correct PF muscle contraction [3]. So pelvic floor muscle assessment and training seem recommended. Below, we address how this can be integrated into women's health by instructors like healthcare professionals, pelvic floor physiotherapists, midwives, or nurses.

An assessment of the PF muscle function starts with an inspection followed by palpation. Specialized pelvic physiotherapists often have other diagnostic tools like biofeedback and ultrasound. These tools provide more specific, detailed information, but inspection and palpation are usually sufficient to determine the function of the PF muscles.

10.4.1   Inspection

During contraction, the vagina closes, and the vagina and perineum move inward. During relaxation, the vagina and perineum move back to their original position. At the Valsalva manoeuvre, the PF muscles have to relax unconsciously, and the perineum should descend a bit. Unfortunately, many women are not able to perform a Valsalva manoeuvre correctly. Instead of relaxing their PF muscles, they squeeze them and push simultaneously ('paradoxically pushing'). Proper pushing makes stool or child pass outside. So, paradoxical pushing is a serious disadvantage. The woman must be able to squeeze, relax, and push properly. If she cannot do so, she should learn those skills.

10.4.2   Palpation

One must prepare carefully for palpation, including consent and a good lubricant. Gently introduce one finger (in the primipara) or two fingers (in the multipara) into the vagina. This manoeuvre should never be painful in a healthy vulva with a well-lubricated finger!

Start with determining the resting tone. With a good resting tone, the finger can be introduced easily and without any resistance, and the PF muscles softly enclose the examining finger. Ask her to contract: the finger will be firmly enclosed, pulled inward, and ventralward.

Ask her to relax: the muscles and the finger will move back to the original position. Ask her to perform the Valsalva manoeuvre: the muscles relax unconsciously and move downward, by which the enclosing of the finger decreases, and the finger partly is pushed out of the vagina.

The next part of the examination deals with coordination: the woman should be able to squeeze and relax the PF muscles with proper strength, timing, and duration.

A woman should be able to make 10–15 fast contractions in a row without losing strength and relax completely after each contraction. Furthermore, she should be able to squeeze the PF muscles for 30 s continuously at 50–70% of her maximal strength. After this endurance contraction, she should be able to relax immediately and completely. We test this in several series with different ways of squeezing and relaxing. One should always be aware that both contraction and relaxation are important. The emphasis in pelvic floor muscle training should therefore be on both actions. Only a completely relaxed pelvic floor can be stretched as much as necessary (200–300%) during vaginal birth.

An underactive pelvic floor has a low resting tone, weak contractions, and little endurance. The examining finger is just slightly enclosed. There is little strength and little or no endurance. The woman can not firmly close the genital hiatus. The elevation of the bladder neck is absent or weak. Here, pelvic floor muscle training should focus on gaining strength and endurance without forgetting coordination.

An overactive pelvic floor has a high resting tone, and the relaxation is delayed and incomplete. It firmly encloses the examining finger. Whereas contraction can vary from weak to strong, relaxation can be absent, delayed, or incomplete. Be aware that overactive is not synonymous with strong. There is often a combination of overactive PF with paradoxical pushing. Here, the training should focus on relaxation and coordination.

10.4.3   The PF Muscles During Pregnancy

Due to the release of the hormone relaxin, the connective tissue all over the body softens during pregnancy. Because the PF muscles contain connective tissue, the pelvic floor weakens. Furthermore, due to the growing size of the uterus, the intra-abdominal pressure increases.

Pregnancy itself can lead to disturbances in micturition and defecation, varying from just a bit of inconvenience to real disorders. Due to the imbalance between the increased intra-abdominal pressure and the decreased urethral closing pressure (decreased PF muscle function), stress urinary incontinence (SUI) may occur. Depending on the degree of imbalance, SUI may vary from just a few drops while coughing to severe loss during all activities that increase the intra-abdominal pressure.

Due to the growing uterus, there will be less and less space for the bladder, and the bladder capacity will decrease, which can cause frequency.

The stool can change during pregnancy as well. The imbalance between the intra-abdominal pressure and the anal closing pressure can cause flatal incontinence. Fortunately, there is rarely faecal loss during pregnancy. As written above, incontinence will depend on the degree of imbalance. Constipation is another inconvenience caused by the softening of the connective tissue of the smooth muscles of the colon and rectum.

Besides the weakening of the PF muscles, pelvic floor dysfunctions can occur as a compensation strategy for these complaints. These compensation strategies often may exacerbate the original complaints. Appropriate, tailored coaching is important to cope with these inconveniences or complaints.

10.4.4 The Pelvic Floor Muscles During Birth

During childbirth, the PF muscles are stretched by 200–300%. No other muscle in the human body can stretch that much. Other tissues are also stretched, including the connective tissue that supports the pelvic organs and the nerves. The more relaxed a muscle is, the more stretchable it is. So the woman must be able to relax her pelvic floor muscles and push properly. Pushing on a non-relaxed PF or pushing paradoxically might lead to more PF and perineal damage.

Several authors have described the changes in PF anatomy and function during the women's lifetime. According to DeLancey [4], physiological lifespan of the pelvic floor differs, with PF function being optimal between age 15–25, depending on the age of the first pregnancy and birth [5]. After 20–25, the pelvic floor function decreases slowly. Women (and men) need a minimal function to maintain continence and other pelvic floor functions. That is why the elderly have many pelvic floor dysfunctions like incontinence (Fig. 10.3).

Vaginal birth affects PF anatomy and function but not to the same extent in every woman. Many variables influence changes in anatomy and function. Furthermore, recovering from pelvic floor injuries varies in women. But not just the extent of damage or dysfunction makes women feel impaired. Circumstances, culture, and expectations influence the woman to experience her pelvic floor disorders just as a (temporal) inconvenience or as a real impairment.

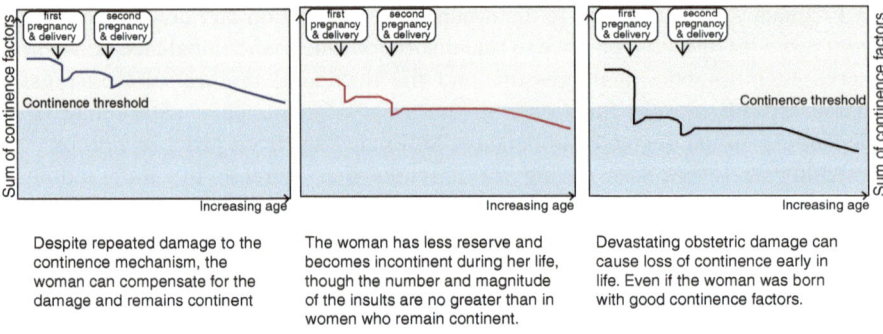

Despite repeated damage to the continence mechanism, the woman can compensate for the damage and remains continent

The woman has less reserve and becomes incontinent during her life, though the number and magnitude of the insults are no greater than in women who remain continent.

Devastating obstetric damage can cause loss of continence early in life. Even if the woman was born with good continence factors.

Perucchini and DeLancey clarified the consequences of pregnancy and delivery and aging on the female continence mechanism. This is an adapted version of their illustration in Chapter 1.1 in 'Pelvic Floor Re-education: Principles and practice' (Springer 2008). [5]

Fig. 10.3 How the female pelvic floor function can change over the lifetime

10.4.5   The Pelvic Floor in the Post-partum Period

After childbirth, all tissues of the PF have to recover. The muscles, the connective tissue, and the nerves have been overstretched and possibly injured. Full recovery usually takes 9 months in physiological conditions, with the most significant recovery occurring in the first three months. For perivaginal tissue recovery, oestrogen is important. So, breastfeeding can delay recovery.

The complaints of decreased PF function and other damage can vary from minor discomfort to serious complaints. Chapter 16 will address the severe problems.

10.5   Prevention and Prehabilitation

Women benefit from being well informed about their pelvic floor and its changes during pregnancy and after childbirth. Unfortunately, most nulliparous women are neither sufficiently informed nor aware of how to squeeze, relax, or push properly (even not during labour and post-partum). As long as pelvic floor awareness is not taught in schools or by mothers, the midwife could take this role and teach how to use the PF muscles to enjoy sex and optimize their function in preparation for childbirth. It seems wise to start that process early in pregnancy because already throughout pregnancy, the PF is changing.

Next to explaining anatomy with images or models, for increased awareness, it is also relevant to touch and maybe massage the PF muscles, which will optimize bladder and bowel control and improve sex life as well. Learning how and when to squeeze or relax or push will, on the one hand, benefit sexuality ('love muscles') and will, on the other hand, prepare for a better functioning PF during the birth. An easy way to increase awareness and learn relaxation might be to apply a warm compress to the perineum. The warmth will make the woman more aware of the PF muscles' localization and help her relax.

Here, we will address two prehabilitation measures: perineal massage and PF muscle training.

10.5.1   Perineal Massage

We recommend perineal massage during pregnancy [6]. Correctly performed massage will make the woman aware of her pelvic floor tone, teach her how to relax it, and allow passage through her vagina (penis, baby, or dildo). It can be pleasant and rewarding for both partners as a joint action. In primiparous women, it diminishes perineal trauma and episiotomy [6]. It is generally well accepted by women.

Although pregnancy softens the connective tissues and weakens the PF muscles, this does not automatically mean that they are relaxed. First, one must relax the muscles since stretching is not possible when tensed. Warmth or a gentle massage can help to achieve relaxation.

We recommended such a massage at least 1–2× per week from week 34 (see Fig. 10.4 for explanation).

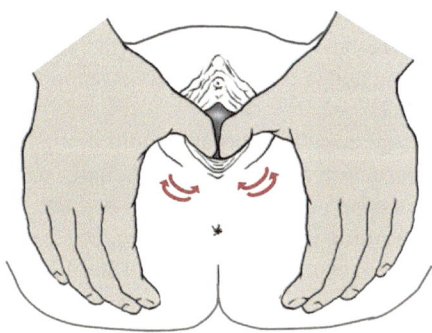

1	Make sure that hands are clean and nails short
2	Choose a quiet place and posture in which legs can be bend and opened in a relaxed way
3	If nesseccary lubricate thumbs and / or perineal tissues (for instance KY jelly)
4	Insert both thumbs about 3–4 cm into the vagina, press down in the direction of the anus and to both sides until a stretching sensation is felt, hold this 1–2 minutes
5	Massage the lower half of the vagina by making a U-shaped movement, stretching the vagina wall dorsally and laterally during 2–3 minutes

Fig. 10.4 Steps in perineal massage

One can also relax and stretch the pelvic floor with the Epi-No®. That is an inflatable balloon coupled to a pressure display hand pump for gradual stretching of the vagina and perineum in late pregnancy [7]. Applied correctly, it might teach women to relax the PF. The Epi-No® does not prevent intrapartum levator ani damage or anal sphincter and perineal trauma. The literature shows conflicting evidence about the effectiveness in preventing PF disorders. In our view, its use has to be coached by trained midwives/HCPs.

10.5.2   PF Muscle Training (PFMT)

PFMT can prevent the detrimental negative effect of a poorly functioning pelvic floor on women's participation in sports and physical activity. In systematic reviews, PFMT during pregnancy and after childbirth improved urinary continence because of better PF function [8, 9].

A systematic review of prenatal and postnatal PFMT showed positive effects on sexual function and female sexuality with post-partum improvements in desire, arousal, orgasm, and satisfaction [10].

An Example of a PFMT Schedule
Start with making an assessment, which guides the training schedule. When the woman can contract for instance for 4 s, that four-second period is the basis of the schedule (as in Table 10.1).

To improve muscle function, the woman should do this daily. After a while, she should increase the contraction and rest time gradually to 6–8 s. Once the woman can perform three series of ten contractions of 6–8 s, she can downgrade to 2–3×/ week. One can do this training lying down, sitting, or standing. It is best to do it in the position in which the woman is most aware of her PF.

Table 10.1 PFMT schedule (based on an assessment of 4 s)

4 s contraction and 4 s rest: to be done 10×
Then 6 fast contractions
Then 1½–2 min pause
This series to be repeated twice

References

1. Jelovsek JE, Piccorelli A, Barber MD, et al. Prediction models for post-partum urinary and fecal incontinence in primiparous women. Female Pelvic Med Reconstr Surg. 2013;19:110–8.
2. Jelovsek JE, Chagin K, Gyhagen M, et al. Predicting risk of pelvic floor disorders 12 and 20 years after delivery. Am J Obstet Gynecol. 2018;218:222.
3. Neels H, De Wachter S, Wyndaele JJ, et al. Common errors made in attempt to contract the pelvic floor muscles in women early after delivery: a prospective observational study. Eur J Obstet Gynecol Reprod Biol. 2018;220:113–7.
4. Delancey JO, Kane Low L, Miller JM, et al. Graphic integration of causal factors of pelvic floor disorders: an integrated life span model. Am J Obstet Gynecol. 2008;199:610.
5. Perucchini D, DeLancey JOL. Functional anatomy of the pelvic floor and lower urinary tract. In: Baessler K, Burgio KL, Norton PA, et al., editors. Pelvic floor re-education; principles and practice. New York: Springer; 2008. p. 3–21.
6. Beckmann MM, Stock OM. Antenatal perineal massage for reducing perineal trauma. Cochrane Database Syst Rev. 2013;4:CD005123Br.
7. Kamisan Atan I, Shek KL, Langer S, et al. Does the Epi-No® birth trainer prevent vaginal birth-related pelvic floor trauma? A multicentre prospective randomised controlled trial. BJOG. 2016;123(6):995–1003.
8. Woodley SJ, Lawrenson P, Boyle R, et al. Pelvic floor muscle training for preventing and treating urinary and faecal incontinence in antenatal and postnatal women. Cochrane Database Syst Rev. 2020;5(5):CD007471.
9. Mørkved S, Bø K. Effect of pelvic floor muscle training during pregnancy and after childbirth on prevention and treatment of urinary incontinence: a systematic review. J Sports Med. 2014;48:299–310.
10. Sobhgol SS, Priddis H, Smith CA, Dahlen HG. The effect of pelvic floor muscle exercise on female sexual function during pregnancy and postpartum: a systematic review. Sex Med Rev. 2019;7:13–28.

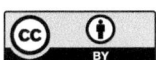

Part III

Introduction to Module 3: 'Nature Losing Its Way'

Woet L. Gianotten, Ana Polona Mivšek, and Sam Geuens

Module 2, with the name 'Nature taking its course', successively addressed sexual aspects in each of the various phases from conception to young parenthood, focusing on the physiological, in other words, uncomplicated or 'healthy' situations.

Module 3, called 'Nature losing its way', follows the same structure but will now address those situations where nature has taken another track, away from the healthy, physiological process. This is, of course, an artificial distinction. Sometimes there is an obvious difference between the natural and the problematic course. However, the reader should be aware that there is a smooth transition area between the two.

The module will successively cover the sexual aspects of the same phases as in Module 2: child wish, conception, pregnancy, labour and childbirth, the postpartum period and young parenthood, breast and breastfeeding, and the pelvic floor.

We have added two chapters that concentrate on the sexual consequences of the most common mental health disturbances and chronic diseases. Those situations can be the direct result of the pregnancy, pre-dated from before the pregnancy or accidentally developed during the pregnancy. The module closes with a chapter on the sexual effects of medication, commonly used in midwifery and obstetric practice.

Especially for the midwifery student, who uses this book as a textbook, the editors recommend starting with Chap. 26, dealing with how to communicate about sexuality, an essential skill that must be mastered before counselling a woman with complicated pregnancy or postpartum with regard to sexuality.

Chapter 11: Sexual Aspects of Fertility Disturbances

Where Chap. 5 addressed 'conception inefficiency' in potentially fertile couples, this chapter concentrates on the situations with actual subfertility or infertility. The message to be infertile or subfertile is usually a severe blow to a person's (sexual) identity, easily impacting, e.g. sexual desire.

The majority of people will continue towards medically assisted forms of reproduction in trying to become pregnant. That phase of examinations and treatments tends to have extensive short-term and long-term sexual consequences.

This chapter will elaborate on those elements inherent to medically assisted forms of reproduction that negatively influence sexuality, such as loss of privacy, demolished intimacy, painful vaginal examinations, and hormonal disturbances. The chapter will also indicate ways to diminish negative impacts on sexual satisfaction and pleasure. Maintaining sexual satisfaction and pleasure during such treatments will keep couples less stressed, positively influencing their conception chances. Also, less stress will keep the woman more relaxed when undergoing pregnancy checks and during childbirth. The amount of stress experienced during ART treatment (Artificial Reproductive Technique) will influence the couple's sexual life in the subsequent phases of pregnancy and young parenthood.

The information in this chapter is, on the one hand, relevant for the midwives and HCPs who are involved in such fertility treatment processes and, on the other hand, for all HCPs by explaining the long-term effects fertility treatment can have on the couple's sexuality.

Chapter 12: Sexual Aspects of High-Risk and Complicated Pregnancy

In a healthy pregnancy, the best response to sexual insecurity is reassurance and telling the couple that they can continue to be sexually active. When the situation gets complicated, things could be different. This chapter elaborates on the sexual risks in conditions such as premature birth, shortened cervix, placental abnormalities, and multiple gestation. It will delineate the relationship between various sexual activities and their potential influence on the uterus and the pregnancy. The chapter will also address how to communicate when specific sexual acts should be discouraged (or forbidden) and simultaneously give room for other sexual acts (the sexual do's and don'ts). Midwives and HCPs have to be aware of the cultural taboos among women and couples. It is a common finding in research that patients have many questions related to sexuality but don't ask those questions. The consequence is that the professional must anticipate when providing information, as it were by 'answering the not-asked questions'. This chapter provides the background information needed to do just that in high-risk and complicated pregnancies.

Chapter 13: Sexual Aspects of Labour/Childbirth Induced Trauma

Especially the first childbirth is a major life event, with far-reaching consequences when things go wrong. This chapter will address the various sexual implications of that 'going wrong'. It will start with the physical troubles of genital tract trauma, perineal damage, and pain.

The chapter will also include psychological trauma. That can, for instance, result from long-lasting consequences of labour pain. Trauma here can also be the disillusionment when a smooth-flowing process suddenly has to be turned into an instrumental delivery; the shock when the baby is not healthy or dies; the disappointment for the partner when the woman in labour completely disconnects, or the bewilderment of the husband, when confronted with his wife's body, after mechanical and possibly bloody procedures. All those situations can have sexual consequences for the woman, the partner, and the couple. And they can call for elements of mourning, readjusting, and renegotiating before a couple can reestablish a healthy sexual relationship.

Chapter 14: Sexual Aspects of Problems in the Postpartum and Early Parenthood (1st Year)

This period, especially after the first childbirth, is the challenge for young parenthood. The new baby suddenly changed the dyad into a triad. The baby is simultaneously a source of pride and pleasure and a source of extreme fatigue and sleepless nights. That appears regularly to be accompanied by sexual tension between the spouses, with many men having far more sexual desire and many mothers experiencing a drop in self-esteem and body positivity (next to physically being worn out), all resulting in sexual difficulties. Up to 80% of young parents experience sexual problems.

The transition to parenthood can be stressful, where gender and gender role differences become apparent. Whereas men usually can separate fatherhood and partnership, those areas are much more intertwined in women. The grimmest consequences are increased family violence and up to 5% of the young parents who separate/divorce within 2 years after the first baby.

This chapter will address the bio-psycho-social causes of those troubles and cover strategies to prevent or diminish them.

Chapter 15: Sexual Aspects of Problematic Lactation

Lactation can be an extremely beneficial factor in the bonding between mother and baby and can, at the same time, also impair the bond between the woman and her (male) partner. On the other hand, breastfeeding can last longer when the partner is supportive. Therefore it is very important to achieve that breastfeeding becomes a couple's strategy. Good lactation is, for many women, also kind of proof of good motherhood. From that perspective, developments like pain during feeding, mastitis, or early breastfeeding cessation can easily have consequences for female identity and the couple's sexual relationship.

This chapter will elaborate on those areas. It will also provide information on breastfeeding in diseases like multiple sclerosis and spinal cord injury, on breastfeeding after breast surgery, and when there has been depression or abuse in the past. A small piece will elaborate on induced lactation in the woman who did not carry the pregnancy.

Chapter 16: Sexual Aspects of Pelvic Floor Disturbances/Disorders

This chapter will pay attention to the disturbances of the pelvic floor and its sexuality-related consequences, with at first attention to the troubles during pregnancy, followed by the problems after childbirth. For instance, whereas pelvic girdle pain is usually pregnancy-related, pelvic organ prolapse tends to result from childbirth.

This chapter will describe the sexual consequences of urinary incontinence and faecal incontinence. It will also provide limited information on pelvic floor physiotherapy so that the midwife can adequately refer the woman when needed.

Chapter 17: Sexual Aspects of Mental Health Disturbances in Pregnancy and Young Parenthood

This chapter will address the various mental health disturbances in this phase of life and their sexual consequences. On the one hand, some women with a psychiatric disease would like to become mothers. On the other hand, mental health disturbances can be related to reproductive changes. The important ones are depression during pregnancy, then postpartum blues, postnatal depression, and in some women, puerperal psychosis. Especially the medication used to treat those situations tends to have many sexual side effects. With clinical case histories, the chapter will demonstrate the clinical impact and potential solutions for these challenging situations.

Chapter 18: Sex, Fertility, Pregnancy, and Parenthood with a Chronic Disease or Other Health Disturbance

In sexology and sexual medicine, it is common knowledge that nearly every chronic disease and almost every cancer treatment have extensive sexual consequences. This chapter will deal with relevant sexual aspects of the common chronic diseases that predated women's pregnancies or that developed during the pregnancy.

After looking at the sexual consequences of chronic disease in general, the chapter will present various specific conditions: chronic bowel disease, diabetes, rheumatic disease, asthma, congenital heart disease, and breast cancer. This chapter will concentrate on those physical health disturbances and their impact on sexuality that are most relevant for midwifery practice.

Chapter 19: Effects on Sexuality of Medication used in Pregnancy and Childbirth

The final chapter of this module will focus on the sexual side effects of various medications and drugs used in midwifery and obstetric practice. The chapter will start with background information on pharmacokinetics and pharmacodynamics geared to pregnancy and the changing pregnant body. On the one hand, it will give some indication on how to deal with sexual side effects. On the other hand, it will look at how to provide women with information on the possible sexual side effects of medication without amplifying the risk of the sexual side effects occurring.

Sexual Aspects of Fertility Disturbances

11

Woet L. Gianotten ⓘ

11.1 Introduction

Worldwide, infertility affects 8–12% of couples, with significant global disparities in figures, causes, and treatment possibilities. The affluent societies have extensive treatment modalities and relatively high infertility prevalence, with higher female age (causing lower ovarian reserve) as a relevant cause. Most poor regions have higher prevalences. In some countries of the '*Infertility belt*' of sub-Saharan Africa, up to 30% of all couples cannot conceive [1], with male infertility and tubal infertility as the predominant explanations. The treatment for those conditions, the expensive reproductive technologies of assisted reproductive techniques (ART) like in vitro fertilization (IVF) and intracytoplasmatic sperm injection (ICSI), are neither available nor affordable to the majority of those couples.

This chapter will not deal with the situation that quickly can develop when a couple gets confused by the lack of success and enters a vicious circle of '*poor sex → no conception → poor sex*'. Such 'conception inefficiency' will be addressed in Chap. 5 ('Getting pregnant').

This chapter will deal with 'real infertility', sometimes defined as 'the failure to conceive after having tried for a full year'. It will start with the fertility consequences caused by sexual dysfunctions (mainly vaginismus, erectile, and ejaculatory problems) and how to deal with those situations.

The next part will shed some light on the most relevant causes of infertility, the standard diagnostic procedures, and the treatment. The following part will explain the implications for sexuality and the intimate relationship, including practical hints for prevention and solutions. The next part will address the complex situations when the couple has an extra handicap (for instance, vaginismus or sexual abuse) that

W. L. Gianotten (✉)
Department of Gynaecology and Obstetrics, Erasmus University Medical Center, Rotterdam, The Netherlands

emotionally conflicts with the invasiveness and intrusiveness of many fertility procedures. Since infertility trajectories cause much collateral damage to sexuality and intimacy, the last part will pay attention to aftercare.

11.2 Sexual Dysfunctions that Disturb Fertility

Although several sexual dysfunctions in men and women will indirectly influence fertility, treating those problems belongs to clinical sexology or sexual medicine [2]. This part will address the most relevant sexual disturbances related to not conceiving (vaginismus, serious dyspareunia preventing penetration, failing erection when penetration is needed, and no ejaculation).

11.2.1 Vaginismus

Some couples with vaginismus conceive without any penetration (but apparently with very fertile sperm). Most couples, however, will not. Many of those couples lived for years in a relationship without having intercourse. A good part of them has a satisfying sexual life (which clashes with our standard frame of reference). So, when a couple with vaginismus seeks fertility treatment, it is crucial to understand their wishes clearly. When there is no intention to have intercourse but only to become pregnant, they usually can be helped with good instructions for bedside insemination (see Table 11.1). For couples who, on the other hand, will use this moment to (finally) address the vaginismus, referral to sexology seems appropriate. A similar approach could be used for a few women with dyspareunia (painful intercourse), although serious dyspareunia usually needs sexological and gynaecological attention.

Table 11.1 Practical aspects of bedside insemination in case of vaginismus

- Give in advance clear oral and written instructions on the optimal elements for conceiving (see Chap. 5)
- Let the woman familiarize herself with vaginally inserting a 1 cc syringe or a thin catheter connected to a 2 cc or 5 cc syringe
- Recommend proper timing for the sexual encounter (optimal is two days and maybe again one day before ovulation)
- Keep the syringe at hand and create good sexual arousal for both (by whatever acceptable method)
- With the man in the supine position, stimulate him till he ejaculates on his belly (warm and no soap)
- Suck the seed in the syringe and insert it deep into the vagina (with the woman in the supine position)
- Stay a while like that and enjoy the intimacy of being together

11.2.2 Failing Erection

The pattern of failing erections is rather diverse.

When never getting an erection (even not when waking up), the man could need a referral to a physician. When he never has an erection with his partner, he probably needs a referral to a sexologist.

Erections can also disappear because of the challenge of wishing a child. Such fertility-related loss of erection can indicate ambivalence about becoming a father, usually in men who already have children from a previous relationship, but sometimes in other men. In those situations, the man, and sometimes the couple, may need some timeout for renegotiating parenthood.

Different is the situation where erections disappear because of the stress of the moment, as can happen during the IVF trajectory ('*This is the night syndrome*'). That stress can be very high when ovulation induction in his partner has been very troublesome. The man needs explanation, reassurance, and maybe some help from an 'erection pill' in such nervousness.

11.2.3 Ejaculation Disturbances

Several ejaculation disturbances belong to specialized care, for instance, retrograde ejaculation (the seed then gets into the bladder) in a man with spinal cord injury or diabetes mellitus. For this book, anorgasmia ('not getting an orgasm') and premature ejaculation ('far too fast') are more relevant.

Stress and inhibition can cause anorgasmia, but most cases result from antidepressant sexual side effects. More than half of the patients taking the common SSRI/SNRI antidepressants cannot reach orgasm [3]. Unfortunately, many antidepressant-prescribing HCPs do not mention this to the patient. Then, consultation with or referral back to the prescribing physician appears necessary.

Premature ejaculation is frequently disturbing for sexual pleasure and is sometimes a conception-disturbing factor. It happens relatively more in societies with a strong taboo on masturbation. Without masturbation, it is difficult to learn ejaculation control. When the man, without such control, meets on their wedding night a bride who is very scared of pain, and when they also have to prove her virginity, the stress can become so high that he ejaculates even before entering the vagina, which can be the start of a sad vicious circle.

Education and other non-pharmaceutical interventions form the usual treatment for the common premature ejaculation. For the severe pre-penetration type, one can delay ejaculation with the same drugs that cause anorgasmia. A dose of 20 mg oral paroxetine (4 h before sexual contact) will delay ejaculation, enabling intravaginal ejaculation (and maybe conception).

11.3   Some Basics of Disturbed Fertility

Infertility patterns vary over the globe and change over time. In many affluent societies, couples are older at the start of a family when fertility is already declining. The ovarian reserve drops rapidly from age 30 to 35, and sperm quality diminishes from age 40 to 45. In the less affluent societies, the leading causes are different. STIs cause high percentages of male and female infertility, and poor contraceptive opportunities cause unwanted pregnancies and septic abortions, resulting in extra female infertility. Those factors also explain the difference between primary infertility (globally ±2% of women) and secondary infertility after having gone through a pregnancy and delivering a live baby (globally ±10% of women).

Among the many different causes of male and female infertility are 'medical factors' and lifestyle-related factors like obesity, malnutrition, tobacco, and marihuana smoking.

Globally, the estimates for infertility causes are:

- Solely male factors (±45%)
- Solely female factors (±40%)
- Combinations of male and female factors (±15%), including cervical factors where a woman's cervical mucus is incompatible with her specific partner's semen.
- A small number of couples with unexplained infertility conceive later without any treatment.

At the start of the trajectory, careful history taking and a thorough physical examination are for both partners more or less the same. After that, the direct burden of investigations and treatment is mainly on the woman's plate.

In men, the most common diagnostic procedures are analysis of sperm after harvesting via masturbation, via epididymal microsurgery (MESA), percutaneously (PESA), or from the testes (TESE). The most common male ART procedures are sperm cryopreservation; using sperm to impregnate a harvested ovum (IVF), and directly injecting sperm into the ovum's cytoplasm (ICSI or IMSI).

In women, the most common diagnostic tests are hysterosalpingography, laparoscopy, cervical mucus testing, and post-coital test. The most common female ART procedures are artificial insemination of partner's or donor sperm into the cervical entrance; intrauterine insemination (IUI); ovulation induction with medication regimes; egg retrieval ('ovum pick-up'); IVF; and embryo transfer.

11.4   Sexual and Emotional Consequences
of Disturbed Fertility

The sexuality of many couples is already compromised when entering the infertility trajectory. Not conceiving easily impairs female and male sexual identity causing low desire. Ovulation-based timing tends to reduce desire and arousal, potentially causing dyspareunia. Subsequent medical interventions add to the decline in sexual quality. Spontaneity disappears when timing and orgasm are dictated by the physician or treatment protocol. Men can be under stress when 'forced' to sexually perform at predetermined times. Sexual intimacy gets reduced by (repeated) genital examination and by having to share details of sexual activities. As a result, the sexual relationship can get under stress. Tension and disappointment can cause mutual irritation. The message that one of them is the cause of infertility can create emotional distance. Besides, the couple's mutual contact might diminish because males and females tend to react rather differently to practical challenges and emotional deceptions.

11.4.1 Male Elements

For most men, physical examination is no big deal, but it is threatening for a small part of men because of sexual abuse experience. Such threat will increase when the sperm has to be collected directly from the epididymis. Whereas masturbation for semen sample collection is in many cultures sufficiently accepted, other cultures restrict that because of shame or religious rules. When the seed is found poor, the 'bad seed'-message is a big blow to most men and an assault on their masculine identity. In part of the men, this will cause sexual dysfunction [4] and it can impair the relationship. Even when entirely accepted, successful masturbation can become problematic when the man has to do it on command. Especially when ovulation induction has been very troublesome, having to perform can be very threatening (with much guilt and sometimes suicidal thoughts when failing to produce sperm). One can diminish the stress of that moment by (in advance obtained) cryopreserved sperm.

11.4.2 Female Elements

Women undergo many more physical examinations and treatment procedures that can interfere with their female identity, bodily integrity, quality of life, and sexuality. Hysterosalpingography, laparoscopy, intracervical insemination, intrauterine insemination, collecting cervical mucus, vaginal ultrasound to monitor the follicle development, and embryo transfer into the uterus are all intrusive and, for the majority of women, also a breach of what belonged to the intimacy between her and her partner. Those procedures are extra troublesome when there is a history of sexual abuse. But also for women from cultures where nakedness is strongly linked to loss of honour. In addition, the combination of stress and (fear of) pain can cause long-standing pelvic floor muscle tension.

Ovulation induction can have many side effects (headache, bloating, nausea, hot flashes), impairing sexuality and intimacy, which is badly needed on those difficult days. Forced ovarian hyperstimulation can have worse side effects, including abdominal pain, fast weight gain, and diarrhoea.

11.4.3 The Couple

The preoccupation with pregnancy and treatment does not help develop pleasure, joy, and relaxed sex. Men feel the imperative to have sex at ovulation, especially when recommended by a fertility specialist. Such 'timed intercourse' imperative can result in sexual dysfunctions and extramarital contact. In one study, 43% of men had erectile disturbances, with a quarter of them having extramarital contact(s) [5]. When ART is decided, having no more imperative to have sex can give relief. But then, with the man in the spectator role, the woman has to undergo treatment with intrusive procedures that easily interfere with her female identity, intimacy, bodily integrity, and quality of life. That is probably one reason for the higher amount of major depressive disorders during this trajectory (39% in women and 15% in men) [6]. ART attacks the relationship, which the HCP should never forget.

11.5 Dealing with the Combination of Severe Sexual Disturbance and Infertility

Whereas in the infertility trajectory, the pleasure element of sexuality becomes less relevant, other aspects of sexual functioning become very important. In IVF, it is vital that the man can produce sperm at the right time and that the woman can open her vagina for a speculum or vaginal ultrasound.

This part deals with such situations where a sexual dysfunction or a past traumatic experience can conflict with the smooth running of the infertility treatment, causing a reduced chance of conception, extra emotional damage to the couple, and frustration for the medical team [7]. Next to various medical precautions, the preparation for assisted reproduction should also anticipate reactions to high stress, such as ejaculatory performance failure and re-experience of sexual abuse.

Here, three possible disturbers will be addressed: male disturbances, vaginismus, and psychotraumatic luggage.

When dealing with such complex cases, the choreography between the couple and the fertility team can be very delicate. Couples desperately wanting a pregnancy sometimes intensely focus on a 'quick fix'. HCPs should refrain from techniques that may speed up the process and cause long-term damage. The anorgasmic man who 'loses' four months in psychosexual treatment but has learned to ejaculate by himself will probably be much happier in the longer term than the man who underwent epididymal aspiration under general anaesthesia. Similarly, the woman with PTSD who 'loses' a year to treatment but then can undergo the procedures fully conscious, without much stress and loss of control, may be more self-satisfied and less damaged than the woman who becomes pregnant through vaginal procedures under general anaesthesia. The final target of an infertility trajectory should be a happy family with happy parenthood. Less stress and a more satisfying sexual life will keep the relationship in better order and benefit both parents' relationship with the new child [8].

11.5.1 Male Disturbances

Whereas erection is not primarily needed in ART, ejaculation is very relevant. For IVF, one prefers fresh ejaculate, so masturbation usually has to occur in a room close to the lab. The stress of that moment can prevent erection and ejaculation. Since many men will be insecure about that, we recommend proactively motivating the man into maximum sexual stimulation (vibrator, X-rated movies of their choosing, et cetera). Real stress can be a good indication for a PDE5-inhibitor ('erection pill') taken one hour before masturbation. Every fertility unit must ensure a special room equipped with vibrators and proper erotic and X-rated stimulation available (or the possibility to access erotic material through their smartphone), where the man can masturbate without or with his partner and where he will not be disturbed.

When the stress of 'having to produce semen' at a given moment is very high, a backup with cryopreserved sperm can sometimes offer sufficient reassurance. There is another reason to pay attention to the man's stress because high stress can negatively influence semen quality. When they introduced counselling, the semen quality tended to stay good on the day of oocyte recovery [9].

11.5.2 Vaginismus

Vaginismus will not be a problem for most couples with child wish because self-insemination is a reliable solution for most. Vaginismus, however, is a significant obstacle when vaginal ultrasound, intrauterine insemination, or embryo transfer are inevitable. It seems wise to refer the woman or the couple to a clinical sexologist or an experienced pelvic floor therapist and treat the vaginismus before starting ART. But how to handle when the couple and the fertility department get caught in a 'Catch 22' situation (for instance, when the treatment has been started, and the vaginismus threatens to disturb the process)? Here are some do's and don'ts.

- General anaesthesia seems logical but tends to be very threatening to many women with vaginismus. The anxiety can go up, and the 'loss of control' easily can prolong 'vaginistic behaviour'.
- Self-hypnosis or self-relaxation techniques usually can be learned in a short period. Especially useful when combined with 'self-management'.
- Self-management. This is a reliable way to have control over the situation. For some women, a feeling of self-competence is more important than a bit of pain. Many times women can learn to introduce the speculum or vaginal probe. Treatment is much easier when the same fertility team always attends the woman (if possible, with very patient female HCPs).
- Neither anxiolytic nor muscle-relaxing drugs tend to help since losing control under medication can be a very frightening experience for many of these women.

11.5.3 Previous Sexual or Physical Abuse

For more details on the effects of trauma experience, see Chap. 24.

When harbouring memories of (sexual) trauma, interventions of assisted reproduction can be very threatening. For a traumatized woman, many terrifying associations can come up during treatment. Like laying down partly undressed, someone standing between her legs, the stress of conception insecurity, the door locked, instruments inserted in her vagina, and eventually suffering pain can suddenly break her resistance and cause vivid flashbacks. We may call the combination of a screaming or crying patient, a confused or angry husband, and a disturbed and maybe guilty team an acute emergency. Besides, this situation will impair the conception outcome [7]. Be aware that men can also be traumatized.

Since a fair amount of women have experienced sexual or physical trauma, the team should properly investigate this area before embarking on ART.

Some abused women have sufficiently addressed the trauma. They can handle everyday life and the stress of ART. Other women have PTSD (usually after chronic or repeated trauma exposure) and need a thorough assessment by a professional with sexual trauma expertise. Here, we will focus on the in-between group that functions well in everyday life as long as there are no substantial factors to create vivid flashbacks.

What can we do to prepare such a patient for ART/IVF?

- We advise against quick-fix approaches such as general anaesthesia or anxiolytics. The woman easily will experience such interventions as re-victimization (because of losing control again).
- Because keeping control is such a woman's key element, we recommend much time counselling the couple and the team on how to handle the stress of the situation. Within such a combined approach, anxiolytic medication can sometimes be helpful.
- Develop a trust-based relationship with one HCP who will be present at every procedure. The patient usually will prefer a female HCP unless a woman has abused her. When possible, we recommend that one trusted member of the fertility team performs all vaginal interventions.
- The process can be facilitated when a female psychosocial HCP counsels the woman, advises beforehand on handling the stress, is present during all procedures, and recognizes the patient's reaction pattern. For some women, the partner can have that role.
- Some patients benefit from the knowledge to control the process and interventions. One way of increasing control is, for instance, by inserting the speculum or ultrasound probe herself (and sometimes when the partner does it).
- Tools for facilitating this process are self-hypnosis (*'going to a safe place'*), imagery exercises, relaxation exercises (breathing exercises), meditation music, and transitional objects (like a cuddly toy) that help the woman feel that she will not be harmed.

- When the woman knows what will happen during the various steps of an intervention and is allowed (as far as feasible) to interfere (f.i. by saying *'Stop'* or *'I need a break'*), her sense of control will increase. Such delicate choreography has to be developed by the physician and the other team members, which means it seems a prerequisite always to have the same team.
- Since control will not be feasible at some moments of the process, the patient should be prepared and learn how to handle the emotions that may surface during such a temporary lack of control. There is no blueprint for when the patient suddenly collapses emotionally. Be prepared for that possibility and inquire if the partner knows the good reaction. Whatever strategy is followed, devote ample time and attention to sorting out what happened, how to proceed, and how to prevent next time.

11.6   Cleaning Up the Mess Caused by the ART Procedures

Once the woman is pregnant, there usually follows a reduction of the emotional, relational, and sexual disturbances. However, these expectant couples remain more than average aware of how precious the pregnancy is, which can influence their sexual well-being and pleasure. After birth, they appear, in general, well-functioning parents not much different from parents with a natural-born child. That can be different regarding sexuality. The roller coaster of fertility workup and treatment, followed by a precious pregnancy, can complicate the redevelopment of sexuality just for pleasure and intimacy. So, we recommend proactively integrating this area in the closing consultation and helping the couple, whenever needed, to rebuild that vital element for their long-term relationship. After all, being 'lovers' is not only luxury but also part of the foundation to cope with the hassles of young parenthood.

Caring attention should go as well to the couples who remain childless. Some of them regain sex and intimacy, which becomes a vital element in continuing their relationship (with more sadness and more freedom). How to deal with childless couples strongly depends on their culture. In part of the globe, childless women are equally accepted and can have a fulfilling social life and career. However, both socially and emotionally, the burden of having no child falls in nearly all cultures on women. In many cultures, childless women will be stigmatized, discriminated against, divorced, and sometimes ostracized, even when their husbands are the cause of infertility. Research in low- and middle-income countries shows that women in infertile couples have a disproportionately high prevalence of intimate partner violence (psychological violence, physical violence, sexual violence, and economic coercion) [10]. On the individual level, childless couples, especially women, deserve gentle care and sometimes psychological expertise. On society's level, midwives appear to be the designated professionals to commit themselves to this social injustice.

References

1. Inhorn MC, Patrizio P. Infertility around the globe: new thinking on gender, reproductive technologies and global movements in the 21st century. Hum Reprod Update. 2015;21:411–26.
2. Berger MH, Messore M, Pastuszak AW, Ramasamy R. Association between infertility and sexual dysfunction in men and women. Sex Med Rev. 2016;4:353–65.
3. Serretti A, Chiesa A. Treatment-emergent sexual dysfunction related to antidepressants: a meta-analysis. J Clin Psychopharmacol. 2009;29:259–66.
4. Saleh RA, Ranga GM, Raina R, et al. Sexual dysfunction in men undergoing infertility evaluation: a cohort observational study. Fertil Steril. 2003;79:909–12.
5. Bak CW, Lyu SW, Seok HH, et al. Erectile dysfunction and extramarital sex induced by timed intercourse: a prospective study of 439 men. J Androl. 2012;33:1245–53.
6. Holley SR, Pasch LA, Bleil ME, et al. Prevalence and predictors of major depressive disorder for fertility treatment patients and their partners. Fertil Steril. 2015;103:1332–9.
7. Gianotten WL. The couple with sexual dysfunction. In: Macklon NS, editor. IVF in the medically complicated patient: a guide to management. 2nd ed. London: Taylor & Francis; 2014. p. 193–203.
8. von Sydow K. Sexuality during pregnancy and after childbirth: a metacontent analysis of 59 studies. J Psychosom Res. 1999;47:27–49.
9. Drudy L, Harrison R, Verso J, et al. Does patient semen quality alter during an in vitro fertilisation (IVF) program in a manner that is clinically significant when specific counseling is in operation? J Assist Reprod Genet. 1994;11:185–8.
10. Wang Y, Fu Y, Ghazi P, et al. Prevalence of intimate partner violence against infertile women in low-income and middle-income countries: a systematic review and meta-analysis. Lancet Glob Health. 2022;10:820–30.

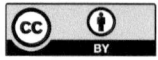

Sexual Aspects of High-Risk and Complicated Pregnancy

Gabrijela Simetinger ⓘ and Woet L. Gianotten ⓘ

12.1   Introduction

Complications during pregnancy tend to create much insecurity, also regarding sexuality. Then, it is tempting for HCPs to advise against 'having sex' or even more veiled to recommend 'pelvic rest'. They are presumably building on a traditional assumption that sex's primary role is to make pregnant and no more needed after reaching that goal. At the same time, we know that sexuality has many functions other than conception. So, in complicated and high-risk pregnancies, HCPs have to balance carefully with their restrictions and recommendations between, on the one hand, damage to the pregnancy, mother or baby and, on the other hand, damage to the sexual health of the woman, her partner, and the relationship. This chapter will start by addressing aspects of this 'balancing approach'.

After that, we will pay attention to the various aspects of sexual behaviour with their potential influence on the health of pregnancy, woman, or baby.

Thereafter, the most relevant disruptions during pregnancy will be reviewed, with some explanation, and with, per disruption, advice/recommendation on what should be discouraged or avoided and what is permissible or recommended. The information relies heavily on an extensive review by MacPhedran [1].

The original version of the chapter has been revised. A correction to this chapter can be found at https://doi.org/10.1007/978-3-031-18432-1_31

G. Simetinger (✉)
Department of Gynaecology and Obstetrics, General Hospital Novo mesto,
Novo mesto, Slovenia
e-mail: gabrijela.simetinger@sb-nm.si

W. L. Gianotten
Department of Gynaecology and Obstetrics, Erasmus University Medical Center,
Rotterdam, The Netherlands

12.2   The Balancing Approach in Communication

Couples and the partners within a couple tend to be different, and so are their sexual needs and their ability to abstain from sexual behaviour when pregnancy gets complicated. Then, some couples can adapt to a reduction or complete absence of sexual contact without really being bothered by it. For many other couples, sexuality is a more relevant or necessary aspect of their life and relationship, and they will have worries and questions about what is allowed and what is or could be dangerous. Most pregnant women will not tell these worries to their HCP, even not to the very trusted midwife. So, in case of complicated pregnancies, the HCP has to 'decide' which strategy to follow. Here are, in short, the essentials of the three strategies.

1. Pay no attention at all. That is not optimal care because it can damage women's and couples' health and sexual health. Besides, it is not suitable for good contact between the HCP and the woman or couple.
2. Pay only attention to what is not allowed and the potential dangers of sex: *'Thou should not have sex!'*. Some HCPs do that more implicit or veiled, for instance, by using the term *'Keep pelvic rest'*. That approach is not quality care either.

Both these strategies can and will have negative consequences. Without explicitly mentioning the discouraged or forbidden elements of sexual behaviour and without mentioning the sexual behaviour that is allowed, the HCP will create insecurity and perpetuate the taboo on openly addressing sexuality. HCPs must be aware of the power of taboo. Besides, the HCP misses an opportunity to establish a trustworthy relationship with the woman and the couple.

3. Pay in detail attention to the discouraged elements of sexuality, and combine that with a proper explanation of the reason for that advice. Moreover, mention explicitly aspects of allowed sexual behaviour.

One could argue that it is the role of the HCP to answer the 'not-asked questions' proactively.

There are smooth transitions between what absolutely should not happen and what better might not occur. There are also smooth transitions between indicating that there is no danger associated with specific sexual acts and, on the other hand, explicitly advising to get started with that way of sex. Sometimes the last seems needed. An example is when penetration can be dangerous, but the male partner is not used to sex without penetration. Then, one can consider mentioning non-penetrative sexuality or masturbation.

On the content aspect: By explicitly mentioning several possibilities, the HCP generates wider sexual choices while at the same time reducing the taboo between the partners.

An example: *'You could cuddle till you feel you need to come. You could continue and bring yourself to orgasm. Many of us learned that masturbation should be done without being seen. However, many also learned that there are other possibilities.*

When your wife feels in the mood, she can help you. Or you can do it yourself with her in your arms. Quite some couples feel that as very intimate!'

On the communication aspect: straightforward advice (e.g. *'Try a vibrator'* or *'Try masturbation on your own or together!'*) can make the HCP virtually enter the woman's or couple's bedroom. It is better to use a detour *(e.g. 'In comparable situations, some couples tried masturbation, and that apparently worked well').*

12.3   The Damaging Potential of Sexuality in Case of Increased Risk

This part pays attention to how various aspects of sexual behaviour could negatively influence the health of the pregnancy, woman, or baby in situations of high-risk and complicated pregnancies. On the one hand, that needs a breakdown of sexuality into separate elements and, on the other hand, a clear explanation of how each part could damage. See Table 12.1.

Table 12.1   Breakdown of sexual behaviour elements and potential influences

Elements of sexual behaviour	Potential influence on pregnancy and health
Experiencing sexually explicit stimuli	→ Arousal??
Kissing	→ Arousal??
Hugging, cuddling without genuine arousal	→ Increased oxytocin levels
Extensive massage/hugging	→ High oxytocin levels
Woman's arousal	→ Increased genital/pelvic circulation
Woman's masturbation	→ Uterine contractions
Woman's orgasm	→ Uterine contractions
	→ Increased circulation and blood pressure
	→ Increased oxytocin levels
Breast/nipple stimulation	→ Increased oxytocin
Oral sex (cunnilingus)	→ Arousal
Oral sex (fellatio) without the intake of semen	→ Arousal
Oral sex with intake/ingestion of semen	→ Idem plus prostaglandin uptake via the mucosa
Vaginal penetration (finger, dildo, penis) without ejaculation	→ Ferguson reflex → oxytocin release
	→ Endogenous prostaglandin release
Direct contact with the cervix	
Vaginal penetration with intravaginal ejaculation	→ Idem with the additional effect of seminal (exogenous) prostaglandins
Pressure on the belly (e.g. in the 'missionary position')	→ Rupture of membranes (esp. when there are vaginal infections)
Anal penetration without ejaculation	→ Ferguson reflex → oxytocin release
Anal penetration with intra-anal ejaculation	→ Idem + prostaglandin uptake through the anal mucosa
Partner's sexual arousal	→ Can increase the woman's arousal
Partner's masturbation	→ Can increase the woman's arousal

Potential risk factors are:

- increased genital/pelvic circulation (as part of sexual arousal),
- increased blood pressure (as part of sexual arousal and orgasm),
- increased oxytocin levels,
- increased prostaglandin levels,
- increased uterine contractions,
- direct mechanical influence.

Although maybe not necessary to mention, let it be clear that none of these phenomena can do any harm in the absence of pathology or pregnancy pathology.

Arousal: When in the non-pregnant situation, the woman perceives sexual stimuli, there is a rapid (within 10–30 s) increase in vaginal circulation. During pregnancy, the genital/pelvic hypercongestion makes it challenging to estimate the additional circulation effects of sexual arousal. It is simply not known if a minor amount of sexual arousal could do any harm. That is different in the high arousal state. Then, the pelvic circulation becomes maximally engorged, and there is a rise in heart rate and systolic blood pressure.

Orgasm: In the third trimester, the clonic orgasm pattern (contract → relax → contract → etc.) can change into a pattern of one tonic spasm, which can last up to a minute, sometimes accompanied by deceleration of the foetal heart rate and recurrent contractions till half an hour after orgasm. There is much inter-individual variety in this orgasm pattern.

Whereas blood pressure and heart rate already can increase during arousal, peak values are found at the start of orgasm.

Oxytocin: causes uterine contractions. It increases at hugging and massage and more at stimulation of breast and nipples. Sexual arousal and orgasm both increase oxytocin levels, which is most clearly seen at orgasm and still is high 5 min. after orgasm. The direct pressure on the cervix and vaginal tissues by the penetrating penis will cause a surge in oxytocin (the 'Ferguson reflex'). This effect is also seen after anal penetration.

There are no research data on the relationship between kissing and oxytocin.

Prostaglandin: PGE and PGF stimulate myometrial activity, can ripen the cervix, and induce labour. Endogenous PG is released when the penis, dildo, or finger touch the cervix. Exogenous PG is deposited with the semen in a higher dose than common cervical ripening agents. It can be found in the vagina up to 12 h after ejaculation. Exogenous PG can cause myometrial activity after being absorbed through the vaginal wall into the woman's circulation, but it can also act directly on cervical ripening.

PGF acts much stronger than PGE. However, semen contains ±20x more PGE than PGF and also ±20x more 19-hydroxy-PGE than 19-hydroxy-PGF [2].

Whereas the PGs deposited at anal ejaculation will not ripen the cervix, they are easily absorbed through the anal mucosa into the woman's circulation.

12.4   The Various Obstetric Disruptions

The rest of this chapter will successively pay attention to the sexual implications of the most common pregnancy disruptions. As far as possible, we will give for each disruption relevant information/explanation and also advice/recommendations on what should be discouraged or avoided and what is permissible or recommended. For part of these recommendations, there is not yet much scientific evidence. More detailed information can be found in the review by Sally MacPhedran [1].

12.4.1 Recurrent Miscarriage: (Habitual or Spontaneous Abortion/Pregnancy Loss)

This is usually defined as three failed clinical pregnancies, confirmed by either sonographic or histopathological examination.

One percent of fertile couples have recurrent miscarriages. Most of these are early losses before 14 weeks of pregnancy. The great majority results from parental chromosomal abnormalities (with many being anembryonic pregnancies that form half of all first-trimester miscarriages) and a small subset of uterine anomalies. Many women with recurrent miscarriages are scared and assume that coitus will harm the foetus or that direct contact between the penis and cervix could trigger a miscarriage. No research data support this possibility. Regarding orgasm: In the first trimester, the oxytocin increase by orgasm will do not harm since the uterus does not yet have enough oxytocin receptors. Regarding the damage of intravaginal ejaculation: the prostaglandin levels of semen are much lower than the high dose of prostaglandins needed for the induction of medical abortion in early pregnancy.

12.4.1.1   Restrictions or Recommendations?

'Can sex cause a miscarriage?' is possibly the most frequently asked (or unasked) question in early pregnancy. Despite even the slightest evidence, HCPs have urged caution (in a review called: 'A concise history of not knowing') [3].

Since the literature does not indicate any adverse effects of the various elements of sexual play in recurrent miscarriage, we can be mild in our recommendations. Maybe most important is a sex-positive approach with, in the discussion, a breakdown of various elements of intimate contact that will be beneficial to the couple and the value of sexual pleasure. Since many women and couples who suffer recurrent miscarriages have esteem issues, the affirmation obtained through sex could be beneficial.

In all literature, we found very few articles that pay any attention to other non-organic aspects of recurrent miscarriage except 'Tender loving care', which is defined as psychological support with weekly medical and ultrasonographic examinations and instructions to avoid heavy work and travel [4]. The authors also indicated avoiding sexual activity. We disagree with the last remark.

12.4.2 Bleeding in First Trimester

Bleeding in the first trimester of pregnancy can signify impending miscarriage, and molar or ectopic pregnancy. Bleeding is the most predictive risk factor for pregnancy loss. Among the other causes of bleeding are vanishing-twin or bleeding unrelated to the pregnancy (including cervical polyp, vaginal infection, rupture of cervical blood vessels, tumour, and trauma). The potential inflammatory consequences of penetration and ejaculation may serve as a secondary insult in an already compromised environment [1].

What Is Allowed: When intrauterine pregnancy is confirmed and no other pathology is found, we believe there is no objection to the full range of penetrative sexuality, excluding the below-mentioned activities.

What Should Not Be Done: We recommend not to have vaginal penetration, vaginal ejaculation, and orovaginal contact at the time of bleeding (because of an already compromised environment).

> Be aware: these precautions of 'no vaginal penetration during bleeding' do not apply during menstruation. Although penetrative sex at that time can be messy or be unacceptable for emotional, cultural, or religious reasons, it does no harm.

12.4.3 Hyperemesis

Whereas 60–75% of pregnant women report usual nausea and vomiting, 0.5–2% report hyperemesis. Among the various causes are high or rapidly rising HCG levels and stress.

What Should Not Be Done: Everything that bothers the woman during nausea.

What Is Allowed/Recommended: Everything that distracts and relaxes her and does not increase nausea. Usually, massage is a good start. The sequel will be determined by the fears and emotional needs of the woman and her partner. And, of course, by how the couple has learned to continue or not to continue after foreplay. Especially when hyperemesis lasts long, it becomes relevant to pay attention to the sexual needs and worries of the partner.

12.4.4 Shortened Cervix

A short cervical length (below 25 mm. measured by transvaginal ultrasound between 16–24 weeks gestational age) developing in this pregnancy is a risk factor for preterm birth. The shorter the length, the greater the risk. Additional risk factors are prior preterm birth, blood loss (even spotting), and uterine contractions.

When there is a short cervix because of earlier conization or large loop excision of the transformation zone (LLETZ) for pre-cancerous cell changes, there seems no reason to abstain from any sexual activity.

What Should Not Be Done: Especially when a short cervix is combined with one or more of the other risk factors, the couple is advised to abstain from all penetrative sex, female orgasm, and other sexual activities that cause or can cause uterine contractions.

It could be wise to recommend that the woman or couple pay attention to the eventual sexual needs of the partner and find ways to deal with that without increasing risk for uterine activity.

12.4.5 Cerclage

The various cerclage types are intended to prevent the cervix from opening too early.

Transabdominal cerclage is done before the pregnancy because of severe cervical anatomy defects. Prophylactic cerclage is done early in pregnancy because of cervical incompetence in former pregnancies. Rescue cerclage is done because the cervix is already flattening or opening in the current pregnancy.

Recommendations: In all cerclage procedures, one should abstain from penetrative sex the week before and the 2 weeks after the procedure.

After prophylactic cerclage, condoms are recommended in penetrative sex because of the risk of infection and chorioamnionitis, leading to preterm birth. The potential inflammatory effect of semen and the penile flora may serve as a secondary insult in an already compromised environment [1]. There are no objections to all other sexual activities.

After rescue cerclage, it is wise to abstain from vaginal penetration, anal penetration, masturbation, and orgasm until approximately 37 weeks. That situation requires extra attention and regular checking if the woman and her partner can handle this situation.

12.4.6 High Blood Pressure and Preeclampsia

Hypertensive disorders complicate 5–10% of all pregnancies and contribute significantly to maternal morbidity and mortality. Part of the pregnant women already had (chronic) hypertension. Hypertension developed after week 20 of the pregnancy (termed *gestational hypertension*) is followed by signs and symptoms of preeclampsia in half of the cases, with preeclampsia in 3.9% of all pregnancies [5].

Which aspects of sexuality are risk factors in the woman with preeclampsia? Physical activity (as in aerobic exercise); autonomous nerve activity; uterine contractions; and increase in blood pressure.

When comparing the woman with a slight increase in blood pressure and the woman with high blood pressure and signs of preeclampsia, it will be apparent that sexual expression will not have the same consequences. That means the HCP should consider which sexual behaviour is still acceptable and which sexual behaviour poses a danger. Next is explaining such information in detail to the couple. And then check in how far the couple can deal with those recommendations.

In gestational hypertension, aerobic exercise is contraindicated, and accordingly, there should be no strenuous sexual activity (for instance, intercourse with the woman on top). When there are signs of preeclampsia, we believe that the woman should refrain from high arousal and orgasm.

There is no objection to gentle kissing, hugging, and cuddling. When penetration appears very needed, some couples could consider gentle penetration, tell how much they love each other, and eventually finish the encounter by the partner's masturbation and ejaculation outside the vagina.

12.4.7 Poor Placental Function

Foetal growth restriction can be a sign of poor placental function. When that is related to the hypertension/preeclampsia complex, the woman better refrains from most aspects of sexual behaviour (see above).

Without preeclampsia, we do not know if sexual behaviour yields any risk for the mother or child. Sexual arousal is accompanied by increased uterine circulation. In pregnancy, however, we do not know if it benefices the circulation of the placenta and the foetus.

12.4.8 Urinary Tract Infection (UTI)

Women regularly have asymptomatic bacteriuria. So this is frequently found in prenatal care. When pregnant, the smooth muscles of the ureters relax. The subsequent dilatation and the increased abdominal pressure due to the growing uterus appear to facilitate the ascent of bacteria from the bladder to the kidney. That creates a dilemma. On the one hand, untreated bacteriuria is associated with more pyelonephritis and an increased risk of preterm birth, low birthweight, and perinatal mortality. On the other hand, treatment with antibiotics creates antibiotic resistance. That is a real disadvantage during pregnancy since several teratogenic antibiotics may not be used. Research focuses strongly on hygienic measures to prevent urinary tract infections. More urinary tract infection was found with sexual activity >2–3x per week and when the bladder was not voided after intercourse [6].

Non-sexual recommendations are as follows: wipe/wash the genital area from front to back after going to the toilet; do not delay when having to pass urine; and drink enough.

Sexual recommendations: void the bladder after intercourse; wash the genital area after intercourse [6]. In addition, we recommend not to have intercourse too frequently (when the need is high, consider having non-penetrative sex). After having anal sex, pay extra attention to perineal washing/cleaning; do not combine any anal activity with vaginal penetration.

12.4.9 Colpitis/Vaginal Infection

The microbiome in the healthy female genital tract is dominated by bacteria that produce lactic acid, maintaining a low pH and protecting against infections. Pregnancy influences that microbiome, resulting in more genital tract infections [7] with, in its wake, an increased risk of preterm birth and pelvic infections.

Pregnancy changes the woman's microbiome. It can also influence her male partner's sexual behaviour, sometimes resulting in extramarital contact and an increased risk of STI or trichomonas [8].

To varying degrees, vaginal infections are relevant because of the complaints (discharge, itching, dyspareunia, burning sensation in the vulva, and burning at passing urine) influencing sexuality and the increased risk for preterm birth and neonatal consequences.

Bacterial vaginosis (BV) is a misdistribution of the normal vaginal flora, resulting from high colonization of anaerobic organisms (Gardnerella vaginalis and others) and increased vaginal pH. BV prevalence among women of reproductive age varies from 5 to 60%, depending on the geographic area and diagnostic criteria. About half of the women with BV are symptomatic, with a fish-smelling discharge as the most common complaint. Although sexual intercourse appears to be a risk factor, there is no evidence that BV is an STI. Women using petroleum jelly as a lubricant have more BV [9]. BV early in pregnancy is a vital risk factor for preterm birth and spontaneous abortion [10]. Treatment of bacterial vaginosis during pregnancy improves symptoms but does not reduce the risk of preterm birth [11].

Candida albicans commonly colonizes the vagina of pregnant women. That can be asymptomatic or cause symptoms like pruritis of vaginal discharge. Reinfection is common without simultaneous treatment of the sexual partner(s). Vulvovaginal candidiasis is found more in women who receive oral sex and when using vaginal lubricants containing glycerine/glycerol because candida thrives on that.

Trichomoniasis is characterized by a foul-smelling discharge. Treatment must include the sexual partner(s).

Aerobic vaginitis shows an increase in mucosal inflammation with subsequently more dyspareunia [12].

GBS or streptococcus agalactiae is one of the potential microorganisms of aerobic vaginitis. Colonization with Group B streptococcal infections (GBS) is often asymptomatic and may cause UTI and PPROM (preterm premature rupture of membranes). Heavy maternal colonization with GBS at birth can be associated with fulminant neonatal infection.

Sexuality: In many couples, the complaints (discharge/smell) will prevent sex and especially the cunnilingus part. Since these troubles frequently are accompanied by dyspareunia, it seems wise to inform the couple that this could be the entrance to a long-lasting vicious circle of 'pain → no desire → pain' and recommend looking for non-penetrative ways of sexual interaction.

Since there are associations between the male-superior position, PPROM, and infections [13], it seems wise to recommend replacing the male-superior with other positions.

12.4.10 Uterine Contractions

Especially for the primigravid woman, uterine contractions may be frightening. The majority are Braxton–Hicks contractions that do not relate to the start of childbirth. They are uncomfortable but tend not to be painful (in contrast to labour pain). They can appear more frequently with sexual activity.

During an orgasm, the woman also has contractions. In the last weeks of pregnancy, some women experience a change in orgasm. The typical clonic pattern of 'contract → relax → contract' turns into a pattern of one strong tonic contraction. That appears to be enhanced by the oxytocin increase and intravaginal deposition of seminal prostaglandin. In a healthy pregnancy that neither does any harm nor causes preterm labour.

Recommendations: As long as the pregnancy is healthy and without signs of preterm birth, there are no contraindications to the whole gamut of sexual play.

However, when painful contractions seem to transition into signs of preterm birth (bleeding, shorter cervix, persisting contractions), the couple should refrain from such sexual activities.

12.4.11 Premature Rupture of Membranes

Preterm premature rupture of membrane (PPROM) refers to chorioamniotic membrane rupture before 37 weeks of gestation. Women with PPROM are at an increased risk of preterm birth because of infection or chorioamnionitis, progression of preterm labour, or placental abruption because of a change in uterine pressure with loss of amniotic fluid. Vaginal penetration, anal penetration, and orovaginal contact increase the risk for ascending infection and chorioamnionitis. Since, in PPROM, the uterus is prone to start labour, the couple/woman should refrain from all sexual/erotic activities that can cause uterine contractions.

What Should Not Be Done: vaginal penetration, anal penetration, orovaginal contact, nipple stimulation, female masturbation, and female orgasm.

What Is Allowed: Kissing, hugging, gentle massage, partner orgasm.

12.4.12 History of Preterm Birth (PTB)

A history of PTB poses an increased risk for recurrent spontaneous PTB. So, many couples will be concerned about the potential dangers of sexual contact. There are, however, no reliable research data to help us in this discussion [1].

In the absence of a short cervix or other obstetric risks, there appear no reasons to abstain from any sexual activity.

When this pregnancy has/had an episode with symptoms indicating preterm labour, it is better to avoid any sexual activity that causes an increase in frequency or intensity of uterine contractions.

After a detailed search, MacPhedran says: "Individualise recommendations based on consideration of obstetric history and comorbidities as well as patient and partner fears and emotional needs" [1].

12.4.13   Bleeding in the Second Half of Pregnancy

There are many reasons for blood loss, including impending preterm birth, placenta previa, vasa previa, abruptio placentae, and uterine rupture. There are also some non-pregnancy-related causes (cervical polyp or tumour, vaginal infection, or trauma). The couple should abstain from sexual activities until a proper diagnosis is made (and treatment started). After that, the HCP should give detailed recommendations. First, we will address placenta previa and then solutio placentae (placental abruption).

Placenta Previa: is an important cause of bleeding in the third trimester. When the placenta is implanted low, the development of the lower uterine segment and the accompanying mechanical separation between the placenta and lower segment can cause (painless) bleeding. Such first ('sentinel') bleeding warrants abstaining from aerobic exercise and all sexual acts that cause uterine contractions or that mechanically influence the lower segment, so no woman-on-top position, no nipple stimulation, no vaginal or anal penetration, and no orgasm.

The same seems recommendable in the case of vasa previa.

Solutio Placentae-Placental Abruption: is the situation where already, before birth, the placenta separates from its implantation site. Total separation is a life-threatening emergency. In partial ('chronic') placental abruption, there is very little scientific information available on how to advise [1]. In a stable chronic placental abruption, it seems wise to recommend abstaining from all sexual activities that result in frequent, intense, or painful uterine contractions and from sexual activities that result in bleeding.

12.4.14   Multiple Gestation

A twin pregnancy differs little from a singleton pregnancy, except for the duration, with childbirth on average taking place at 37 weeks. According to the limited research in this area, sexuality does not influence the onset of birth [14]. So, without complications, the instructions and recommendations on sexuality can be the same.

In affluent societies, some 20% of twin pregnancies result from in vitro fertilization. Those parents tend to have less sex because the pregnancy is so precious (and maybe also by the knowledge that these pregnancies have more obstetrical complications).

Multiple pregnancies (triplets or more) have more prematurity. There are no data on the influence of sexuality on such pregnancies.

Recommendations in twin pregnancy: there are no restrictions.

Recommendations in triplets or more: we guess it wise to inform about the potential consequences of labour-inducing sexual activities and look with the couple for a good balance between safety for pregnancy and baby and, on the other hand, sexual/emotional satisfaction.

12.4.15 Presence of Uterine Scars

In the great majority (>99%) of caesarean sections (CS), there is a transverse incision in the lower part of the uterus. Without other obstetric complications, such a scar does not risk uterine rupture. That is different from the 'classical CS' with a longitudinal midline incision, usually to allow more space to deliver the baby. That scar has a 2% risk of uterine rupture pre-labour and 6% during labour [1]. Comparable risks exist after extensive uterine surgery, for instance for uterus duplex or intramural myomata. In all these women, a contraction stress test is contraindicated, and elective CS is indicated.

Recommendations: we should explicitly and repeatedly explain that any sexual stimulation causing prolonged or painful uterine contractions must be abandoned, indicating the risk of uterine rupture. These are the situations where the partner's sexual needs deserve extra attention.

12.5 Conclusion

When dealing with threatening pregnancy complications, the essential message of this chapter is to proactively address the not-asked questions in the area of sexuality and intimacy. It then seems sensible to clarify which elements of sexual behaviour in their situation are dangerous for the mother-pregnancy-child unit. However, it is also relevant to proactively address what is 'allowed' or 'recommended'. Balancing is needed between the consequences for the pregnancy and the child, and the consequences for the woman, her partner, and their sexual relationship.

References

1. MacPhedran SE. Sexual activity recommendations in high-risk pregnancies: what is the evidence? Sex Med Rev. 2018;6:343–57.
2. Bendvold E, Gottlieb C, Svanborg K, et al. Concentration of prostaglandins in seminal fluid of fertile men. Int J Androl. 1987;10:463–9.
3. Moscrop A. Can sex during pregnancy cause a miscarriage; a concise history of not knowing. Br J Gen Pract. 2012;62:e308–10.
4. American Society for Reproductive Medicine. Evaluation and treatment of recurrent pregnancy loss: a committee opinion. Fertil Steril. 2012;98:1103–11.

5. Cunningham FG, et al., editors. Williams obstetrics. 25th ed. New York: McGraw Hill Medical; 2018.
6. Ghouri F, Hollywood A, Ryan K. A systematic review of non-antibiotic measures for the prevention of urinary tract infections in pregnancy. BMC Pregnancy Childbirth. 2018;18:99.
7. Han C, Li H, Han L, et al. Aerobic vaginitis in late pregnancy and outcomes of pregnancy. Eur J Clin Microbiol Infect Dis. 2019;38:233–9.
8. Whisman MA, Gordon KC, Chatav Y. Predicting sexual infidelity in a population-based sample of married individuals. J Fam Psychol. 2007;21:320–4.
9. Brown JM, Hess KL, Brown S, et al. Intravaginal practices and risk of bacterial vaginosis and candidiasis infection among a cohort of women in the United States. Obstet Gynecol. 2013;121:773–80.
10. Leitich H, Bodner-Adler B, Brunbauer M, et al. Bacterial vaginosis as a risk factor for preterm delivery: a meta-analysis. Am J Obstet Gynecol. 2003;189:139–47.
11. Paladine HL, Desai UA. Vaginitis: diagnosis and treatment. Am Fam Physician. 2018;97:321–9.
12. Donders G, Bellen G, Grinceviciene S, et al. Aerobic vaginitis: no longer a stranger. Res Microbiol. 2017;168:845–58.
13. Ekwo EE, Gosselink CA, Woolson R, et al. Coitus late in pregnancy: risk of preterm rupture of amniotic sac membranes. Am J Obstet Gynecol. 1993;168:22–31.
14. Stammler-Safar M, Ott J, Weber S, Krampl E. Sexual behaviour of women with twin pregnancies. Twin Res Hum Genet. 2010;13:383–8.

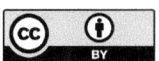

Sexual Aspects of Labour/Childbirth Induced Trauma

13

Petra Petročnik (ID) and Ana Polona Mivšek (ID)

13.1 Introduction

The period after birth is challenging for couples, as childbirth itself may impact everyday life activities and the care for the newborn and might also affect their sexual life after childbirth. This chapter provides detail on physical and psychological trauma related to the process of labour and birth. It addresses various consequences that may impact their future relationship, such as perineal trauma, instrumental labour, the loss of the baby, loss of contact with the partner, or disappointment about the mode of birth. Alongside the theoretical notions, the chapter provides examples from clinical practice. This chapter aims to empower midwives in their important role in recognizing and helping the couple re-establish a healthy sexual relationship after birth.

13.2 Physical Birth Trauma

Several physiological changes in the woman's body (in detail described in Chap. 8) influence postpartum sexuality. In brief, according to O'Malley et al. [1], almost 50% of women reported a lack of sexual interest in sexual activity, whereas 43% experienced a lack of vaginal lubrication, and 37.5% reported dyspareunia in the first 6 months after childbirth. In case of suffering birth trauma, these changes might

P. Petročnik (✉) · A. Polona Mivšek
Faculty of Health Sciences, University of Ljubljana,
Ljubljana, Slovenia
e-mail: petra.petrocnik@zf.uni-lj.si; polona.mivsek@zf.uni-lj.si

© The Author(s) 2023
S. Geuens et al. (eds.), *Midwifery and Sexuality*,
https://doi.org/10.1007/978-3-031-18432-1_13

be topped up with additional fears and potential pains that influence the frequency and quality of their postpartum sexual activity. Many women rarely seek help regarding sexuality since they tend to be more preoccupied with the newborn and self-care. Healthcare professionals (HCPs), including midwives, are the ones that have to initiate the conversation about sexuality. To provide efficient counselling, they must know about perineal and other injuries during childbirth.

13.2.1 Genital Tract Trauma

Up to 85% of women are estimated to sustain some form of genital tract trauma during childbirth [2]. That can be attributed to a certain degree of laceration of the cervix, vagina, perineum, or other parts of the genitalia. Perineal trauma may also result from episiotomy and an operative birth, such as vacuum or forceps labour, just as the abdominal wound after caesarean section (CS). Spontaneous perineal trauma may result in perineal tears, which can be mild, such as first- and second-degree tears, and extend into severe injury involving the anal sphincter, such as third- and fourth-degree tears. The last detailed statistics on perineal trauma during childbirth in European countries were given by the EuroPeristat Report from 2010 [3]. The incidence for first and second-degree tears was 4–58% and for third and fourth-degree tears was 0.1–5% [3].

The extent of the genital tract trauma influences postpartum recovery and impacts both the time of resuming vaginal intercourse and the possible development of dyspareunia. Even though the prevalence of dyspareunia in women is already relatively high, the incidence in the postpartum period is even higher, especially in association with perineal injuries. However, the condition often stays undiagnosed and is therefore undertreated. Women who sustained a second-degree tear or episiotomy experience lower arousal, orgasm, and sexual satisfaction and more dyspareunia at 12 weeks postpartum [4]. Globally, there are different practices regarding stitching or not stitching minor perineal lacerations. Leeman et al. [4] compared the results between no tear, tears with stitching and tears without stitching. At 12 weeks postpartum, they found no differences in urinary incontinence, anal incontinence, sexual activity, and sexual function [4]. Quite different is the situation in major injuries. In a Danish study, 50% of primiparous women with third or fourth-degree perineal tears reported dyspareunia even at 12 months postpartum. As expected, the best overall outcomes after 12 months were reported by those with no tears, tears of labia, or first-degree tears of the perineum [5].

Episiotomy is an iatrogenic perineal trauma. This 'perineal cut', the most frequent intervention during childbirth, is closely connected with perineal pain beyond the postpartum period and hinders women in resuming vaginal penetration. A Cochrane review comparing selective versus routine use of episiotomy found no benefits of routine use of this procedure, neither for the mother nor for the baby [6]. Therefore, according to the professional guidelines, the routine use of episiotomy is not recommended. Studies show that the intensity of postpartum pain is not affected by the mode of episiotomy (mediolateral or median). However, episiotomy causes more perineal pain than spontaneous second-degree perineal tears, even though the same anatomical structures are affected. After an episiotomy, women indeed reported more perineal pain, less sexual satisfaction, and a delayed sexual restart [7]. The anxiety of anticipated pain might also be the case of the delayed re-establishment of desired sexual encounters.

13.2.2 Trauma, Related to the Mode of Birth

Evidence suggests a link between the mode of birth and the impact on postpartum sexual function. Operative deliveries (by vacuum extraction, forceps, and CS) are associated with increased dyspareunia. Moreover, especially vacuum extraction and CS lead to increased rates of persisting dyspareunia up to 18 months postpartum.

The most common operative way of birth is CS, a major abdominal surgery and, as such, a vast physical trauma for women. The incidence of CS varies globally. Even though the WHO [8] recommends a CS rate of 10–15%, in some countries like Cyprus, Brazil, and Turkey, the CS rates exceed 50%. Besides the abdominal wound that is a significant source of pain, CS can also cause certain complications, including infection, haemorrhage, and incidental surgical injuries. Even though the perineum stays intact with a primary CS, a study by Blomquist et al. [9] reports that CS does not protect against postpartum dyspareunia. Women resume sexual intercourse quicker after the CS. However, a systematic review and meta-analysis by Fan et al. [10] reports no differences in postpartum sexual satisfaction between women after CS and women after vaginal birth.

A recent Danish study [11] looked at >43.000 women, on average 16 years after the first birth. CS was shown not to protect against long-term sexual problems. Vaginal birth (even after a previous CS) was associated with fewer long-term sexual problems. An important possible consequence of vaginal birth is trauma to the pudendal nerve. That is why some authors emphasized the potential protective role of CS as it will cause less pudendal nerve injury, less trauma to the pelvic floor, and no perineal damage [12]. This has been one of the controversial facts that led to the dilemma of whether women should be offered the choice of elective CS to avoid the development of pelvic floor dysfunction and possible postnatal sexual dysfunctions. However, both pregnancy and birth are significant factors for changes in the pelvic floor function; therefore, a routine caesarean section is not a solution to preserve the pelvic floor function.

Trauma related to childbirth may affect women as well psychologically, sometimes as a consequence of pain and occasionally independent of pain. On the one hand, the midwife plays a vital role in preventing soft tissue ruptures and unnecessary episiotomy. On the other hand, the midwife should provide the woman with information regarding pain management and wound care and address the topic of sexuality after birth, including the resumption of intercourse. It is important to discuss sexuality face to face with the woman or the couple and have that information also recorded in the discharge protocol. Community midwives should address this topic when caring for women in the postpartum phase at home.

13.3   Psychological Consequences of Physical Trauma

Childbirth may affect women psychologically, for instance, in the case of physical trauma, for example, the psychological damage of labour pain for which the woman was not prepared, totally unexpected pain or pain experienced as intolerable. That can also happen to the partner. While midwives have become familiar with people in pain, this is not the case for most partners, especially not when the loved person seems to be in severe pain.

Due to dyspareunia, the woman might avoid sexual intercourse. If she does not openly discuss that, the partner might not understand her avoidance, with the risk of extended avoiding any form of intimacy altogether.

Studies confirm that perineal trauma as an obstetric complication can result in psychological distress that can manifest in similar symptoms as post-traumatic stress disorder (PTSD) [13]. Besides psychological distress, it might affect partnership by diminishing the quality of sexual and marital interactions. Fear of pain when having intercourse and insecurities about body image is sometimes hard to discuss, especially if communication about sexuality was not well established before or during the pregnancy. In the case of major perineal tears, many women in the study by Skinner et al. [14] exhibited adverse coping behaviours. These authors have reported anxiety, avoidance, detachment from babies/partners, and numbing. There was distress that sexual relations were almost impossible and that involved unwelcome flashbacks of the birth and feelings of the stigma that their bodies were not adequate [14]. Crookall et al. [15] report less desire to be held or touched by her partner when the woman suffered more extensive lacerations during childbirth. Severe perineal trauma can result in many complications (such as urinary or faecal incontinence) that deeply affect a woman's everyday life, impacting her self-esteem. In that case, the partnership (and, consequently, sexuality) come under pressure.

13.4   Psychological Trauma

As a consequence of childbirth, the woman, her partner, or both may experience several other birth-related psychological traumatic experiences. We should not underestimate that psychological trauma of the woman may arise from feelings of failure because the birth was not experienced as they expected and hoped for or did not take place within her 'childbirth value system' (like not giving birth vaginally). Women who see their birth as a traumatic experience might face long-lasting psychological effects [16].

Even when the midwife or any other HCP labels the birth as 'normal', the woman can undergo her labouring experience as traumatic. Indicated risk factors for experiencing birth as traumatic include: negative subjective birth experience, operative delivery, lack of support, and dissociation [17].

On the other hand, the woman's partner may experience some form of psychological trauma as not being prepared for seeing some procedures or consequences of birth. Partners who experienced witnessing a traumatic birth of their woman reported this to negatively impact themselves and their relationship [18, 19]. Antenatal preparation for childbirth is important, just as good cooperation with the couple at the time of birth and in the postpartum period. When couples feel they are prepared for the challenges of labour and childbirth together, this can strengthen their bond through a period of major changes, thus creating an optimal relational context to start up intimacy and sexuality again postpartum.

Here, we successively address some traumatic experiences with their potential sexual consequences.

(a) *Loss of the baby.* Sometimes this is preceded by an emotional rollercoaster of fear and nagging insecurity, but sometimes it is a sudden fact. The sexual consequences partly depend on how the couple's sexuality has been developed. It also depends on the role sexuality has for each of them. For some couples, this experience becomes (also sexually) a strong bonding factor. However, other partners can gradually lose each other because of their differences in dealing with the loss and not understanding the other, including losing each other sexually.

(b) *Re-traumatizing of former abuse or sexual abuse.* One may expect that most women will have sufficiently dealt with their negative past and can handle the not too complex situations, whereas others are (still) much more vulnerable. Even with optimal care, the situation can become traumatic, for instance, when suddenly a vacuum or forceps has to be applied, causing loss of control. Good aftercare can restore the disturbed balance in some women/couples, whereas psychological and sexual consequences can be long-lasting in others. Chapter 24 deals with those situations in more detail.

(c) *Loss of self.* For instance, this can happen when the birth experience does not resemble what the woman had in her mind. When she has prepared herself for a natural first childbirth with candles and flowers but suddenly has to be rushed to the theatre for an emergency procedure, she can experience that as 'failing' in her role as 'a natural mother'. Such a lost sense of self can easily reflect psychological issues with self-worth and consequently diminished sexual desire and damaged relationship with her partner.

(d) *Traumatizing of the partner.* Whereas HCPs are used to blood and pain, we should realize that most partners are not! The husband who has seen the havoc of his wife's third-degree tear can lose sexual desire for a long time.

(e) *Lost connection between the partners.* Childbirth is a stressful experience that places high demands on dealing with each other, completely different from daily. The woman can become so introverted that her partner no longer seems to exist. Or she can curse her husband, screaming that she never, never wants to have sex again. Whereas the woman most probably has forgotten that after a week, some men can need months to get rid of those experiences. The man can himself cause the disconnection, for instance, when he arrives just before the birth in all his nervousness, smelling of alcohol. Such experiences can complicate the transition to healthy parenthood and renewed intimacy in the postpartum period.

(f) *Midwife (or other HCP)-related 'damage'*. In a retrospective search among >2.100 Dutch women who had experienced their birth as traumatic, many women indicated that their trauma could have been reduced or prevented with better communication and support by the caregivers. Other causes of 'damage' were mistreatment, verbal abuse, discrimination, and non-consented procedures [20]. Such breaches of mental integrity in women (who are nearly all vulnerable because in labour) easily can cause or intensify a negative sense of self. For some women, sexuality helps them reconnect to their inner selves. Still, this negative sense of self will impair pleasurable sexuality for many.

13.5 The Role of the Midwife

During childbirth, an essential role of the midwife is the prevention of soft tissue ruptures and unnecessary episiotomy. Preventive interventions should start in pregnancy (in the form of perineal massage after the thirty-fourth week) and during childbirth (warm compresses applied on the perineum, upright positions during birth, hands-on technique of perineal protection). When despite all efforts, an episiotomy is needed or lacerations occur, the wound should be adequately cared for, and the woman should receive unbiased and detailed information on the injury and its care.

Women often say that they did not get an explanation of what happened to their genitals during birth [14], and therefore, they might imagine their wounds as more severe than they actually were. Explanation from the midwife on what the woman can expect postpartum might help prevent or resolve unfounded fears and anxiety. The midwife should provide information on managing pain, care for the wound, and address the topic of first intercourse after the birth. With the woman's consent, we should include the partner when discussing sexual aspects of recovery and dealing with sexual worries and questions. When we give such information on dyspareunia, we should do that without increasing the woman's feelings of fear or anxiety. The couple should be encouraged to discuss sexual concerns and agree upon the timing of the first intercourse (both must feel ready). It should be outlined that it is entirely normal that many women (especially when breastfeeding) are not yet really in the mood for penetrative sex in the first period after childbirth. For many women, the focus is on the newborn baby. Therefore, it is crucial that both partners feel ready and choose the sexual activity that suits them both. Perhaps in the first days or weeks following childbirth, this should include cuddling without penetration, with the latter only added when the woman feels ready for it.

In postpartum sexuality problems, the midwife can determine which role to choose in caring for the couple's postpartum sexual health (for instance, which level to pick up from the extended PLISSIT model, described in Chap. 3). However, in severe perineal trauma, the midwife must be alert and consider possible physical complications that might need a referral to other specialists. When the midwife cannot provide continued care after discharge from the maternity unit, the provided information on sexuality must be forwarded to the next HCP.

13.6 Conclusion

Midwives and other HCPs should understand possible changes in sexual life based on the mode of birth. They should give realistic information on the physical consequences of the interventions during birth and inform how to deal with pain. Besides, they should proactively address potential sexual effects and indicate possible ways to handle that. After birth, the midwife should offer proper consultation to all women who sustained childbirth-related trauma.

Therefore, health professionals who take care of women in the postpartum period must also address the topic of sexuality and intimacy in case of possible physical or psychological trauma. Sexuality issues should be dealt with and recorded in the discharge protocol for both the woman and her partner. Community midwives should address this topic when caring for women in postpartum home care. Since an open conversation between partners on sexuality and intimacy appears beneficial, the midwife should promote this from early pregnancy.

References

1. O'Malley D, Higgins A, Begley C, et al. Prevalence of and risk factors associated with sexual health issues in primiparous women at 6 and 12 months postpartum; a longitudinal prospective cohort study (the MAMMI study). BMC Pregnancy Childbirth. 2018;18:196.
2. Brandie K, Mackenzie A. Perineal trauma following vaginal delivery. J Assoc Chart Physiother Women's Heal. 2009;105:40–55.
3. EuroPeristat European perinatal health report: health and care of pregnant women and babies in Europe in 2010. 2010.
4. Leeman LM, Rogers RG, Greulich B, Albers LL. Do unsutured second-degree perineal lacerations affect postpartum functional outcomes? J Am Board Fam Med. 2007;20:451–7.
5. Gommesen D, Nøhr E, Qvist N, Rasch V. Obstetric perineal tears, sexual function and dyspareunia among primiparous women 12 months postpartum: a prospective cohort study. BMJ Open. 2019;9:e032368.
6. Jiang H, Qian X, Carroli G, Garner P. Selective versus routine use of episiotomy for vaginal birth. Cochrane Database Syst Rev. 2017;2:CD000081.
7. Yıldız H. The relation between prepregnancy sexuality and sexual function during pregnancy and the postpartum period: a prospective study. J Sex Marital Ther. 2015;41:49–59.
8. World Health Organization. WHO statement on caesarean section rates. Geneva: World Health Organization Human Reproduction Programme; 2015.
9. Blomquist JL, McDermott K, Handa VL. Pelvic pain and mode of delivery. Am J Obstet Gynecol. 2014;210(423):e1–6.

10. Fan D, Li S, Wang W, et al. Sexual dysfunction and mode of delivery in Chinese primiparous women: a systematic review and meta-analysis. BMC Pregnancy Childbirth. 2017;17:408.
11. Hjorth S, Kirkegaard H, Olsen J, et al. Mode of birth and long-term sexual health: a follow-up study of mothers in the Danish National birth cohort. BMJ Open. 2019;9:e029517.
12. Johnson CE. Sexual health during pregnancy and the postpartum. J Sex Med. 2011;8:1266–7.
13. Ayers S, Bond R, Bertullies S, Wijma K. The aetiology of post-traumatic stress following childbirth: a meta-analysis and theoretical framework. Psychol Med. 2016;46:1121–34.
14. Skinner EM, Barnett B, Dietz HP. Psychological consequences of pelvic floor trauma following vaginal birth: a qualitative study from two Australian tertiary maternity units. Arch Womens Ment Health. 2018;21:341–51.
15. Crookall R, Fowler G, Wood C, Slade P. A systematic mixed studies review of women's experiences of perineal trauma sustained during childbirth. J Adv Nurs. 2018;74:2038–52.
16. Murphy H, Strong J. Just another ordinary bad birth? A narrative analysis of first time mothers' traumatic birth experiences. Health Care Women Int. 2018;39:619–43.
17. Hollander MH, van Hastenberg E, van Dillen J, et al. Preventing traumatic childbirth experiences: 2192 women's perceptions and views. Arch Womens Ment Health. 2017;20:515–23.
18. Inglis C, Sharman R, Reed R. Paternal mental health following perceived traumatic childbirth. Midwifery. 2016;41:125–31.
19. Daniels E, Arden-Close E, Mayers A. Be quiet and man up: a qualitative questionnaire study into fathers who witnessed their partner's birth trauma. BMC Pregnancy Childbirth. 2020;20:236.
20. Bohren MA, Mehrtash H, Fawole B, et al. How women are treated during facility-based childbirth in four countries: a cross-sectional study with labour observations and community-based surveys. Lancet. 2019;394:1750–63.

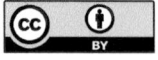

Sexual Aspects of Problems in the Postpartum and Early Parenthood (1st Year)

14

Deirdre O'Malley ⓘ, Valerie Smith ⓘ, and Agnes Higgins ⓘ

14.1 Introduction

The first year postpartum for new parents, whether first-time or non-first-time parents, may be complicated by many psychosocial issues, for example, challenges associated with transitioning and adapting to parenthood, the stress related to baby care, and changes to the couple's intimate relationship (see also Chap. 8). For some women, new physical and mental health morbidities can also occur, including leaking urine, faecal incontinence, pelvic girdle pain, anxiety, depression, and sexual health problems, which can negatively impact the woman's quality of life. In addition, pre-existing physical and mental health problems can be exacerbated during pregnancy or postpartum resulting in long-term sexual health problems, which may cause significant distress to women and couples during the first year postpartum.

14.2 Postpartum Sexual Health Problems

Postpartum sexual health problems can be diverse. Women experience a wide array of postpartum sexual health problems, including dyspareunia, lack of vaginal lubrication, difficulties with orgasm, and lack of sexual desire. Although these problems can self-resolve early in the postpartum period, health professionals (HCPs) must

D. O'Malley (✉)
Department of Nursing, Midwifery and Early Years, Dundalk Institute of Technology, Dundalk, Co Louth, Ireland
e-mail: deirdre.omalley@dkit.ie

V. Smith · A. Higgins
School of Nursing and Midwifery, University of Dublin, Trinity College, Dublin, Ireland

© The Author(s) 2023
S. Geuens et al. (eds.), *Midwifery and Sexuality*,
https://doi.org/10.1007/978-3-031-18432-1_14

address them. Many postpartum sexual health problems can persist a year or many years after birth causing women and their partners great distress and, in some cases, relationship breakdown. The prevalence of different sexual health problems 1 year after birth varies. For example, 9% of a sample of 832 nulliparous women reported vaginal looseness, whereas 40% of these women reported a loss of interest in sex [1]. Studies indeed indicate that women experience sexual health problems during the first year after birth. These may be new-onset, associated with underlying medical or mental health illness or exacerbated by birth and the postpartum period [2, 3]. Before we discuss these issues, it is important to realize that many studies apply the Female Sexual Function Index (FSFI) to measure the prevalence of sexual problems. Therefore, we will first pay some attention to the challenges and limitations of the studies that use the Female Sexual Function Index (FSFI) to measure prevalence.

14.3   The Complexities of Diagnoses of Postpartum Sexual Health Problems

Estimating the prevalence of postpartum sexual health problems is complex and challenging. Numerous papers and reports label postpartum women as sexually dysfunctional or having sexual health problems. They base that on the results of studies that utilize the FSFI scale. The FSFI measures sexual arousal, vaginal lubrication, achieving orgasm, dyspareunia, and sexual satisfaction [4], with lower scale scores (<26) used as markers of sexual dysfunction. Using the FSFI, however, is problematic for several reasons. The scale originated from the dated and disputed Master and Johnson's Sexual Response Cycle [5], that is now obsolete. Their response cycle described a linear model progressing through four phases: excitement, plateau, orgasm, and resolution, and it was fundamentally identical in men and women. Thus, it took no account of women's motivation for sex, sexual desire, relational dynamics, or emotional intimacy needs, all considered important to women's sexual response [6].

Since the FSFI scale was neither developed for postpartum sexual health nor validated with postpartum women, using the FSFI for this discrete population is questionable and problematic. Classifying women as being sexually dysfunctional on the FSFI results alone ignores the complexity of postpartum sexual well-being and the potential influence of the broader context of women's lives and relationships, including the impact that adapting to parenting roles, extreme tiredness, and concern over baby's well-being may have on sexual function and intimate relationships.

The subsections below examine some of the commonly experienced new-onset sexual health problems encountered in the first year after birth. We also look at common pre-existing conditions affecting sexual well-being after birth.

14.3.1 Persistent Dyspareunia

Many primiparous women experience dyspareunia in the initial months postpartum.[1] In many cases, it will resolve itself, or the couple can manage it with some simple strategies. However, there is evidence that some women may experience distressing and long-term dyspareunia that can negatively impact their quality of life and relationships with their partners. An Australian cohort study demonstrated that 28% (333/1184) of primiparous women continued to experience dyspareunia 12 months postpartum and 23% (261/1155) at 18 months. One in ten of the women with dyspareunia described the pain as '*distressing*', '*horrible*', or '*excruciating*' [7]. While it is difficult to identify risk factors for intense dyspareunia, McDonald and colleagues report that caesarean section birth was associated with intense pain 6 months after birth when they considered other maternal and obstetric factors [7]. However, the study did not report whether the caesarean section was an elective or emergency procedure. We believe that relevant since an emergency caesarean section and possible protracted labour might influence the association with the intense pain reported in McDonald's study. There is evidence that severe perineal trauma increases the likelihood of experiencing 'difficulty with coitus'. This difficulty was explained as a lack of sexual desire, pain at the vaginal orifice during penetration, and/or pain during deep penetration [8]. While it may be challenging to identify women who are at risk of developing intense dyspareunia, it is important that maternity HCPs provide woman and couple-centred support and advice for these women and their partners.

In the first instance, women need to be supported and encouraged to talk to their partner about their experience of pain, how it makes them feel, and how it affects their desire for sexual activity. We may advise the couple to try different sexual positions, lubricants, and alternative sexual activities. When these strategies have been unsuccessful, we recommend advising the couple to make an appointment with their general practitioner (GP) or gynaecologist. We suggest that the couple attends as the problem is a couple's issue, not solely a postpartum woman's issue.

The detailed assessment by the HCP should include information on pre-pregnancy sexual activity and sexual intercourse, mode of birth, traumatic birth, perineal trauma, infant feeding method, use of contraceptives, time of resumption after birth, and type of resumed sexual activities. The woman's age, the possibility of perimenopausal symptoms, and the side effects of prescribed medication contributing to the experience of pain need to be considered. The HCP should ask about the experience of pain, including whether it is a new-onset pain post-birth, where and when precisely the pain is felt, for example, on penile entry, during deep penetration or both, and whether the pain is superficial and isolated to the vulva or vaginal entrance or felt in a particular area of the vagina only. The woman should describe any sensation associated with the pain, for example, feelings of spasm, burning, tightness, or friction. Vaginal and urinary tract infections will need to be ruled out as causative factors of pain. Especially in intense dyspareunia, psychosocial issues,

---

[1] For a more in-depth look, see Chap. 8.

such as relationship problems, mental health issues, drug and alcohol misuse and current or past physical, emotional or sexual trauma, need to be addressed. The HCP has to perform such a thorough assessment sensitively, aware of the potential for embarrassment and couple distress. Likely, the woman's partner may also be experiencing distress at the notion that he may be causing his partner to experience intense pain during vaginal penetration. Thus, a good strategy is asking for permission to talk about this sensitive topic, starting with the least sensitive questions and progressively moving to more sensitive areas of inquiry, meanwhile explaining the rationale for each question (see Chap. 26 on 'talking sexuality'). Recognizing the need for help and making an appointment to see their HCP are significant steps for many couples. Still, the HCP needs to remain cognisant of the sensitive nature of the conversation by using language that the couple understands, explaining professional terms, and avoiding euphemisms, such as 'down below' when referring to the vagina or penis.

Depending on the findings from the assessment and the available services, the HCP may advise the couple to attend a women's health physiotherapist or pelvic floor therapist. They can teach strategies to ease sensations of tightness and spasms, such as how to stretch pelvic floor muscles. Some couples need a referral to a clinical sexologist or sex therapist may be warranted for couples who require support to discuss and resolve possible underlying relationship issues, traumatic birth experiences, or past trauma. See details in Chap. 29. A psychosexual therapist may educate the couple on how sex therapy works, relaxation therapy and hypnotherapy as tools to help in instances of sexual pain problems or vaginismus. Psychosexual therapy may include developing a programme with the couple involving progressive touching, kissing, and exploring each other's bodies but avoiding vaginal penetration.

Some women/couples need a referral to a gynaecologist to investigate the physical source of the pain. For example, persisting pain after the repair of a severe perineal tear may need close examination under general anaesthetic (GA) and maybe minor surgery to repair scar tissue. Some women have found relief from using a local anaesthetic during penetration, such as lignocaine, when pain is localized and accessible. We should adapt any referral or strategy to the couple's needs and be assured they agree.

14.4   Adapting to Parenthood

In much of the discussion on sexual well-being after birth, we identify that the relationship between the couple is paramount: a relationship of trust, which facilitates vulnerability and is characterized by good communication. However, the stress associated with adapting to parenthood can cause conflict in a relationship. Adapting to parenthood has been described as a serious drain on couples' emotional, physical, and material resources [9], which ultimately can result in relationship breakdown. In their 8-year follow-up study of new parents, Hansson and Ahlborg [10] determined that a couple's sensual and sexual satisfaction levels decreased in the first 4 years after birth and had not returned to early postpartum levels 8 years after the birth of the first child. It is likely that couples need support and help to adapt to parenthood while maintaining a satisfying intimate and sexual relationship. This help might take the form of preparing for potential changes to sexual well-being commonly experienced, as outlined in Chap. 8. Strategies to support maintaining sexual well-being in the long term might include planning time alone as a couple away from family and home, scheduling time for intimate touch and sex if they wish, expanding their sexual repertoire beyond penetrative sex, opening a dialogue on sex, communicating other needs, such as support with childcare, household chores, or financial strains. Psychosexual therapy and couple therapy might also be an option for some couples.

14.5   Pre-Existing and Perinatal Mental Health Issues

Some women who become pregnant and give birth have underlying or pre-existing mental health conditions. While it is not within the scope of this chapter to review how all these conditions impact postpartum sexual well-being, it would be remiss not to address some of the more common mental health conditions in maternity care, namely, depression, anxiety, and post-traumatic stress disorder. Chapters 17 and 18 address, in detail, several pre-existing medical and mental health conditions and how they may impact sexual well-being.

14.5.1 Postnatal Depression

Postnatal depression (PND) is estimated to affect 10–15% of women in the months after birth. Symptoms may vary from poor appetite (or comfort eating), guilt or negative thoughts, inability to enjoy things, difficulty looking after the baby and self, to feeling that life is not worth living. Depression (in general) and PND are associated with sexual health problems. In PND, the symptoms of mood disorders such as low self-esteem, feelings of helplessness, and fatigue negatively impact women's sexual well-being. Furthermore, many antidepressants can cause or exacerbate existing sexual health problems.[2] Between 50–70% of people with depression and antidepressants experience iatrogenic sexual dysfunction such as low sex drive, arousal, and orgasm [11]. The most commonly reported adverse sexual effects in women taking antidepressants are problems with sexual desire (72%), sexual arousal (83%), and orgasm (42%) [12]. Yet, the relevant HCPs neither tell women how depression can impact their sexual well-being, nor that prescribed antidepressant medication can impair their sexual function.

  Chapter 8 mentioned that women in same-sex couples are absent from the discussions on postpartum sexual well-being. This is also the case in the literature on

---

[2] For more information on the impact of antidepressants on sexual functioning, see Chap. 19.

mood disorders and women in same-sex relationships, even though depression appears more prevalent in same-sex couples than in opposite-sex couples [13].

A multidisciplinary team approach to caring for a woman experiencing PND is important. Care and treatment plans should take a holistic view of the woman, her family life, her working life, her support systems, and her relationship with her partner. Strategies to manage the sexual problems associated with PND may include behavioural approaches (exercising before sexual activity, scheduling sexual activity, vibratory stimulation, psychotherapy), complementary and integrative therapies (acupuncture, nutraceuticals), or a combination of these modalities. If sexual dysfunction associated with antidepressant medication is an issue, strategies may involve dose reduction, drug discontinuation or switching, augmentation, or using medicines with lower adverse effect profiles. Sexual well-being is an essential aspect of a couple's intimate relationship. Sexual well-being between couples enables a unique closeness and vulnerability within the couple-dyad that is not shared by anyone else.

For some women with depression, sex is the only domain of their life that is less or not affected by their depression. That reality can be helpful as a wellbeing-anchor or even a tool for looking at depression.

14.5.2 Postnatal Anxiety

The literature on postnatal anxiety appears less conclusive, with discrete prevalence rates difficult to source because anxiety frequently merges with PND in discussions on mental health after birth. Nonetheless, a systematic review and meta-analysis (102 studies, $N = 221,974$ women) demonstrated that 15% of women had self-reported anxiety symptoms 6 months after childbirth, and 9% had a clinical diagnosis of any anxiety disorder [14]. Postnatal anxiety symptoms include constant or near-constant feelings of nervousness or panic, persistent worries about self, baby or relationship, and being prone to panic attacks. Self-confidence, self-esteem, perception of body image, feelings of sexual desire, and arousal may all be negatively impacted. The experience of postnatal anxiety and sexual problems can become a cyclical response. Feelings of anxiety may lead to worsening vaginismus and dyspareunia due to muscle tension. This can aggravate feelings of stress, isolation, and worry about self and relationship. Managing anxiety is a priority, but we should as well address the woman's concerns and symptoms. Among the possible tools to manage anxiety are medication, psychotherapy, and mindfulness. The last two are valuable strategies to deal with anxiety-related sexual health problems. Additionally, communication within the couple, planning alone time as a couple, exploring what activities give pleasure without the pressure of sexual activities experienced as threatening. Issues around body image and self-esteem may need exploration by a psychotherapist.

When the couple feels ready, they can try to redevelop via prolonged foreplay, sex toys, lubricants, masturbation, oral sex, et cetera, and a gradual build-up towards penetrative sex.

14.5.3 Post-Traumatic Stress Disorder and Birth Trauma

A traumatic birth experience or birth trauma can have a lasting impact on a woman and her entire family. Birth trauma might result from an obstetric emergency, an instrumental birth, emergency caesarean section, or long, painful labour. Equally, factors not associated with 'clinical' issues per se can also be causal, including feeling ignored or not being listened to by caregivers during birth or feeling powerless and a sense of loss of control. The impact of birth trauma can result in post-traumatic stress disorder (PTSD). Estimates of clinically diagnosed PTSD following childbirth range from 5.6% to 9%. However, the rate of women with post-traumatic stress symptoms but not meeting the complete PTSD diagnosis is 18% [15]. Women with PTSD are sometimes misdiagnosed as depressed or anxious, although these can present as co-morbidities. Symptoms of birth trauma can be severe and vary from feelings of anxiety, panic, and fear to nightmares and flashbacks, triggered by smells, images, and sounds, resulting in reliving the traumatic experience. Some women describe difficulty coping and bonding with their baby, and some experience feelings of guilt, shame, and worthlessness. Notwithstanding the personal distress women with birth trauma experience, there is also evidence that explores the impact of birth trauma on a couple's relationship. Women have described their relationship with their partners as being '*shattered*' [16]. A Norwegian cohort study ($N = 1,480$) showed poor relationship satisfaction in women with postpartum PTSD at 2 years after birth [17]. In postpartum PTSD, sexual relationships are frequently affected, with loss of intimacy and reduced sexual activity. Women reported having flashbacks when initiating sex or avoiding sexual intercourse due to fear of becoming pregnant and going through childbirth again [18]. Much of the advice and support offered to women, in this case, is similar to what we have described earlier: communicating fear and worries with their partner, planning intimacy, extended foreplay, and agreeing where touch is welcome on the body, birth debriefing, psychotherapy, and survivor support groups.

14.5.4 Past Sexual Trauma

Global estimates vary, but approximately one in five women experience some form of sexual trauma/violence from 16 years. Sexual trauma or sexual abuse is sexual contact or behaviour that occurs without the explicit consent of the victim. It may range from attempted rape, unwanted sexual touching, forcing a victim to perform sexual acts, such as oral sex or penetrating the perpetrator's body or penetration of the victim's body, also known as rape in many countries.

Estimates of the incidence of rape are difficult to obtain. The proportion of women who reported rape lies between 8% and 12% in Western countries. International trends demonstrate an annual increase in reported cases. With most sexual abuse in women occurring before age 24, many of these women will have pregnancies and birth experiences that will be influenced by that sexual trauma. Postpartum care practices, such as examining the perineum and breasts, exposing their body to the gaze of others, and triggering language, for example 'lie still', are issues that women who have experienced sexual trauma have identified as being challenging for them and potential triggers to flashbacks of trauma. For some women, breastfeeding may be rife with triggers. For others, it can become a healing process. Since many of these issues can potentially re-traumatize the woman, we must provide sensitive, individualized, trauma-informed care. More on this issue can be found in Chap. 24.

It is important to consider women who got pregnant due to rape and how we should support these women in adjusting to motherhood and baby care. The juxtaposition of emotions is complex and unique to each woman. Depending on the legislation in their country, an abortion may not be an option. Then, the woman may feel further trapped and traumatized by continuing the pregnancy and birthing the baby. They may choose not to care and hand the baby in for adoption. Women may disclose or not disclose reasons for putting their baby up for adoption. HCPs should, either way, provide non-judgemental care supporting women in the choices they make.

On the other hand, some women may decide to continue with the pregnancy, believing that something positive and life-affirming can come from the trauma. Though the woman actively decided to continue the pregnancy, the childbirth may re-traumatize and impose a visual reminder of the past sexual abuse. A baby boy may be significant to the woman, with physical features that remind the woman of the perpetrator. We recommend HCPs ask about infant feeding choices and about support with baby care. We should explain to the mother that attachment between mother and child can be a complex and rewarding process for all women, irrespective of how conception occured. The woman may wish to speak to whoever has supported her in her recovery from the sexual abuse, family, friend, therapist, or support group facilitator. We must respect her wishes, document them, and communicate them to all care-team members.

14.5.4.1   Interventions to Support Women and Partners

It sometimes takes months or even years to recover from PTSD, birth trauma, and sexual trauma. Women might need the support of specialist professionals, which would likely include birth debriefing, psychotherapy, and survivor support groups. Women may experience PTSD, depression, and anxiety due to the trauma. Maternity care providers must recognize their limitations in supporting these women and know the referral pathways available in their maternity services. Maternity care providers must ensure that women are not lost in these pathways by following up on any referrals made via phone calls or confirmatory emails and incorporating trauma-informed care in each woman's pregnancy and birth journey.

14.6   Addressing Diversity

Women in same-sex relationships, single women, young women, women with multiple partners, and women from smaller cultural communities (e.g. Roma community) are absent from the literature and discussions on postpartum sexual well-being. While some of the discussion in Chap. 8 on everyday postpartum sexual well-being might well apply to these groups of women, we cannot state this with confidence about problematic postpartum situations. The nuances of these women's intimate relationships and their relationship priorities during the first year postpartum may differ from the standard population participating in research on sexual health after birth. Study samples tend to be heterosexual, in long-term relationships, over 30 years, and well educated to a degree level or above. To ensure inclusive and truly woman-centred care, there is an urgent need to develop strategies that include these women groups in research.

Key Points of Note from the Chapter
- Many women experience sexual health problems in the months and years after birth.
- There is difficulty in interpreting prevalence rates of postpartum sexual health problems due to the overreliance on FSFI, a partially obsolete measurement tool.
- One-fifth of women continue to self-report dyspareunia 12–18 months after birth, with 10% of them describing their pain as *'distressing'*, *'horrible'*, or *'excruciating'*.
- Identifying risk factors for persistent dyspareunia is difficult, but severe perineal trauma may be a risk factor.
- If different sexual positions, lubricants, and alternative sexual activities do not resolve persistent dyspareunia, the couple deserves referral to a sexuality-positive GP for a detailed assessment and management plan.
- Additional referral may be needed to a psychosexual therapist, women's health physiotherapist, or a gynaecologist.
- Some parents struggle to adapt to parenthood. If left unattended, this has the potential to cause a broken relationship.
- Postnatal depression and the medications used to treat postnatal depression can complicate postnatal sexual health problems.
- Postnatal anxiety and the complexity of symptoms experienced by women can lead to a cyclical response whereby sexual pain problems worsen, and women's anxiety increases.
- Women with PTSD and birth trauma may experience co-morbidities of depression and anxiety. The trauma experience can harm the couple's relationship and sexual relationship.
- One in five women globally experiences some form of sexual violence.

- In a woman with past trauma, aspects of postpartum care, body exposure, and inappropriate language can re-traumatize her.
- When the pregnancy resulted from rape, the woman deserves extra attention regarding attachment to the baby.
- Maternity care providers must recognize their limitations in supporting women with PTSD, birth trauma, and past sexual abuse. They need to be familiar with their local services and available referral pathways.
- Women in same-sex relationships, single women, young women, women with multiple partners, and women from smaller cultural communities are all absent from the literature and discussions on postpartum sexual health problems.

References

1. O'Malley D, Higgins A, Begley C, Daly D, Smith V. Prevalence of and risk factors associated with sexual health issues in primiparous women at 6 and 12 months postpartum; a longitudinal prospective cohort study (the MAMMI study). BMC Pregnancy Childbirth. 2018;18:196.
2. Lipschuetz M, Cohen SM, Liebergall-Wischnitzer M. Degree of bother from pelvic floor dysfunction in women one year after first delivery. Eur J Obstet Gynecol Reprod Biol. 2015;191:90–4.
3. Galbally M, Watson SJ, Permezel M, Lewis AJ. Depression across pregnancy and the postpartum, antidepressant use and the association with female sexual function. Psychol Med. 2019;49:1490–9.
4. Rosen R, Brown C, Heiman J, et al. The female sexual function index (FSFI): a multidimensional self-report instrument for the assessment of female sexual function. J Sex Marital Ther. 2000;26:191–208.
5. Masters W, Johnson V. Human sexual response. New York: Little Brown; 1966.
6. Basson R. Are our definitions of women's desire, arousal and sexual pain disorders too broad and our definition of orgasmic disorder too narrow? J Sex Marital Ther. 2002;28:289–300.
7. McDonald EA, Gartland D, Small R, Brown SJ. Frequency, severity and persistence of postnatal dyspareunia to 18 months post partum: a cohort study. Midwifery. 2016;34:15–20.
8. Fodstad K, Staff AC, Laine K. Sexual activity and dyspareunia the first year postpartum in relation to degree of perineal trauma. Int Urogynecol J. 2016;27:1513–23.
9. Pacey S. Couples and the first baby: responding to new parents' sexual and relationship problems. Sex Relationship Ther. 2004;19:223–46.
10. Hansson M, Ahlborg T. Quality of the intimate and sexual relationship in first-time parents—a longitudinal study. Sex Reprod Healthc. 2012;3:21–9.
11. Rothmore J. Antidepressant-induced sexual dysfunction. Med J Aust. 2020;212:329–34.
12. Lorenz T, Rullo J, Faubion S. Antidepressant-induced female sexual dysfunction. Mayo Clin Proc. 2016;91:1280–6.
13. Pakula B, Shoveller JA. Sexual orientation and self-reported mood disorder diagnosis among Canadian adults. BMC Public Health. 2013;13:209.
14. Dennis CL, Falah-Hassani K, Shiri R. Prevalence of antenatal and postnatal anxiety: systematic review and meta-analysis. Br J Psychiatry. 2017;210:315–23.
15. Beck CT, Gable RK, Sakala C, Declercq ER. Posttraumatic stress disorder in new mothers: results from a two-stage U.S. national survey. Birth. 2011;38:216–27.

16. Fenech G, Thomson G. Tormented by ghosts from their past': a meta-synthesis to explore the psychosocial implications of a traumatic birth on maternal well-being. Midwifery. 2014;30:185–93.
17. Garthus-Niegel S, Horsch A, Handtke E, et al. The impact of postpartum posttraumatic stress and depression symptoms on Couples' relationship satisfaction: a population-based prospective study. Front Psychol. 2018;9:1728.
18. Delicate A. The trauma between us. AIMS. 2019;30(4).

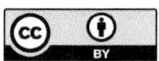

Sexual Aspects of Problematic Lactation

15

Dilek Uslu ⓘ and Serena Debonnet

15.1 Introduction

Whereas Chap. 9 addressed various sexual aspects of the healthy breast and successful breastfeeding, this chapter will deal with the more challenging and problematic situations.

The relationship with sexuality is 'the Red Thread' throughout this chapter.

It will start with the situation when breastfeeding does not develop properly because of challenges experienced by many women, including pain. After that, we will highlight conditions where breastfeeding cannot or should not develop. We will then address situations where for various medical reasons, breastfeeding can be troublesome. Finally, we will focus on the more complex emotional connections interfering with breastfeeding, including depression and past traumatic experiences. We will devote a small part to lactation induction in the non-birthing woman, a possibility for a lactation stand-in when the mother cannot nurse or the co-mother in a lesbian relationship who opts for co-nursing. For more insight, we start with a short intermezzo about endocrinology and its implications.

The original version of the chapter has been revised. A correction to this chapter can be found at
https://doi.org/10.1007/978-3-031-18432-1_31

D. Uslu (✉)
Doctor's Center, Nisantasi, Istanbul, Turkey

S. Debonnet
Federal Public Service: Public Health, Brussels, Belgium

© The Author(s) 2023, corrected publication 2024
S. Geuens et al. (eds.), *Midwifery and Sexuality*,
https://doi.org/10.1007/978-3-031-18432-1_15

15.2   Endocrinological Aspects of Breastfeeding

During full breastfeeding, female sexual function is under the influence of hyper-prolactinemia, which is necessary to maintain milk production. The high prolactin levels cause a generalized suppression of ovarian functioning with a decrease in oestrogen levels (hypo-estrogenism) and testosterone levels.

The physiological hypo-estrogenism causes a situation comparable to menopause with high vaginal pH, increased parabasal and intermediate cells, and decreased superficial cells. Next to these atrophic changes, there is also a decrease in genital vasocongestion and dry vaginal mucosa.

The lowered testosterone levels cause fatigue, reduced mood, low sexual desire, and decreased arousability. The combination of these endocrinological factors can negatively affect the woman's sexual life and satisfaction, independent of additional factors like perineal trauma, motherhood's responsibilities, and childcare demands. Many other factors influence the resumption of sexuality and how sexuality and intimacy will redevelop. While some new mothers feel a loss of femininity by stretch marks and weight gain, others shine through motherhood. Breastfeeding itself is also experienced differently. For some as a very tiresome task; for others, it is close to experiencing sheer happiness. And last but not least, the sexual needs of the partner will influence when and how postpartum sexuality will get shaped.

15.3   When Breastfeeding Does Not Develop Properly for 'Normal' Reasons, Including Pain

15.3.1 Pain During Breastfeeding

During the first year of the life of their infants, about 50% of breastfeeding mothers have reported breastfeeding pain. The most common causes of breastfeeding pain include nipple pain, mastitis, candida infection, engorgement, and clogged milk ducts.

The incidence of each cause may vary from study to study in relation to the mother's and the infant's risk factors. Persistent nipple pain is one of the reasons for consultation in around 40% of cases due to incorrect positioning, infection, palatal anomaly, flat or inverted nipples, tongue tie, mastitis, and vasospasm [1]. Infectious skin disorders of the breasts can also cause physical discomfort, poor quality of life, and sexual problems for nursing mothers. It is important to diagnose them at an early stage. Pain is a relevant factor to decrease sexual desire and pleasure and, when experienced for a more extended period, can influence the couple's relationship.

15.3.2 Mastitis

Mastitis is an inflammation of the breast, sometimes related and sometimes not to a bacterial infection. The clinical findings show up as wedge-shaped, hot, swollen, and tender areas of the breast with a temperature over 38 °C. Prospective studies estimate the incidence of mastitis in breastfeeding from 3% to 20%. Main factors related to mastitis include a history of mastitis, university education, blocked duct, and cracked nipples. The majority of cases appear during the first 6 weeks postpartum.

Good healthcare support will identify lactation mastitis early and make a full recovery possible. In general, the healing does not involve medical intervention and can be resolved by self-management through feeding, cold compresses for soothing, and massaging the affected breast area. Nonetheless, some cases may require antibiotic treatment. If under-treated, it can result in a breast abscess and may cause hospitalization and surgery. For the woman with mastitis, the sexual consequences will depend on how much the breasts are part of her erotic identity, and for both partners, it will depend on how much the breasts were an integrated part of initiating sexual contact and lovemaking.

15.3.3 Candida Infection

Candida infection (also known as thrush) is a fungal infection that also can develop on the breast and the nipples. It manifests clinically by stabbing and radiating pain through the breast tissue. White patches in the baby's oral cavity and a white coating on the tongue are diagnostic signs. Maternal risk factors are recent antibiotic use and recurrent yeast infections. It is found more after vaginal candida and vaginal birth. The treatment of Candida mastitis involves topical antifungal application on the nipples after each breastfeeding session.

In recurrent candida infection of the nipple/breast, it is wise to consider candida transfer from the vulva to the nipples, either via the woman's masturbating fingers or via the partner's tongue.

15.3.4 Psychological Stress Associated with Breastfeeding Pain

Postpartum, there can be close encounters between breastfeeding and psychological stress. Mothers who were not depressed during pregnancy and intended to breastfeed have lower risks of depression postpartum. However, mothers who had that intention but did not succeed have a higher risk for depression. Therefore, conditions causing substantial breastfeeding pain and causing early weaning might increase the chances of postpartum depression and stress.

Providing specialized support to young mothers largely diminishes that risk [2].

Another factor affecting breastfeeding cessation is the mode of birth. After emergency or planned Caesarean section, women delay the initiation of breastfeeding and are less likely to breastfeed. Those deliveries influence, in some way, the physiology of lactogenesis resulting in more lactation difficulties. Research indicated the surgery-related decreased oxytocin secretion and increased maternal stress as factors disrupting the hormonal pathway for lactogenesis [3].

Breastfeeding is important for the infant's health and is also a way for the mother to bond with her baby. So HCPs must be aware of the effect of early cessation of breastfeeding on the sexuality of the mother. Besides causing stress, involuntary early cessation has a higher risk for mastitis and pain.

In addition to parenting duties, having pain might cause a decrease in sexual desire and the quality of life and cause difficulties in concentrating on sexuality and self-esteem. Although there are barely any studies on breastfeeding disturbances and sexuality, we may say that it is paramount to prevent these conditions and, if they do arise, to treat them appropriately.

15.4   When Breastfeeding Cannot Develop or Should Not Develop

15.4.1 Sheehan Syndrome

Sheehan syndrome is a hormonal disturbance that develops when massive blood loss during childbirth causes shallow oxygen levels and necrosis in the anterior pituitary gland, later resulting in low levels of various hormones, including gonadal hormones. Among the consequences are no or poor development of breastfeeding and low androgen levels needed for energy and sexual desire. The psychotraumatic impact of such a sudden life-threatening experience will probably influence both partners and their sexuality. Nowadays, this Sheehan syndrome relatively seldom happens in more affluent medical care.

15.4.2 When Breastfeeding Is (Nearly) Impossible or Contraindicated

Lactation can be impossible when severe trauma or burns have damaged the breasts and sometimes after cosmetic breast surgery.

Breastfeeding can also be contraindicated. The mother needs, for instance, a treatment necessary for her health (e.g. chemotherapy) but dangerous for the baby because being passed into breastmilk. Or the mother has a high viral load (with HIV, HTLV-1, or cytomegalovirus) that reach the baby via breast milk.

Those situations can ask for pharmacological suppression with cabergoline or bromocriptine. These dopaminergic drugs are also in use for patients with pituitary failure, where they are known sometimes to cause a substantial increase in sexual desire ('hypersexual side effects').

A study comparing oral cabergoline (1× 1 mg) and oral bromocriptine (2× daily 2.5 mg for 14 days) for lactation suppression did not mention sexual side effects [4].

For some women, not being able or 'not being allowed' to breastfeed their baby can mean a real blow to her 'maternal identity' or her 'female identity', thus potentially diminishing her sexual identity. Whereas for other women, that will have far less emotional and sexual consequences.

15.5 Relevant Aspects of Breastfeeding Related to Some Medical Conditions

Chapter 18 will address various medical conditions that indirectly influence breast-feeding and sexuality. This paragraph will focus on three conditions with a more direct influence: spinal cord injury, multiple sclerosis, and breast eczema, followed by some relevant consequences of breast surgery.

15.5.1 Spinal Cord Injury (SCI)

Although women with SCI experience many sexual difficulties, there usually is no problem becoming pregnant. For these mothers, breastfeeding is more than average essential to develop an optimal bonding with the baby. But lactation goes accompanied by several difficulties.[1]

One of the complexities is breastfeeding positioning [5].

People with an SCI have lower systolic blood pressure. Knowing that breast-feeding is accompanied by lowered blood pressure and heart rate, SCI women who breastfeed (and their HCPs) should be aware of developing low blood pressure and orthostatic hypotension. Women with a cervical or high thoracic level lesion deserve extra attention. During breastfeeding (or breast engorgement), they can face autonomous dysreflexia (with very high, dangerous systolic blood pressure) [5].

Another primary factor in women with an SCI is a non-functional let-down reflex essential for providing milk to a nursing infant. The infant's suckling activates tactile receptors on the breast. Via sensory nerves and the T4–6 posterior root centres in the spinal cord, the signal goes to hypothalamic neurons, which release oxytocin to the bloodstream. That oxytocin release is required for milk ejection. In women with SCI above T4, the first step of this pathway is absent, meaning that the tactile receptors are not activated. Thus, the let-down reflex is not present. In women with SCI between T4 and T6, the reflex is reduced [6].

With a complete SCI above T4, the woman will have no tactile sensation in the breasts nor any other lower part of the body. That should not be a reason for the partner to abstain from playing with breasts and nipples and everywhere else. Whereas that might not serve as direct neurological stimulation, the woman can experience such loving touch as an indication of still being attractive, and even it can arouse her into feeling a tactile sensation, a process called sensory integration.

---

[1] Extra care information via 'Bring Home Baby' project. http://sci-pregnancy.org/pamphlets/Bringinghomebaby.pdf

15.5.2 Multiple Sclerosis (MS)

In MS patients, sexuality and sexual relationship are affected in multiple ways. The brain damage, the lesions in the sexuality-orchestrating centres in the spinal cord, and the peripheral neuropathy can directly damage sexual function. In addition, spasticity, fatigue, lethargy, urinary, and sometimes faecal incontinence are major symptoms interfering with sexual well-being.

MS causes many sexual worries about 'being a good lover', performance anxiety, and also insecurity because she can never be sure how her body will react this time during the sexual encounter.

When pregnant, the woman may not use the most current MS medication. However, relapses are significantly reduced during pregnancy, especially in the last 3 months, because of higher levels of oestrogen and progesterone in the cerebrospinal fluid. So above-mentioned sexual insecurity and distraction can diminish.

Since postpartum gonadal steroids go down, relapses are common, making disease-modifying medication recommended after childbirth. That, however, passes into breastfeeding. Gradually, it is becoming clear that (especially exclusive) breastfeeding is protective against postpartum MS relapses [7].

15.5.3 Eczema

We define the clinical presentation of several types of dermatitis eczema. Eczema in breastfeeding patients presents itself mainly on the areola, occasionally extending to the breast, with the nipple much less affected. Patients with these eczema lesions describe them as pruritic, painful, or burning [8]. Identifying a maternal history of eczema, atopic, and allergic dermatitis can prevent eczema cases in breastfeeding mothers.

For treatment, we use topical corticosteroids and antibiotics [8]. To prevent endocrine disturbances in the nursling, the woman should breastfeed the baby before applying the corticosteroids. Remember that neither the woman nor her partner should develop an aversion to the breast. Some couples prevent this when the partner applies the ointment while gently massaging the breast. Regarding other skin diseases, there is minimal scientific data on the various associations between eczema, hidradenitis suppurativa, prurigo, blistering disorders, psoriasis, urticaria, skin infections, and pruritus with sexual health, although the impact on sexual difficulties seems relatively high.

15.5.4 After Breast Surgery

Most breast surgery concerns aesthetic breast implant augmentation, the number one popular plastic surgery worldwide. Reports show that breast augmentation surgery can improve women's sexual satisfaction and self-confidence by 80%. Since many women undergo these operations relatively young, many will bear childbirth later. A meta-analysis of studies showed that fewer women reach exclusive breastfeeding after this surgery [9]. Thus, when women want to proceed with this, the plastic surgery team should fully inform women of the negative influence of the operation on breastfeeding. Surgery can damage glandular tissue and the innervation of the breasts. The pressure made by implants on breast tissue may also affect lactation by damaging the breast tissue or blocking lactiferous ducts [10]. The authors remark that the lower breastfeeding rate after implants should not be a contraindication for aesthetic surgery but rather a stimulus for good breastfeeding counselling.

Although many studies deal with women's sexuality after breast augmentation surgery, they do not target women with actual breastfeeding difficulties. Future research will lighten the effects of implants on lactation and sexual dysfunctions.

In breast reduction surgery, the surgical technique is essential. Preservation of the column of subareolar parenchyma does not impair lactation [11].

Unilateral mastectomy (e.g. for breast cancer) is no reason not to breastfeed since one breast can perfectly supply enough milk.[2]

15.6   Emotional Connections Interfering with Breastfeeding

15.6.1 Depression and Breastfeeding

Breastfeeding may mediate the association between pregnancy and postpartum depression (PPD). A systematic review of several studies showed that postpartum depression predicts and is predicted by breastfeeding cessation [12]. Both pregnancy depression and postpartum depression are associated with shorter breastfeeding duration.

The estimated effect of breastfeeding on PPD differed according to whether women had planned to breastfeed their babies and whether they had shown signs of depression during pregnancy. For mothers who were not depressed during pregnancy, the ones who had planned to breastfeed, and who had actually breastfed had the lowest risk of PPD. Those who had planned to breastfeed but without continuation had the highest PPD chance [13]. Several studies report that women who are not breastfeeding are more likely to have depressive symptoms than breastfeeding women. A longitudinal Japanese study found that at 5 months postpartum, breastfeeding mothers had fewer signs of PPD compared to women who were formula-feeding ($p = 0.04$) [14].

That seems at odds with the information from the beginning of this chapter about lactation-related low oestrogen levels causing an atrophic vagina and low testosterone levels causing fatigue, lowered mood, less sexual desire, and less arousability. The likelihood that lactation-related dyspareunia and decreased sexuality contribute to the development of depression is apparently counterbalanced by other factors like the joy of parenthood and the bonding with the baby.

For the sexual consequences of depression and antidepressant medication, see Chap. 17.

---

[2] See http://sci-pregnancy.org/pamphlets/Bringinghomebaby.pdf

15.6.2 Dysphoric Milk Ejection

Dysphoric milk ejection reflex (D-MER) is a relatively new phenomenon, described as an overwhelming flow of negative emotions during breastfeeding that corresponds precisely to the milk ejection. Some researchers find it common among breastfeeding mothers [15].

It occurs just before the milk is released and continues for a few minutes. A drop in the dopamine level and the release of oxytocin during the let-down is one of the explanations [15]. But many other elements seem to play a role, including hormonal, psychological, and neurobiological mechanisms. Due to the modern media, the sexualization of the female breasts influences the thoughts and fantasies about breastfeeding with a wide range of emotions between mystification of the nursing mother, high levels of modesty, and embarrassment about the carnal aspects (with self-objectification and 'reproductive shame'), all influencing both the willingness to breastfeed, the success of it, and sexuality. In other words, D-MER is a bio-psycho-socio-cultural phenomenon needing a BPSC-approach and BPSC-aware research. That research should also include attention to the influence of D-MER on sexuality.

15.6.3 Past Traumatic Experiences

Child sexual abuse (CSA), with or without physical and emotional abuse, can have many consequences for the woman's sexual life and her sense of safety and integrity. In various ways, it can also influence breastfeeding. A US representative sample on breastfeeding compared women with and women without CSA. With CSA, women were more than twice likely to initiate breastfeeding [16]. The authors' explanation for this somewhat surprising finding is that these women appear to be more attentive to good parenting. The breastfeeding experience boosts the sense of having value for some women and it can be a discovery (or rediscovery) of sensuality.

Other women cannot handle the physical connection with the baby. Breastfeeding, requiring an intimate touch between the mother's breast and the baby's mouth, might feel uncomfortable. Some mothers indeed experience the sucking baby nearly as a sexual aggressor.

Narratives indicate that a few women do not want to breastfeed because their breasts have become a no-go zone, having been part of the abuse.

In women with CSA, unintended pregnancies or a low socioeconomic situation may also decrease the likelihood of breastfeeding.

15.7   Induced Lactation in Another Woman

In some situations, the need arises for a woman to breastfeed a baby she is not carrying. Examples of such lactation stand-in are as follows: when adopting a newborn baby; when the mother died; when the mother is under chemotherapy treatment or too weak; or when another woman carried the pregnancy. In the ideal situation, a protocol (e.g. the Newman-Goldfarb protocol)[3] should start already 6 months before expected childbirth with combined oral contraceptives and domperidone, a peripheral dopamine antagonist. In the last 6 weeks, that should change to domperidone combined with breast stimulation and pumping the breast. The milk quality is just as good as the milk on the normal tenth postpartum day. Only a minority of women will be able to produce all the milk the baby will need. However, it will facilitate emotional bonding with the child and transmit extra protection from antibodies, other proteins, and immune cells with the milk.

The domperidone will increase the prolactin level, potentially diminishing sexual desire. However, the lactation stand-in woman will not suffer from vaginal atrophy and low testosterone levels, the common reasons for dyspareunia in postpartum women.

Induced lactation in a newer form is becoming common in lesbian relationships when the co-mother wants to co-nurse the baby. For more details on lesbian motherhood, see Chap. 21.

15.8   Conclusions

Pregnancy comes with many changes affecting the physical health and well-being of mothers. When a mother has planned to breastfeed but is unable because of illness and pain, many consequences will affect the mother–infant dyad, the mother and her sexuality, and the woman–partner dyad, including their mutual sexuality.

Disordered sexual function postpartum is highly affected by the lack of appropriate sexual health counselling in prenatal and postnatal care. Better qualified professionals can help maintain or improve the sexual life of breastfeeding mothers by guiding them through topics such as lubrication and breastfeeding periods. Furthermore, during months of lactation, professional guidance of the woman and her sexual partner can help readjust their sexual relations.

References

1. Kent JC, Ashton E, Hardwick CM, et al. Nipple pain in breastfeeding mothers: incidence, causes and treatments. Int J Environ Res Public Health. 2015;12:12247–63.
2. Borra C, Iacovou M, Sevilla A. New evidence on breastfeeding and postpartum depression: the importance of understanding women's intentions. Matern Child Health J. 2015;19:897–907.
3. Evans KC, Evans RG, Royal R, et al. Effect of caesarean section on breast milk transfer to the normal term newborn over the first week of life. Arch Dis Child Fetal Neonatal Ed. 2003;88:F380–2.

[3] A good example is: http://www.canadianbreastfeedingfoundation.org/induced/regular_protocol.shtml

4. Single dose cabergoline versus bromocriptine in inhibition of puerperal lactation: randomised, double blind, multicentre study. European Multicentre Study Group for Cabergoline in lactation inhibition. BMJ. 1991;302(6789):1367–71.
5. Holmgren T, Lee AHX, et al. The influence of spinal cord injury on breastfeeding ability and behavior. J Hum Lact. 2018;34:556–65.
6. Cowley KC. Psychogenic and pharmacologic induction of the let-down reflex can facilitate breastfeeding by tetraplegic women: a report of 3 cases. Arch Phys Med Rehabil. 2005;86:1261–4.
7. Krysko KM, Rutatangwa A, Graves J, et al. Association between breastfeeding and postpartum multiple sclerosis relapses: a systematic review and meta-analysis. JAMA Neurol. 2020;77:327–38.
8. Barankin B, Gross MS. Nipple and areolar eczema in the breastfeeding woman. J Cutan Med Surg. 2004;8:126–30.
9. Cheng F, Dai S, Wang C, et al. Do breast implants influence breastfeeding? A meta-analysis of comparative studies. J Hum Lact. 2018;34:424–32.
10. Schiff M, Algert CS, Ampt A, et al. The impact of cosmetic breast implants on breastfeeding: a systematic review and meta-analysis. Int Breastfeed J. 2014;9:17.
11. Kraut RY, Brown E, Korownyk C, et al. The impact of breast reduction surgery on breastfeeding: systematic review of observational studies. PLoS One. 2017;12:e0186591.
12. Dias CC, Figueiredo B. Breastfeeding and depression: a systematic review of the literature. J Affect Disord. 2015;171:142–54.
13. Matthies LM, Wallwiener M, Sohn C, et al. The influence of partnership quality and breastfeeding on postpartum female sexual function. Arch Gynecol Obstet. 2019;299:69–77.
14. Nishioka E, Haruna M, Ota E, et al. A prospective study of the relationship between breastfeeding and postpartum depressive symptoms appearing at 1-5 months after delivery. J Affect Disord. 2011;133:553–9.
15. Ureño TL, Berry-Cabán CS, Adams A, et al. Dysphoric Milk ejection reflex: a descriptive study. Breastfeed Med. 2019;14:666–73.
16. Prentice JC, Lu MC, Lange L, et al. The association between reported childhood sexual abuse and breastfeeding initiation. J Hum Lact. 2002;18:219–26.

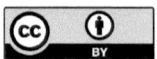

Sexual Aspects of Pelvic Floor Disturbances/Disorders

16

Liesbeth Westerik-Verschuuren (ID),
Marjolijn Lutke Holzik-Mensink, Marleen Wieffer-Platvoet,
and Minke van der Velde (ID)

16.1 Introduction

Whereas Chap. 10 looked at the sexual aspects of the pelvic floor (PF) in healthy pregnancy and postpartum, this chapter will address how various PF disorders influence sexuality. The chapter will successively pay attention to urinary problems, defecation problems, pelvic organ prolapse, and pelvic girdle pain and how they relate to sexuality. We start with the pregnancy-related situations and then the postpartum situations.

16.2 Pelvic Floor Disturbances/Disorders During Pregnancy

16.2.1 Introduction

PF disorders are common during pregnancy. The increased intra-abdominal pressure and the relaxation of the PF connective tissues can disturb micturition and defecation and cause pelvic organ prolapse [1]. Those are embarrassing complaints

L. Westerik-Verschuuren (✉) · M. Lutke Holzik-Mensink
Bekkenfysiotherapie Twente, Expertise Center for Pelvic Floor Physiotherapy,
Enschede, The Netherlands

SOMT University of Physiotherapy, Master Pelvic Physiotherapy,
Amersfoort, The Netherlands
e-mail: l.westerik-verschuuren@somt.nl

M. Wieffer-Platvoet
Bekkenfysiotherapie Twente, Expertise Center for Pelvic Floor Physiotherapy,
Enschede, The Netherlands

M. van der Velde
Seksuologiepraktijk Twente, Center for Sexology, Enschede, The Netherlands

© The Author(s) 2023
S. Geuens et al. (eds.), *Midwifery and Sexuality*,
https://doi.org/10.1007/978-3-031-18432-1_16

185

that decrease quality of life, including sexual life. The range of disturbances goes from a slight inconvenience to severe disorders. Factors such as shame in the woman and her partner influence the degree of impact on sexuality and sexual well-being, just as the importance they attach to sexuality.

16.2.2 Urinary Disorders During Pregnancy

Both pregnancy and childbirth are risk factors for developing urinary incontinence.

Stress urinary incontinence (SUI) is the involuntary loss of urine on effort or physical exertion. SUI can already develop before childbirth and happens in 38% of nulliparous [pregnant] women [2]. With the potential damage caused by delivery added, SUI occurs in 42% of multiparous women [3].

Urgency urinary incontinence (UUI or urine leakage at urgency[1]) also increases during pregnancy but less frequently.

The amount of urine loss differs. Whereas some women lose some drops, the bladder empties entirely in others. It can be experienced as embarrassing, diminishes the woman's self-esteem and self-worth, and impairs her sexuality.

SUI and UUI can also happen during sexuality, with SUI occurring relatively more frequently during penetration and UUI relatively more frequently at orgasm. The last, called 'climacturia', is especially disturbing during cunnilingus (oral sex to the woman's genitalia), a standard part of the sexual script for couples in many parts of the globe.

Urinary tract infections (UTI) affect up to 10% of pregnant women. Although some people consider sexual intercourse to cause recurrent UTIs, (un-)hygienic measures and dysfunctional voiding seem more relevant. Some women appear to avoid sexuality to prevent UTIs with dysuria and the continuous urge to void as additional reasons to abstain from penetrative sex.

16.2.2.1 Treatment Aspects

During pregnancy, urinary incontinence (UI) is associated with an underactive pelvic floor, and is a risk factor for developing postpartum UI. So the woman should train her PF muscles (PFMT as described in Chap. 10), focusing on contraction (increasing strength and endurance), relaxation and coordination. The most important aspect of PFMT is learning to squeeze the PF muscles when the abdominal pressure increases and consciously relax them when no contraction is needed. A correct function and good awareness of the PF will allow penetration and intensify sexual feelings.

In case of recurrent urinary tract infections, adequate toilet technique needs attention.

With a completely relaxed PF, voiding can take place spontaneously without pressing. The woman should also take time to empty the bladder completely.

---

[1] Urgency is 'having difficulty to postpone a sudden or unstoppable sensation to urinate or defecate'.

16.2.3 Defecation Disorders During Pregnancy

In pregnancy, defecation disorders include anal incontinence, involuntary loss of faeces or flatus, and constipation. Anal incontinence and constipation are highly distressing and negatively impact sexuality.

Although pregnant women rarely report the involuntary loss of solid or liquid faeces (out of shame?), the research found incidences between 2% and 9.5% [4]. Involuntary loss of flatus ('flatal incontinence') affects 12–35% of pregnant women and is especially embarrassing during intercourse. As a result, some women seem to avoid sexuality, others avoid genital contact, and nearly all abstain from receptive oral sex.

The causes of constipation during pregnancy are manifold. In constipation, defecation is infrequent or incomplete, or there is a need for frequent straining or digital assistance to defecate. The relaxation of the connective tissues of the bowels increases the 'colon transit time', increasingly solidifying the stool. The woman then strains to defecate, which can cause haemorrhoids and painful and incomplete evacuation. Oral anaemia-related iron supplementation can aggravate this process.

Constipation can cause abdominal pain, reduced appetite, and reduced well-being, negatively affecting sexuality. In addition, the rectum filled with faeces can cause an unpleasant sensation of urgency during sex.

16.2.3.1 Treatment Aspects

In case of anal or flatal incontinence, PFMT (pelvic floor muscle training) is recommended (as described in Chap. 10). In case of constipation, osmotic laxatives can soften the stool. Furthermore the position during a bowel movement is important.

For proper defecation, the position is essential. The knees should be placed higher than the hips. In this 'squatting' position, the PF (especially the puborectal muscles) relaxes and enhances free passage (Fig. 16.1).

16.2.4 Pelvic Organ Prolapse During Pregnancy

Pelvic organ prolapse (POP) is the descent of the anterior vaginal wall, posterior vaginal wall, uterus, or combinations. Since the connective tissues relax and the intra-abdominal pressure increases, one may expect a descent of the pelvic organs during pregnancy. In contrast, there is a cranial shift from the pelvic organs from mid- to late pregnancy [5]. So, a pelvic organ prolapse is not expected in the primigravid woman. Pregnant women, however, report a heavy, dragging sensation in the vaginal area. Most probably, circulatory changes, particularly reduced venous backflow with perivaginal varicose and venous congestion, are responsible for this heavy sensation. Combined with the increased vaginal blood circulation of sexual arousal, this can increase the feeling of prolapse. In some women, that might be a reason to avoid sexual activities. The decreased function of the pelvic floor muscles might be another part of the explanation for the 'prolapse sensation'.

Be aware that in threatening premature labour, the woman can also experience the sensation of prolapse.

Fig. 16.1 Position for easily passing stool. (Illustration by Corine Adamse)

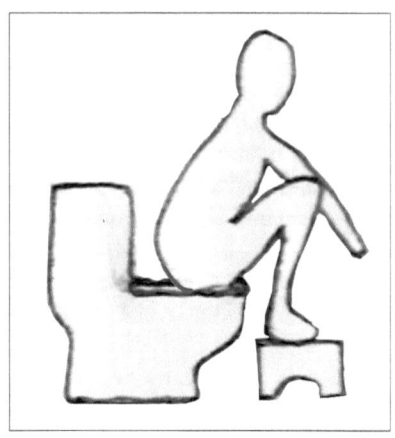

16.2.4.1 Treatment Aspects

Without other signs of threatening premature labour, it seems relevant to reassure pregnant women that the sensation of prolapse is just part of the pregnancy and that sexual activities, including penetration, will not worsen this condition. On the other hand, the woman could diminish the sensations by limiting her standing time to decrease the pressure on the lower belly.

Improving the PF function will create better support for the pelvic organs and be, in that way, effective. Training of the PF muscles, performed in the supine position, will activate the muscle pump and relieves by diminishing the venous congestion.

16.2.5 Pregnancy-Related Pelvic Girdle Pain (or Pregnancy-Related Low Back Pain)

The definition of pelvic girdle pain (PGP) is: pain experienced between the posterior iliac crest and the gluteal fold, particularly in the vicinity of the sacroiliac joint. The pain may radiate in the posterior thigh and occur in the symphysis [6]. It generally develops during pregnancy or the first 3 weeks postpartum. PGP affects up to 45% of pregnant women and causes multiple limitations in daily life activities [7]. Musculoskeletal pain can limit sexual activities as well [8].

Furthermore, PGP can be considered a motor control impairment of the lumbar spine and the pelvis, leading to several compensation strategies. One of those compensation strategies is using the pelvic floor muscles to improve motor control. Many women unconsiously develop an overactive pelvic floor. Such PF muscle overactivity can cause dyspareunia [9].

16.2.5.1 Treatment Aspects

Counselling, explaining the pain, and training to improve motor control of the lumbar spine and the pelvis can reduce this pain and be sufficient to resume sexual activities. Here, it can be helpful to recommend trying adapted positions for

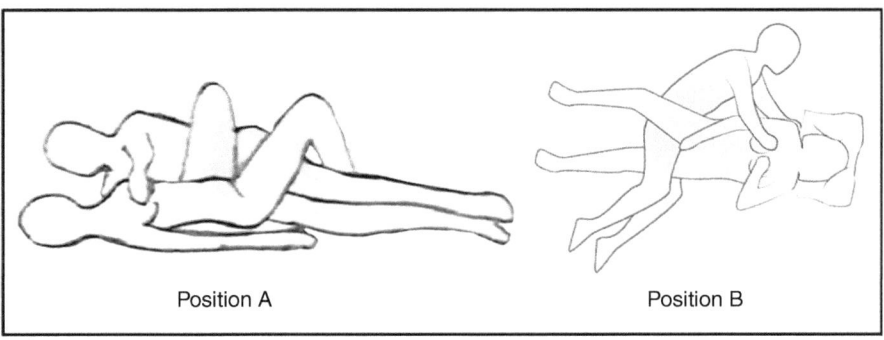

Fig. 16.2 Sexual positions to be recommended in Pelvic Girdle Pain. Position A: woman supine, man on his side, penis towards the vagina. Position B: scicoors position. (Illustration by Corine Adamse)

penetrative sex, for instance, the man on his side and the woman on her back with knees bent and vagina towards the penis (position A) (Fig. 16.2a). The woman's pelvis is spared in this position, just as in the 'scissors position' (position B). When advising couples on such pelvis-sparing positions for penetration, it is necessary to be very concrete and detailed to minimize any hesitation to implement these tips at home because of doubts about the 'How?'. Here, hand-out illustrations can be beneficial.

16.3 Pelvic Floor Disturbances/Disorders in the Postpartum Period

16.3.1 Introduction

Pregnancy and vaginal birth are the most common risk factors for postpartum PF disorders: stress urinary incontinence, overactive bladder syndrome, pelvic organ prolapse, and anal incontinence [1]. This might sound like pathologizing birth. However, HCPs tend to underestimate the rates of obstetric (anal) injury, and in most textbooks, levator ani avulsion is not even mentioned. In an Australian study with 483 patients, only 33–40% of primiparous women achieved an atraumatic normal vaginal birth [10].

These disorders develop by various combinations of damaged PF muscles, damaged PF nerves, and damaged connective tissues, all potentially influencing sexuality. This part will first address perineal pain, vaginal laxity, and overactive pelvic floor, followed by urinary incontinence, anal incontinence, pelvic organ prolapse, and pelvic girdle pain.

16.3.2 Perineal Pain

Perineal pain can happen because of episiotomy, lacerations, or (over)stretching of the perineum. Nine out of ten women report this pain, with a third of the women experiencing moderate-to-severe pain and one in seven women still suffering 9 weeks after childbirth [11]. Perineal pain can limit daily life activities. It can also impair sexual life and sexual pleasure with, especially in couples with poor communication, the risk that dyspareunia develops into long-standing sexual and relationship problems.

16.3.3 Vaginal Laxity

One of the effects of childbirth PF injuries is a reduced strength of the PF muscles. When the strength has decreased too much, the woman cannot close the genital hiatus sufficiently. This symptom is called vaginal laxity. With such laxity, there is no or little friction between the penis and the vagina during penetration. This laxity diminishes sexual pleasure for both partners. Furthermore, it can cause vaginal noise or 'vaginal flatus' during intercourse, which is embarrassing for most people. Because of the entrance's insufficient closure, air enters the vagina and is noisily pushed out by the intercourse movements. Though laxity does not physically hurt, it means, for some couples, a serious sexual disorder needing counselling with practical recommendations on how to avoid vaginal flatus during penetrative sex.

Couples could try another position. Unfortunately, literature does not offer solution of 'noise-free' positions. One could try minimally moving the penis after penetration and use other stimulation like kissing, caressing the breasts, stimulating the clitoris, or whatever a couple prefers. Some couples use loud music and orchestrate penetration on the beats of the music.

Vaginal laxity is frequently linked to an avulsion of the levator ani muscle, meaning that the muscle is partly (and sometimes wholly) torn away from the pubic bone. In a multicentre study on women with first deliveries, the prevalence of levator ani avulsion was 18.8% (with 8% in spontaneous, 29% in vacuum-assisted, and 51% in forceps–assisted delivery) [12].

16.3.3.1 Treatment Aspects

PFMT, creating a kind of hypertrophy of the puborectal and pubococcygeus muscle, will decrease the cross-sectional area of the genital hiatus and thus improve the closure of the genital hiatus and increase the friction between the vaginal wall and the penis with a more intense sexual sensation [13].

16.3.4 Overactive Pelvic Floor

Overactivity is the opposite of laxity. The PF has an increased tone and is not able to relax when needed. This can be caused by perineal pain and fear of (urinary or anal) incontinence or prolapse. The overactivity causes the PF nods and closes the vagina, resulting in a short and narrow vagina, as described in Chap. 10. The consequences are difficulties in penetrating, dyspareunia, and the risk of developing a vicious circle of 'dyspareunia → no desire → dyspareunia'.

16.3.4.1 Treatment Aspects

PFMT should focus on relaxation and coordination. In perineal pain, the woman needs reassurance that squeezing the PF will not cause harm. On the contrary, alternately, maximum squeezing and complete relaxation of the PF will decrease the pain. Especially here, be aware of the risk of developing long-standing vicious circles of pain, poor sexual pleasure, and relationship problems. Having couples avoid all potentially painful sexual activities is often considered an excellent start to treatment and a way of preventing the development of more permanent pain associations [11].

16.3.5 Urinary Incontinence

Urinary incontinence affects up to a third of women in the first 3 months after childbirth. Unfortunately, 1 year after birth, that has barely changed.

Urinary incontinence is a burdensome condition affecting the quality of life, often causing shame and loss of one's self-perceived sexual appeal.

Vaginal birth is particularly associated with stress urinary incontinence (SUI). It is caused by injuries to the PF muscles (reduced strength), connective tissues (weakened support of the bladder neck), and the pudendal nerve. SUI limits all 'abdominal pressure increasing' activities like coughing, running, jumping, bending, and carrying the baby. During sex, it occurs with pressure on the belly and when the penetrating penis pushes against the bladder. So urinary incontinence can affect personal, work, and leisure activities.

There is no difference between vaginal and caesarean delivery regarding urgency urinary incontinence [14].

Urinary incontinence can also lead to coital incontinence (as described in Chap. 10), diminishing sexual activity in some couples.

16.3.5.1 Treatment Aspects

Part of these injuries will heal but not recover completely. Well-functioning PF muscles can partly compensate for this damage [15].

They can improve the closure of the urethra.

To close the urethra optimally, a contraction of the diaphragm pelvis and the urogenital diaphragm, in particular the external urinary sphincter, is required. Actually, the external urethral sphincter is not really a sphincter, but a horseshoe-shaped muscle that closes the urethra by pressing it against the fascia.

The closure of the urethra should be emphasised. With your palpating finger against the bladder neck, ask the woman to contract her PF. A proper contraction will lift the urethra ventralward ('bladder neck elevation').

Following the advice given in Chap. 10, (healthy) women can expect improvement by PFMT after 6 weeks. Recovery of the pelvic floor muscles will take more time in the breastfeeding woman because of her low oestrogen levels.

Practical aspects: empty the bladder before sexual activity.

Adjust urine production to desired sexuality (food that makes the urine smell, timing, the diuretic effect of caffeine, et cetera).

16.3.6 Anal Incontinence

Anal incontinence is a rather embarrassing condition, more bothersome and burdensome than urinary incontinence. After vaginal childbirth, 14% of women suffer from anal incontinence [16].

Anal incontinence is associated with third- and fourth-degree anal sphincter tears [17]. Women with anal sphincter tears often have injuries to the perineal muscles (pubovaginalis, puborectalis) and the pudendal nerve as well. Like urinary incontinence, anal incontinence limits all 'abdominal pressure increasing' activities. With a sphincter tear, women have less resumption of sexual activities [18]. Because of the extent of the injury, there can be a decrease in sensations during sexual activities. Fear of losing stool or gas does neither make a woman feel feminine nor attractive.

16.3.6.1 Treatment Aspects
Practical aspects: Work with quality and timing of food intake and defecation training towards regular daily bowel movements. With such regularity, the rectum will be empty for the rest of the day, and one will not lose stool. Training of strength and coordination of both the anal sphincter and the puborectal muscle is vital to maintain anal continence. Both aspects will improve sexuality as well.

16.3.7 Pelvic Organ Prolapse

Over her lifetime, pelvic organ prolapse (POP) affects 50% of all women who have had at least one vaginal birth [19]. Women with prolapse experience various pelvic floor symptoms depending on the localization and prolapse stage. The most apparent sign of POP is a bulge descending into the vagina. This bulge can be the descending bladder, uterus, or rectum. Sometimes, the vagina seems blocked by the bulge. However, during sexual activities, the bulge can easily be pushed aside.

Damage to the PF muscles and connective tissues causes the prolapse. Sometimes the pudendal nerve is damaged as well. Many women with POP cannot sufficiently close the genital hiatus. During childbirth, the PF muscles, specifically the pubovaginal and puborectal muscles, have to stretch with a factor of 3–4. Since striated muscles cannot stretch more than a factor of 1.5, it is not surprising that these PF muscles get injured during childbirth. Such an overstretching can result in a partial or complete avulsion of the levator ani muscle or traumatic overstretching. Levator ani muscle avulsion is not reversible and has a 13–36% incidence [20]. After a first vaginal birth, the next vaginal deliveries are unlikely to cause avulsion [12].

An open or insufficiently closed genital hiatus can lead to vaginal noise or 'vaginal flatus' and low friction between the vagina and the penis [21]. POP affects the quality of life, particularly the woman's self-image or self-esteem. Mechanically, sexual intercourse is, in general, not impaired. In other words: penetration stays possible.

16.3.7.1   Treatment Aspects

For sexual contact and intercourse, the couple can choose positions in which gravity does not push the prolapse into the vulva, which makes penetration easier. In urogenital prolapse, training of the PF muscles (PFMT) is the first treatment option. Another frequently used strategy is a pessary [3]. PFMT will improve the closure of the hiatus and will increase the friction between the vagina and the penis creating a more intense sexual sensation [22]. The levator ani, bulbospongiosus, and ischiocavernosus muscles are important in sexuality by clasping what enters the vagina, increasing the clitoral circulation, and experiencing orgasm contractions.

If PFMT, a pessary, or the combination does not yield effect, the next option is surgery, aiming to repair the disturbed anatomical structures.

16.3.8 Pelvic Girdle Pain (PGP)

Though postpartum PGP prevalence decreases, it still affects a quarter of women 1 year postpartum [9]. Pelvic girdle pain (formerly sometimes called pelvic instability) is usually caused by impaired motor control of the lumbar spine and the pelvis.

Since the PF muscles connect the pelvic bones and can increase the abdominal pressure, they can give an increased feeling of motor control. When experiencing a lack of motor control, the woman will unconsciously compensate for this with her pelvic floor. Though that will partly contribute to the stiffness of the predominantly bony pelvic ring, it does not lead to optimal motor control. As a result, the PF muscles gradually become overactive without improving the pain. Then, a vicious circle can develop with the pain stimulating the PF muscles to keep trying improved motor control. The overactive pelvic floor impedes sexual reflexes and nods and closes the vagina. Sexual well-being is thus harder to attain.

16.3.8.1   Treatment Aspects

Teach proper techniques to improve motor control without excessively squeezing the PF. After achieving effective motor control, one should learn PF relaxation. See also Chap. 10 or refer to a PF physiotherapist. As in prepartum PGP, being aware of specific positions for penetrative sex is valuable.

16.4   Conclusion

Sexual disorders related to pregnancy and childbirth can be due to PF disorders and dysfunctions. Women need more information about their PF muscles and their changes during pregnancy and after birth [23]. Increasing PF muscle awareness and improving PF muscle function can contribute to more satisfying sex. Though sexuality will always be different after childbirth, it does not mean that a woman cannot enjoy sex anymore. On the contrary, the woman who, in the course of the pregnancy, becomes more aware of her pelvic floor and learns how to use those muscles as 'love muscles' can benefit tremendously.

References

1. Handa VL, Blomquist JL, McDermott KC, et al. Pelvic floor disorders after vaginal birth: effect of episiotomy, perineal laceration, and operative birth. Obstet Gynecol. 2012;119:233–9.
2. Moossdorff-Steinhauser HFA, Bols EMJ, Spaanderman MEA, et al. Long-term effects of motherfit group therapy in pre-(MOTHERFIT1) and postpartum women (MOTHERFIT2) with stress urinary incontinence compared to care-as-usual: study protocol of two multi-centred, randomised controlled trials. Trials. 2019;20:237.
3. Thom DH, Rortveit G. Prevalence of postpartum urinary incontinence: a systematic review. Acta Obstet Gynecol Scand. 2010;89:1511–22.
4. Johannessen HH, Wibe A, Stordahl A, et al. Anal incontinence among first time mothers— what happens in pregnancy and the first year after delivery? Acta Obstet Gynecol Scand. 2015;94:1005–13.
5. Reimers C, Staer-Jensen J, Siafarikas F, et al. Change in pelvic organ support during pregnancy and the first year postpartum: a longitudinal study. BJOG. 2016;123:821–9.
6. Vleeming A, Albert HB, Ostgaard HC, et al. European guidelines for the diagnosis and treatment of pelvic girdle pain. Eur Spine J. 2008;17:794–819.
7. Lawson S, Sacks A. Pelvic floor physical therapy and women's health promotion. J Midwifery Womens Health. 2018;63:410–7.
8. Mens JM, Damen L, Snijders CJ, Stam HJ. The mechanical effect of a pelvic belt in patients with pregnancy-related pelvic pain. Clin Biomech (Bristol, Avon). 2006;21:122–7.
9. Faubion SS, Shuster LT, Bharucha AE. Recognition and management of nonrelaxing pelvic floor dysfunction. Mayo Clin Proc. 2012;87:187–93.
10. Caudwell-Hall J, Kamisan Atan I, Guzman Rojas R, et al. Atraumatic normal vaginal delivery: how many women get what they want? Am J Obstet Gynecol. 2018;219:379.e1–8.
11. Neels H, De Wachter S, Wyndaele JJ, et al. Does pelvic floor muscle contraction early after delivery cause perineal pain in postpartum women? Eur J Obstet Gynecol Reprod Biol. 2017;208:1–5.
12. Cassadó J, Simó M, Rodríguez N, et al. Prevalence of levator ani avulsion in a multicenter study (PAMELA study). Arch Gynecol Obstet. 2020;302:273–80.
13. Kolberg Tennfjord M, Hilde G, Staer-Jensen J, et al. Effect of postpartum pelvic floor muscle training on vaginal symptoms and sexual dysfunction—secondary analysis of a randomised trial. BJOG. 2016;123:634–42.
14. Memon H, Handa VL. Pelvic floor disorders following vaginal or caesarean delivery. Curr Opin Obstet Gynecol. 2012;24:349–54.
15. Mørkved S, Bø K. Effect of pelvic floor muscle training during pregnancy and after childbirth on prevention and treatment of urinary incontinence: a systematic review. J Sports Med. 2014;48:299–310.
16. Schei B, Johannessen HH, Rydning A, et al. Anal incontinence after vaginal delivery or cesarean section. Acta Obstet Gynecol Scand. 2019;98:51–60.
17. Bols EM, Hendriks EJ, Berghmans BC, et al. A systematic review of etiological factors for postpartum fecal incontinence. Acta Obstet Gynecol Scand. 2010;89:302–14.
18. Gommesen D, Nøhr E, Qvist N, Rasch V. Obstetric perineal tears, sexual function and dyspareunia among primiparous women 12 months postpartum: a prospective cohort study. BMJ Open. 2019;9:e032368.
19. Hagen S, Stark D. Conservative prevention and management of pelvic organ prolapse in women. Cochrane Database Syst Rev. 2011;12:CD003882.

20. Friedman T, Eslick GD, Dietz HP. Delivery mode and the risk of levator muscle avulsion: a meta-analysis. Int Urogynecol J. 2019;30:901–7.
21. Neels H, Mortiers X, de Graaf S, et al. Vaginal wind: a literature review. Eur J Obstet Gynecol Reprod Biol. 2017;214:97–103.
22. Braekken IH, Majida M, Ellström Engh M, Bø K. Can pelvic floor muscle training improve sexual function in women with pelvic organ prolapse? A randomised controlled trial. J Sex Med. 2015;12:470–80.
23. Neels H, Wyndaele JJ, Tjalma WA, et al. Knowledge of the pelvic floor in nulliparous women. J Phys Ther Sci. 2016;28:1524–33.

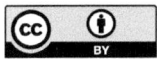

Sexual Aspects of Mental Health Disturbances in Pregnancy and Young Parenthood

17

Mijke Lambregtse-van den Berg (ID) and Hester Pastoor (ID)

17.1 Introduction

Some women with psychiatric diseases would like to have children. Pregnancy and childbirth can aggravate mental health disorders and induce them, while there is little evidence that this period is protective against mental health disorders. Psychiatric disorders usually also have an impact on sexuality and the partner relationship. In addition, the medication used to treat these disorders might have sexual side effects. This chapter will address the various mental health disorders in the period of pregnancy and postpartum and their sexual consequences. It will provide guidelines for diagnosing sexual disorders and for treatment interventions. Cases will illustrate the text.

17.2 Psychiatric Disorders During and After Pregnancy

Psychiatric disorders are among the common morbidities during and after pregnancy. They can have adverse effects on the mother, her child, and the family and influence sexuality and partner relationships. Research in childbirth-related mental disorders mainly focused on postpartum depression. However, it becomes increasingly clear that other psychiatric disorders are also prevalent and relevant in this period. This chapter will review the available evidence on symptoms, epidemiology,

M. Lambregtse-van den Berg (✉)
Department of Psychiatry/Child & Adolescent Psychiatry,
Erasmus University Medical Center, Rotterdam, The Netherlands
e-mail: mijke.vandenberg@erasmusmc.nl

H. Pastoor
Division Reproductive Endocrinology and Infertility, Department of Obstetrics and Gynaecology, Erasmus MC, Rotterdam, The Netherlands

© The Author(s) 2023
S. Geuens et al. (eds.), *Midwifery and Sexuality*,
https://doi.org/10.1007/978-3-031-18432-1_17

and treatment options for psychosis, depression, anxiety disorders, and post-traumatic stress disorder (PTSD), as well as the common consequences for sexuality and sexual relationship.

17.2.1 Psychosis

Among peripartum psychiatric disorders, postpartum or puerperal psychosis is the most severe condition. The prevalence of postpartum psychosis is 1–2 in 1000 deliveries, with an increased risk for women with a history of bipolar disorder or a previous postpartum psychosis. Postpartum psychosis nearly always requires admission to a psychiatric ward, as it is associated with an increased risk of suicide and infanticide. Postpartum psychosis usually develops within 2 weeks after birth, with rapidly growing symptoms such as insomnia, irritability, and mood fluctuation, with mania, depression, or a combination of those two ('mixed state'). Core features of psychosis are delusions and hallucinations, often related to the theme of childbirth. Women might also have delirium-like symptoms, such as disorientation, confusion, derealisation, and depersonalisation. As part of a manic episode, women might have increased sexual desire and loss of sexual decorum [1].

Postpartum psychosis is primarily treated with medication. The sequential administration of benzodiazepines, antipsychotics, lithium, and electroconvulsive therapy (ECT) leads to almost 100% recovery [2]. Women with a history of bipolar disorder or a previous postpartum psychosis are treated with prophylactic medication immediately after birth to minimise the risk of relapse [3].

17.2.2 Depression

Depressive disorders are common during and after pregnancy, with a prevalence rate of approximately 10% of women, making it the most common peripartum complication [4]. Whether the incidence of depression is higher after birth is still not clear. Poor identification and diagnosis of depression during pregnancy could lead to many women being misclassified with postpartum onset [5].

A low mood, irritability, or sudden mood changes affect around 50% of the women in the first 2 weeks after birth (so-called baby blues). These symptoms are usually mild and transient and probably related to physiological changes, including abrupt changes in reproductive hormones after birth. When depressive symptoms persist after 2 weeks postpartum, one should be aware of a depressive disorder. The use of a validated screening instrument like the worldwide most used Edinburgh Postnatal Depression Scale (EPDS) is helpful in the detection of peripartum depression [6]. The symptoms of peripartum depression resemble depressive symptoms outside the peripartum. They include at least a depressed mood and loss of interest and pleasure. Other symptoms are weight changes, loss of energy, feelings of worthlessness and guilt, diminished concentration, and recurrent thoughts of death. There is significant overlap in sexual aspects of depression since reduced interest or pleasure in almost all activities, including sex and loss of sexual desire, is highly prevalent in depression.

Since pharmacological treatment in peripartum depression can affect foetal and infant health, it needs careful evaluation. Therefore, as a general principle, non-pharmacological interventions are the first choice. Most evidence exists for inter-personal and cognitive behavioural therapy. The efficacy of other types of non-pharmacological interventions such as massage, acupuncture, bright light, and omega-3 oils reported inconsistent results [7, 8]. If non-pharmacological treatments are not available or the severity of the depression asks for immediate action, for example, because of suicidal thoughts or actions, antidepressants are indicated.

17.2.3 Anxiety

Anxiety disorders in the peripartum period are more often overlooked and less stud-ied than depression. Nevertheless, they are common, with self-report prevalence rates varying from 18% to 25% during pregnancy and 15% after postpartum. The overall prevalence of a clinical diagnosis of any anxiety disorder is around 15% dur-ing pregnancy and 10% after pregnancy [9]. A meta-analysis reported a signifi-cantly higher risk of obsessive-compulsive disorder in pregnant women (2,1%) and postpartum women (2,4%) than in non-pregnant women in the general population (1,1%) [10].

Tocophobia is a severe fear of pregnancy and childbirth. There is no exact defini-tion as it is not considered a separate psychiatric diagnosis. However, the overall prevalence is estimated at 14% of pregnant women [11].

Vaginismus, the fear of being penetrated often combined with the fear of giving birth, is another anxiety that interferes with conception or pregnancy. These fears can cause avoidance of becoming pregnant, severe anxiety during pregnancy, and avoidance of natural birth by asking for a caesarean section. These women might also avoid gynaecological or midwife consultations or continue requesting consul-tations to feel reassured. Biofeedback, hypnosis, Internet-based cognitive behav-ioural therapy, and antenatal education are promising treatments for fear of childbirth [12].

Cognitive behavioural therapy is the treatment of preference for other anxiety disorders, including obsessive-compulsive disorder. When resources are limited, and the anxiety is disabling, antidepressant medication is a practical option [1].

17.2.4 Post-Traumatic Stress Disorder (PTSD)

PTSD in the peripartum period can result from sexual abuse, abuse in general, or other traumatic experiences before or during pregnancy or childbirth. The preva-lence of PTSD during pregnancy is 3.3%, and postpartum PTSD related to birth has a mean prevalence of 4.0% [13]. Typical symptoms of PTSD are intrusions (such as flashbacks and nightmares), hyperarousal, avoidance, and feelings of guilt and shame. Peripartum PTSD is highly comorbid with depression. HCPs easily miss this diagnosis since, in PTSD, women tend to avoid sharing their traumas due to the disorder. Therefore, it is essential to actively ask about traumatic experiences before, during, or after pregnancy.

Although the efficacy of treatment of PTSD in the peripartum period is scarce, evidence-based trauma-focused psychotherapies for PTSD outside the peripartum period also seem to be effective and safe during pregnancy and after childbirth [14, 15]. The first-choice trauma-focused therapies are trauma-focused cognitive behavioural therapy (TF-CBT) and eye movement desensitisation and reprocessing (EMDR) therapy. Such TF-CBT typically includes 8–12 sessions with a psychotherapist. It includes psychoeducation about reactions to trauma, strategies for managing arousal flashbacks and safety planning; elaboration and processing of the trauma memories and trauma-related emotions (i.e. shame, guilt, loss, and anger); restructuring trauma-related meanings and helps to overcome avoidance; re-establishing adaptive functioning (i.e. example work and social relationships) [16]. EMDR is a highly protocolled therapy in which traumatic memories are recalled while the person simultaneously focuses on an external stimulus (i.e. therapist-directed lateral eye movements or taps and tones) until the memories are no longer distressing (www.emdr.com).

17.3   Psychiatric Disorders, Partner Relationship, and Sexual Function

When, during or after pregnancy, the woman has a psychiatric disorder, the risk increases that the partner will suffer the same fate. It is less studied, but men can also have or develop a psychiatric disorder during or after pregnancy. From pregnancy until 1 year after childbirth, 8% of men suffer from depression [17]. For 'any' anxiety disorder, this ranges between 4.1% and 16.0% during pregnancy and 2.4–18.0% after childbirth [18].

Psychiatric disorders are known to impact sexual function in women and men [19]. This is true for all psychiatric disorders, with depression and anxiety disorders probably as the most known. A prospective study among pregnant women with depressive/anxiety symptoms showed that more than 20% of these women perceived a decline in sexual life [20].

In depression, lack of sexual desire is common. In anxiety disorders, avoiding sex because of fear of having a panic attack (panic disorder), fear of being judged by the sexual partner (social phobia), or PTSD symptoms are common.

In some cases, like borderline personality disorders, sexuality can be an important way to establish and maintain a sense of security and attachment, applying pressure on the partner to reciprocate these sexual desires.

In conclusion, when one of the partners has a psychiatric disorder or sexual dysfunction, the partner will suffer also. Relevant factors are the change in partner roles, and the distress and concerns, with a major impact on both partners and the relationship. Relationship problems and sexual problems influence each other. Male partners of women with sexual dysfunction have a threefold risk of developing sexual dysfunction [21]. Especially when communication between the partners is problematic or stuck in a pattern of blaming, the (sexual) relationship will be under a lot of pressure.

17.4   Sexual Side Effects of Psychiatric Medication

Sexual dysfunction is a common problem in psychiatry and can be related to the psychiatric disorder itself or be a side effect of the prescribed medication. The incidence of sexual side effects can be up to 70–100%, with several drugs reporting a 50–70% incidence [19]. Almost all psychotropic drugs influence overall sexual function and all three phases of the sexual response cycle (i.e. desire, arousal, orgasm/ejaculation). However, there are some distinctions to be made. Antidepressants most of all influence the ability to orgasm or ejaculate. Antipsychotics influence sexual desire more than other functions. Especially, the older generation of antipsychotics can negatively influence fertility. Anxiolytics and mood stabilisers influence all sexual response phases equally. Experiencing sexual side effects can be very distressing and even interfere with treatment compliance. Patients with depression mention decreased desire and orgasmic dysfunction as the most common reasons to stop taking their medication [19].

Depending on the cause of the sexual dysfunction, there are several possible interventions [19]. However, determining the most likely cause of sexual dysfunction can be difficult. As sexuality is a biopsychosocial phenomenon, many factors might influence and interact with each other. The best way to determine if the medication causes the sexual dysfunction is to establish a thorough timeline concerning the development of the psychiatric disorder, the development of the sexual dysfunction, the start of pharmacological treatment, and other potentially influencing factors, like, for example, changes in the partner relationship or general health.

Usually, sexual dysfunctions caused by medication tend to develop very soon after starting and subside very soon after stopping the medication. In general, the influence of physical disease on sexual function usually develops slowly over time, whereas a fast decline usually is a sign of a 'sudden' physical change (e.g. medication, surgery) or a psychological change (e.g. psychiatric disorder, relationship issues).

17.5   Diagnosis and Treatment of Sexual Dysfunctions Related to Peripartum Psychiatric Disorders

One needs a thorough evaluation before being able to treat a sexual problem properly [22].

Here are the most relevant questions in diagnosing sexual problems or dysfunctions: when did it start (lifelong or secondary), in what situations is it present (situational or generalised), and in what phase of the sexual response cycle can we put it (desire, arousal, orgasm, recovery). The answers give much information on what causes the problem and how to deal with it. Besides this, it is also essential to ask about sexual repertoire, sexual behaviour, and sexual stimulation. Limited stimulation or repertoire is often a significant and common cause of sexual dysfunction. It is a professional error not to ask this since it can completely change the choice of intervention. How to diagnose sexual dysfunction will be described in Chap. 29.

The main sexual dysfunctions during pregnancy and postpartum are a lack of sexual desire and dyspareunia [23]. For professionals not trained in sexology, the PLISSIT model (with Permission; Limited Information; Specific Suggestions; and Intensive Therapy) is a useful stepped care model for Treatment [24]. This model (explained in Chap. 3) is helpful in the general population and the psychiatric population of peripartum and young parenthood.

Advising or treating sexual dysfunction in a psychiatric population during the peripartum and young parenthood period is not very different from advising or therapy in other people. Of course, one has to investigate what caused the sexual dysfunction and adjust one's psychoeducation to contain information about the effect of psychiatric illness or medication. Besides this, a lot of interventions could be pretty similar. For midwives, advice and treatment should stay within their own expertise and within the PLISS of the PLISSIT model. We will demonstrate this with some cases with the PLISSIT elements (P, LI, SS, & IT) indicated in brackets.

17.6   Cases

Case 1 Amy
Amy (31, nurse) has had multiple traumatic sexual experiences in her teens and adult years. She has difficulty trusting other people, and she got treatment for PTSD. Amy has also had very exciting sexual experiences, but always with 'bad boys'. By now, she has a loving husband, John (39, account manager), and a very committed relationship, but she doesn't feel like having sex with him.

Because of John's low sperm count, Amy has become pregnant through IVF. During the gynaecological exams, the retrieval of oocytes, and the embryo implantation, Amy was very anxious. Because of her strong wish to become pregnant, she struggled through it all, though she had preferred to have everything done under anaesthesia. She doesn't dare to think about giving birth and avoids discussing the topic.

Amy consults her midwife, who starts with psychoeducation (LI) about the effect of the traumatic experiences on her fears and her pelvic floor. Amy needs to know that it is normal to have these fears since they can remind her of being 'out of control'. Amy finds this very useful, but her fears are still there. She expresses the need for more security during gynaecological examinations and childbirth. The midwife then switches to inquiring about what things are essential for Amy to feel safe during the gynaecological examinations and birth. She marks this information in Amy's file for the professionals who will be on duty during Amy's childbirth. Besides, Amy is allowed the opportunity to bring someone she completely trusts for emotional support during the examinations and the birth (SS). Amy also gets information about plan B, in case this will not be sufficient. An experienced gynaecologist or sexologist will 'practice' the gynaecological examination with her, during which Amy receives information on how to handle her fears (IT). With this knowledge, Amy starts feeling more in control, and she is less scared. Her birth goes without any additional psychotrauma.

Case 2 Julie

Julie (28, teacher at a primary school) is married to Thomas (30, manager at a big supermarket). Three months ago, their first baby was born. Julie is not very self-assertive and has trouble expressing her wishes. On the other hand, Thomas is a very assertive man, controlling many aspects of their relationship. However, their sexual relationship is not thriving, with a low frequency of sexual contact.

Sexual desire appears to be the only aspect under Julie's control. Since the baby is born, Julie feels down. She is becoming increasingly inactive and unresponsive to the baby. Thomas is very concerned and has contacted their family physician, who diagnosed Julie with depression.

Julie contacts the midwife who supervised her pregnancy and tells her about the depression. The midwife gives Julie some psychoeducation (LI) about possible causes of feeling down when being a young mother and all the changes in her life and the attached new responsibilities. She adds that the depressed feelings could also be related to changing hormones or her low self-assertiveness. Julie realises that with a newborn baby having any control in her life is difficult, combined with the relationship pattern she is in, both influencing her mood and her sexual desire.

To improve her mood, Julie then gets instructions (SS) to establish a daily routine as far as possible. In addition, Julie tries to enjoy some activities without the baby (or at least not as a mother) and share her feelings with people she trusts. Unfortunately, this is not effective enough, after which her family physician refers Julie to a psychologist for cognitive behavioural therapy (IT) combined with medication. There, she also gets sensate focus exercises to improve her sexuality. That turns out to be a good way to re-establish intimate physical contact with Thomas. Julie then starts daring to be more self-assertive and discovering what she herself wants and likes.

Case 3 Fatima

Fatima (25, who finished her master's in psychology at the beginning of her first pregnancy) developed a postpartum psychosis. Her psychiatrist prescribed antipsychotic medication. Soon after starting the medication, Fatima noticed that her sexual desire had 'disappeared'. Sexuality had always been vital for her and her husband Arthur, a 28-year old engineer.

Of course, the pregnancy and giving birth had changed their sexuality, but Fatima still wanted to be close, intimate, and even sexual with Arthur. After starting the medication, she does not feel anything sexual anymore. For Fatima, this is an extraordinary and undesired situation.

The psychiatrist starts with psychoeducation (LI) about the effect of antipsychotic medication on sexual function in general. That already turns out to be a real relief for both Fatima and Arthur. Now they understand that those changes have nothing to do with their relationship. They learn that Fatima should not wait until feeling desire (because it will not come as spontaneous as it used to), but that they have to just start with physical contact and intimacy to 'awaken' sexual desire as a reaction to pleasurable touch and experiences (SS). Experiencing this indeed works makes them very happy. They also change their sexual routine and apply more direct stimulation to Fatima's clitoris (sometimes even with a vibrator), which improves the physical part of her sexual response. Altogether the results are so positive that there is no more need for the eventual next step of changing Fatima's medication (IT).

17.7 Conclusions and Clinical Recommendations for Midwives

Pregnancy, the postpartum period, psychiatric disorders, and sexual function are interrelated. As we demonstrated, addressing sexuality is important. In this chapter, we have described some topics and guidelines. We conclude with some clinical recommendations.

- It is essential to involve the partner from the start of treatment. As mentioned, a psychiatric or sexual disorder will also influence the partner. The partner could be the one with the disorder. So, actively ask for both partners' distress, traumatic experiences, or psychiatric symptoms. Additionally, discuss sexuality and its importance for both partners. Since sexual fears or fears of giving birth are common, assess if these are present.
- When confronted with a woman or a couple with a psychiatric disorder and sexual dysfunction, it is essential to address sexuality early. Ask about the effects on the partner relationship, sexual function, and well-being of both partners. Start with educating the couple about common psychiatric symptoms and disorders in the peripartum and young parenthood period. If they are already using medication, inform the couple about possible sexual side effects of medicines and the impact of the psychiatric disorder on sexual function. Check if this affects treatment compliance.
- Interventions and advice for improving sexual function can often be similar to those in other populations. They can be related to medication, mental health, sexuality, or lifestyle. The PLISSIT model is very beneficial for this purpose. For general advice, see Chaps. 3 and 29. Specific advice or interventions for the population in this chapter is related to counselling on sexual side effects of psychiatric problems and psychiatric medication. Advise the couple to discuss this with the prescribing healthcare professional to decide on a strategy to reduce

these side effects (e.g. wait for spontaneous remission, lower the dose, change the medication, change the timing of the medication, or add a drug to counter the side effects).
• Finally, we should not forget that psychiatric disorders can interfere with the postpartum bonding with the child. Be aware of signs of disturbed bonding to the child in both parents. If this is the case, discuss this with the couple and refer them to a healthcare professional, like a psychologist or psychiatrist, with experience in infant mental health.

References

1. Meltzer-Brody S, Howard L, Bergink V, et al. Postpartum psychiatric disorders. Nat Rev Dis Primers. 2018;4:18022.
2. Bergink V, Burgerhout KM, Koorengevel KM, et al. Treatment of psychosis and mania in the postpartum period. Am J Psychiatry. 2015;172:115–23.
3. Wesseloo R, Kamperman AM, Munk-Olsen T, et al. Risk of postpartum relapse in bipolar disorder and postpartum psychosis: a systematic review and meta-analysis. Am J Psychiatry. 2016;173:117–27.
4. Woody CA, Ferrari AJ, Siskind DJ, et al. A systematic review and meta-regression of the prevalence and incidence of perinatal depression. J Affect Disord. 2017;219:86–92.
5. Howard LM, Molyneaux E, Dennis CL, et al. Non-psychotic mental disorders in the perinatal period. Lancet. 2014;384(9956):1775–88.
6. Cox J, Holden J, Sagovsky R. Detection of postnatal depression: development of the 10-item Edinburgh postnatal depression scale. Br J Psychiatry. 1987;150:782–6.
7. van Ravesteyn LM, Lambregtse-van den Berg MP, Hoogendijk WJ, Kamperman AM. Interventions to treat mental disorders during pregnancy: a systematic review and multiple treatment meta-analysis. PLoS One. 2017;12:e0173397.
8. Dennis CL, Hodnett E. Psychosocial and psychological interventions for treating postpartum depression. Cochrane Database Syst Rev. 2007;4:CD006116.
9. Dennis CL, Falah-Hassani K, Shiri R. Prevalence of antenatal and postnatal anxiety: systematic review and meta-analysis. Br J Psychiatry. 2017;210:315–23.
10. Russell EJ, Fawcett JM, Mazmanian D. Risk of obsessive-compulsive disorder in pregnant and postpartum women: a meta-analysis. J Clin Psychiatry. 2013;74:377–85.
11. O'Connell MA, Leahy-Warren P, Khashan AS, et al. Worldwide prevalence of tocophobia in pregnant women: systematic review and meta-analysis. Acta Obstet Gynecol Scand. 2017;96:907–20.
12. Badaoui A, Kassm SA, Naja W. Fear and anxiety disorders related to childbirth: epidemiological and therapeutic issues. Curr Psychiatry Rep. 2019;21:27.
13. Yildiz PD, Ayers S, Phillips L. The prevalence of posttraumatic stress disorder in pregnancy and after birth: a systematic review and meta-analysis. J Affect Disord. 2017;208:634–45.
14. Baas MA, van Pampus MG, Braam L, et al. The effects of PTSD treatment during pregnancy: systematic review and case study. Eur J Psychotraumatol. 2020;11:1762310.
15. de Bruijn L, Stramrood CA, Lambregtse-van den Berg MP, Rius ON. Treatment of posttraumatic stress disorder following childbirth. J Psychosom Obstet Gynaecol. 2020;41:5–14.
16. NICE—National Institute for Health and Care Excellence. Treating posttraumatic stress disorder in adults. http://pathways.nice.org.uk/pathways/posttraumatic-stress-disorder. NICE pathway last updated: 04 November 2020.
17. Cameron EE, Sedov ID, Tomfohr-Madsen LM. Prevalence of paternal depression in pregnancy and the postpartum: an updated meta-analysis. J Affect Disord. 2016;206:189–203.

18. Leach LS, Poyser C, Cooklin AR, Giallo R. Prevalence and course of anxiety disorders (and symptom levels) in men across the perinatal period: a systematic review. J Affect Disord. 2016;190:675–86.
19. Lew-Starowicz M, Giraldi A, THC K, editors. Psychiatry and sexual medicine. A comprehensive guide for clinical practitioners. Cham: Springer; 2020.
20. Faisal-Cury A, Huang H, Chan YF, Menezes PR. The relationship between depressive/anxiety symptoms during pregnancy/postpartum and sexual life decline after birth. J Sex Med. 2013;10:1343–9.
21. Chew PY, Choy CL, Bin Sidi H, et al. The association between female sexual dysfunction and sexual dysfunction the male partner: a systematic review and meta-analysis. J Sex Med. 2020;18(1):99–112.
22. Althof SE, Rosen RC, Perelman MA, Rubio-Aurioles E. Standard operating procedures for taking a sexual history. J Sex Med. 2013;10:26–35.
23. Jawed-Wessel S, Sevick E. The impact of pregnancy and childbirth on sexual behaviors: a systematic review. Ann Rev Sex Res. 2017;52:411–23.
24. Annon JS. The PLISSIT model: a proposed conceptual scheme for the behavioral treatment of sexual problems. J Sex Ed Ther. 1976;2:1–15.

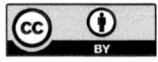

Sex, Fertility, Pregnancy, and Parenthood with a Chronic Disease or Other Health Disturbance

18

Rik H. W. van Lunsen ⓘ

18.1   Introduction

From puberty to old age, sexual functioning is an essential aspect of quality of life (QoL) for almost all women and men. Sexual functioning and the human sexual response are determined by an intricate interplay between biological, psychological, social, and relational factors.

All medical, psychological, social, and relational events throughout the lifespan may impact sexual functioning, sexual well-being, and reproductive health. However, the way women and their partners can adjust their sex lives to critical life events determines whether or not they will be able to enjoy pleasurable sexual encounters irrespective of the difficulties they have to face.

Disease and medical interventions can have profound effects on all aspects of sexuality, and that is certainly the case when procreation, pregnancy, childbirth, and the genitals are involved.

People living with a chronic disease have to cope with the impact of the disease and its treatment on their sexual lives. In addition, they have to deal with the possible effects of the disease and its physical, psychological, and relational ramifications on fertility, pregnancy, parenthood, and offspring.

Sometimes a chronic disease or other serious health disturbance manifests itself during pregnancy, which might have consequences for the pregnancy itself and sexual functioning, future well-being and reproductive choices and possibilities.

However, irrespective of the consequences of medical events, the main predictor for satisfactory sexual functioning after such events is the previous sexual functioning with, on the one hand, a broad repertoire of sexual activities and, on the other

R. H. W. van Lunsen (✉)

Department of Sexology and Psychosomatic Gynaecology (Retired), Amsterdam University Medical Center, Independent Sexual Health Expert, Amsterdam, The Netherlands
e-mail: h.w.vanlunsen@amsterdamumc.nl

© The Author(s) 2023
S. Geuens et al. (eds.), *Midwifery and Sexuality*,
https://doi.org/10.1007/978-3-031-18432-1_18

207

hand, the ability of the couple to adjust their sex lives to changing conditions. Whether or not the sexual ramifications of pregnancy and chronic disease become problematic very much depends on the couple's effectiveness to communicate about wishes, needs, boundaries, and (im-)possibilities concerning sexuality and intimacy. Throughout pregnancy and postpartum, the midwife has the main task to help the woman and her partner communicate effectively about their sexual and intimate needs, expectations, and worries in light of their health disturbances.

Whenever people living with a chronic physical impairment succeed in producing the right stimuli in the right context and communicating effectively about their needs, expectations, and possibilities regarding intimacy and sexuality, they might fulfil the main prerequisites of a healthy sex life (see Chap. 3).

18.2 Health Disturbances, Sexuality, and Childwish

For most people with a chronic disease or a history of cancer who have a childwish, the decision to try to conceive is more complicated than for most others. The disease and its treatment might harm fertility. Couples are not always able to conceive with penis-in-vagina intercourse due to sexual dysfunction or physical disability. Many chronic medical conditions such as diabetes, hypertension, psychiatric illness, and thyroid disease have implications for pregnancy outcomes and need optimal management before pregnancy. Detailed information on medication use, possible teratogenic effects, and the influence on the pregnancy should be part of the preconception counselling. Couples are also in need of counselling about the many worries they might have: Will the disease negatively affect the course of the pregnancy or infant health? Will the pregnancy influence the course and severity of the mother's disease? What is the prognosis of the disease concerning parental functioning? Is there a genetic risk?

Many studies have shown that although women and men with chronic diseases (like inflammatory bowel disease, diabetes, and asthma) have more sexual dysfunctions, they are no less sexually active than others. On the other hand, they have significantly fewer children, mainly because of voluntary childlessness.

The midwife should realise that pregnancy for these couples often results from a long process of contemplating possible advantages, disadvantages, complications, and outcomes. Sexuality often has lost its positive connotations about intimacy and pleasure, either because of a preceding period of sexual behaviour exclusively focusing on conception, or because of a process of medically assisted reproduction through IVF, ICSI, or gamete donation.

18.3 Sexual Sequelae of Chronic Diseases and Other Health Disturbances

Chronic illness can have profound adverse effects on the relationship and sexual satisfaction and also on all phases of the sexual response of both patient and partner. Sexuality is, after all, a complex bio-psycho-social phenomenon. Therefore, the possible effects of chronic disease on sexuality are multifactorial and a result of an interaction of physical, psychological, relational, and social aspects.

On a physical level: Due to diseases such as diabetes and multiple sclerosis (MS), nerves and blood vessels essential for the genital sexual response might have been damaged, resulting in erectile dysfunction in men, and a lack of lubrication, and genital swelling in women or an orgasmic disorder. Hormonal changes, e.g. diminished bioavailability of testosterone and other hormones, might result in reduced responsiveness to sexual stimuli. These sexual dysfunctions also can be the result of medication such as antidepressants, commonly prescribed to people living with a chronic disease.

On a psychological level: Sexual desire might be affected by anxiety, depression, loss of self-esteem, and grief often associated with chronic disease. Surgical procedures and medication (e.g. scarring, amputation, mastectomy, colostomy, and hair loss) can profoundly affect bodily appearance and function, leading to difficulties accepting changes to body image and perceived desirability.

On the relationship level: Chronic illness will also affect the *relationship* between patient and partner. When the lover becomes the carer, it can be hard to keep the flame of sexuality alive. The stress of illness can exacerbate pre-existing relational problems.

On a social level: There is a prevailing view that sex is the prerogative of the young, the fit, and the attractive. Society, including caregivers, often neglect the fact that sex is an essential part of life irrespective of age and health status and that people living with a chronic disease, physical disability, or cancer want them to pay attention to their worries and problems on sexual and reproductive health.

18.4   Sexuality and Specific Chronic Diseases and Other Health Disturbances

Some chronic diseases and health disturbances have a higher prevalence than average in the childbearing years. It is not unlikely that the midwife will head-on meet pregnant women or their partners living with these conditions and who would very much welcome a health professional who pays attention to their specific questions, worries, and problems regarding sexual health. Below, we will address the sexual sequelae of some of these conditions in more detail.

18.4.1 Breast Cancer (BC)

In the Western World, breast cancer is the predominant type of malignancy among women, and 5–15% of women with BC carry the disease in their reproductive years. Because many women postpone childbearing to a more advanced age, an increasing number of women with (a history of) BC have childwish or get the BC diagnosis during pregnancy. Breast cancer can negatively impact sexual functioning in many ways. Research shows that – as in many other situations – the best predictor of the quality of sex life after diagnosis and treatment is the quality of sexual life before the diagnosis [1]. Radiotherapy, chemotherapy, and hormonal therapy all may affect sexual functioning and fertility.

Since the woman should not become pregnant during BC treatment, the couple should use effective contraception. When BC is diagnosed during pregnancy, the woman needs a multidisciplinary approach because of the possible consequences of different treatment modalities for the mother, the pregnancy, and the foetus. Multiple studies showed that pregnancy doesn't increase the recurrence risk after BC and perhaps even has a protective effect.

After BC, many couples get advice to postpone pregnancy until 2 years after treatment because of psychological reasons and recurrence risk, although there usually is no medical rationale for this advice. Since the biological clock is ticking away the reproductive opportunities, couples often make their own plan anyway.

18.4.2 Inflammatory Bowel Disease (IBD)

Crohn's disease (CD) and ulcerative colitis (UC) affect patients' quality of life in many ways, and most patients with IBD will carry the diagnosis during their reproductive years or already since puberty or adolescence.

Body image, sexuality, and relationships are some of the major concerns of IBD patients, but these concerns are rarely spontaneously expressed. Almost half of IBD patients report that their disease prevented them from pursuing intimate relationships. Sexual dysfunctions in IBD are reported by 45–60% of women and 15–25% of men. Depression and exacerbation of the disease increase the likelihood of sexual dysfunction. Women have more concerns about self-image, feeling alone, and being fearful of having children [2]. Especially in women who have had surgery, a negative body image prevents them from entering a relationship and enjoying sexual encounters. Although the rate of sexual activity of IBD patients is similar to healthy individuals, their satisfaction is significantly lower than that of the general population.

IBD is not associated with decreased fertility in patients who have not undergone surgery. Yet these women are significantly more likely to remain (voluntarily) childless compared with the general population. That is due to (often unfounded) fears about the possible impact of IBD and medication on pregnancy and neonatal outcomes, worries about the impact of pregnancy on IBD and maternal health, and fears regarding hereditary transmission [3].

18.4.3 Cervical Cancer

About 75% of cervical cancer cases are detected in women aged 30–40, 20% in women aged 20–29, and only 1–2% of affected women are under 20. The development of cervical cancer is related to exposure to the human papillomavirus (HPV).

The incidence dropped significantly in countries with screening programmes (Pap smears) and HPV vaccination. The HPV infection often occurs shortly after the first sexual activity. HPV infections are more likely to occur in adolescent women than in older women because the transformation zone of the cervix is more vulnerable in young women. In adolescents and young women, most HPV infections are transient and 'cleared' (healed by themselves within 2 years). There is evidence that individuals who have been victims of sexual abuse as children have higher rates of anogenital HPV at a younger age than individuals without such a history [4]. Some 3% of cervical cancer cases are diagnosed during pregnancy. Most of these women have early-stage diseases. Research suggests that cervical cancer diagnosed during pregnancy does not grow faster and does not spread more likely than outside pregnancy. Therefore, in most cases, treatment can be postponed until after childbirth. After cervical cancer treatment, the incidence of sexual dysfunction is high (between 40% and 100%) due to the physical, emotional, and relational impact. Surgery (with the removal of the ovaries), radiotherapy, and chemotherapy may cause loss of ovarian function with far more hormonal implications than natural menopause. The additional loss or threat of losing fertility may profoundly affect identity, self-image, mood, and sexuality.

18.4.4 Diabetes Mellitus (Type 1 DM)

Diabetes mellitus type 1, which usually starts in adolescents and young adults, affects both women and men in many different ways, including effects on sexuality, fertility, pregnancy, and offspring.

Because type 1 DM influences fertility, the patient/couple deserves expert guidance in pregnancy planning and extensive preconception counselling. After conceiving, the main issue is to control the DM in the woman as closely as possible.

Deterioration in sexual functioning is one of the significant and earliest DM complications resulting from combinations of microvascular and/or nerve damage, fluctuating blood sugar levels, hormonal changes, and the psychological effects of having a chronic disease with many implications for QOL. In men, the primary complications are erectile dysfunction, ejaculatory dysfunction, and loss of sexual desire. Although often disregarded, women experience similar sexual problems, including diminished lubrication, dyspareunia, decreased sexual desire, and orgasmic difficulties [5]. Sexual dysfunctions are most prevalent in diabetes patients with vascular (retinopathy) and/or nerve (neuropathy) damage. Young women with type 1 DM using an insulin pump have the same prevalence of sexual dysfunctions as healthy age-matched women. That differs from women using multiple daily insulin injections since their prevalence of sexual dysfunctions is significantly increased, suggesting that fluctuations in glucose levels harm sexual functioning.

Gestational diabetes develops during pregnancy. Whereas it can negatively influence sexual functioning during pregnancy and postpartum, there is no difference with women who have an uncomplicated pregnancy.

18.4.5 Multiple Sclerosis

Multiple sclerosis (MS) is a chronic inflammatory disease of the central nervous system, more prevalent in the northern hemisphere. It is also more prevalent in women and tends to start in the 20–40-year age range, the period with high sexuality and reproduction expectations. The disease usually causes relapsing-remitting attacks of inflammation, demyelination, and axonal damage, leading to various degrees and spectra of neurological symptoms and disability. The literature reports sexual dysfunctions in 45–90% of all MS patients. In a study of people with MS, 63% reported that their sexual activity had declined since their diagnosis. Nerves involved in the sexual response may be damaged, resulting in arousal and orgasm disorders. MS symptoms such as fatigue or spasticity may cause sexual problems. As in other chronic disabilities, the psychological and relational factors contributing to changes in sexual functioning are multifactorial. They may involve loss of self-esteem, depression, anxiety, anger, and the stress of living with a chronic illness.

Although a pregnancy was often discouraged in the past, there is extensive evidence that pregnancy reduces the number of relapses related to high estriol levels during pregnancy [6]. Postpartum, there is an increased risk of relapses. Since breastfeeding reduces the risk of relapses, exclusive breastfeeding should be promoted for at least 3 months as long as no MS therapeutics are used that may be harmful to the baby. Two years after childbirth, there is no difference in disability between women who have been pregnant and those who were not.

18.4.6 Rheumatic Disease

The rheumatic disease group consists of more than 100 different types of conditions that affect joints, tendons, ligaments, bones, muscles, and often other organs. Most of these conditions are autoimmune diseases. Rheumatic diseases that might affect people at a young age are, for instance, juvenile idiopathic arthritis (JIA), rheumatoid arthritis (RA), and systemic lupus erythematosus (SLE).

Sexual problems among patients with rheumatic diseases are common [7]. Lack of mobility and musculoskeletal pain can restrict intercourse and limit sexual activity. Fatigue, mental distress, depression, functional limitations, low levels of self-efficacy, and a negative body image are associated with sexual problems. Many of the drugs used in the treatment of rheumatic disease might affect sexual functioning as well. Patients with RA, JIA, and SLE have a smaller family size. The rate of infertility in young women with rheumatic disease is significantly higher than in women who develop it later in their life. The causes of fewer children include impaired sexual function, decreased gonadal function, pregnancy loss, effects of therapy on pregnancy, and personal choices. Voluntary childlessness is related to disease-related concerns such as deleterious effects of drugs on offspring, ability to care for small children, or fear to transmit the disease to children. Preconception counselling is necessary since drug therapy can influence fertility and obstetric outcomes because of gonadal toxicity and teratogenicity. Often pregnancy has to be postponed, and the woman should keep a safety interval between drug discontinuation and conception. About 75% of women with rheumatic disease experience improving symptoms during pregnancy. Therefore, pregnancy results in better sexual lives for some couples because of reduced pain and improved mobility. After birth, 90% report a relapse within 3 months. Combined with the more common postpartum sexual and relational obstacles, this often has prolonged adverse effects on sexuality. Most, but not all, anti-rheumatic medications are compatible with breastfeeding [8].

18.4.7 Asthma

Asthma is a common chronic condition among women of childbearing age with a 1–13% prevalence. Studies have shown that at least two-thirds of people living with asthma feel that asthma negatively affects their sexual life because of the impact of the physical, practical, psychological, and relational effects of having a chronic disease. Of the people with severe asthma, 10–13% feel the impact of breathlessness and fear it during physical intimacy, kissing, and sexual activity [9]. Chronic fatigue, the side effects of medication, and the necessity to have a nebuliser at hand when being intimate are only some of the factors people with asthma and their partners have to cope with when organising their sexual activity.

Corticosteroid treatment and limited physical ability may influence appearance and body image, causing low self-esteem that often contributes to decreased sexual activity. Corticosteroid treatment might result in decreased sexual responsivity due to decreased bioavailibility of androgens.

Sexual activity in general and especially orgasm can trigger asthma bronchospasms, sometimes even requiring emergency care and hospitalisation, which can induce fear for future sexual activity.

During pregnancy, the course of asthma symptoms is unpredictable, with one-third improvement, one-third no change, and one-third deterioration. Likewise, some women will perceive improvement in sexual functioning, while others experience the opposite. In general, women can continue asthma medication throughout pregnancy. Inhalation corticosteroids are safe for mother and child and are highly effective for controlling asthma and reducing asthma exacerbations. On the other hand, maternal asthma exacerbations are associated with adverse perinatal outcomes such as preeclampsia, preterm birth, and low birth weight. Inhalation corticosteroids are safe for use during breastfeeding. Breastfeeding diminishes infant wheezing and asthma, at least during the first few years.

18.4.8 HIV

The increased access to effective antiretroviral treatment (ART) has made HIV comparable to other chronic diseases. For HIV-positive women, sexual and reproductive health are complex concerning partner relationships, sexual behaviour, reproductive choices, pregnancy, and parenthood. HIV-positive women have more sexual problems than uninfected women and significantly lower sexual desire, activity, and satisfaction scores. Although effective antiretroviral therapy (ART) resulting in an undetectable viral load prevents transmission to one's partner or baby, the fear of viral transmission and feelings of contagiousness often impact sexual behaviour and reproductive choices [10]. Motherhood seems to make the burden of being HIV-positive easier to bear. However, contrary to their wishes, HIV-positive women often have no partner, are not sexually active, and stay childless. Women with an undetectable viral load who daily take their ART and have regular controls can safely breastfeed as long as they exclusively breastfeed for at least 6 months. Mixing breastmilk and other foods before 6 months increases the transmission risk.

18.4.9 Congenital Heart Disease

Approximately 1% of all newborns have congenital heart disease (CHD). In the more affluent countries, 85% of these children survive into adulthood due to successful treatment. Women with CHD have high levels of concern regarding their fertility and risk of genetic transmission of CHD, and concerns about adverse effects of pregnancy on their own health [11, 12]. Pregnancy carries potential risks for these women and their children. Therefore, planning a pregnancy needs careful cardiological and genetic counselling. Although being one of the most important areas of concern for women with CHD and their families, we know little about the impact of pregnancy and childbearing on long-term health. Adolescents and young adults with CHD start later and have less sexual activity than their healthy peers. Women with CHD have more sexually related distress and dysfunctions and decreased sexual activity. However, the risk for adverse cardiovascular events during sexual activity is low. Even lower death rates have been reported for specific groups, such as women in general and asymptomatic young adults with CHD. There is no reason to discourage any form of sexual activity during pregnancy.

18.4.10 Chronic Kidney Disease (CKD)

Most patients with chronic kidney disease have sexual and reproductive problems. Common disturbances include menstrual irregularities, decreased sexual desire, sexual arousal disorders, and decreased fertility. These disturbances are related to psychological distress and depression, body changes and fatigue, organic factors such as uraemia, gonadal irregularities, and many other comorbid conditions and medications. Some of these conditions improve after initiation of dialytic therapy;

others will worsen. In general, advice is given to uraemic women not to become pregnant while on dialysis.

Kidney transplantation improves sexuality, fertility, and reproductive possibilities in women and men with CKD. Although most pregnancies in kidney transplant recipients are successful, comorbidities (such as hypertension or immunosuppression side effects) that are not the result of the transplant itself often complicate these pregnancies. As a result, there is a high rate of preeclampsia, preterm deliveries, Caesarean sections, and small-for-gestational-age babies. We did not find any study on sexual functioning during pregnancy in women with CKD. Since studies have convinced us that most immunosuppressives are safe, the number of breastfeeding mothers on maintenance-immunosuppression after kidney transplantation increases.

18.5   Conclusions

Patients with chronic medical conditions expect their caregivers to proactively discuss uncertainties, worries, and problems concerning sexuality, contraception, fertility, reproduction, pregnancy, and parenthood. Unfortunately, very few professionals do so. Moreover, in obstetrical care, sexuality is a neglected area as well. By raising the topic of sexuality during pregnancy and postpartum in patients with a chronic disease, the midwife may help women and their partners to express their needs, expectations, and worries regarding intimacy and sexuality in the light of their health disturbances, possible comorbid sexual dysfunctions, and their new roles as parenting couple.

References

1. Den Oudsten BL, Van Heck GL, Van der Steeg AF, et al. Clinical factors are not the best predictors of quality of sexual life and sexual functioning in women with early stage breast cancer. Psychooncology. 2010;19:646–56.
2. Leenhardt R, Rivière P, Papazian P, et al. Sexual health and fertility for individuals with inflammatory bowel disease. World J Gastroenterol. 2019;25:5423–33.
3. Selinger C, Ghorayeb J, Madill A. What factors might drive voluntary childlessness in women with IBD? Does IBD-specific pregnancy-related knowledge matter? J Crohns Colitis. 2016;10:1151–8.
4. Unger ER, Fajman NN, Maloney EM, et al. Anogenital human papillomavirus in sexually abused and nonabused children: a multicenter study. Pediatrics. 2011;128:e658–65.
5. Enzlin P, Mathieu C, Van den Bruel A, et al. Prevalence and predictors of sexual dysfunction in patients with type 1 diabetes. Diabetes Care. 2003;26:409–14.
6. Finkelsztejn A, Brooks J, Paschoal F Jr, et al. What can we really tell women with multiple sclerosis regarding pregnancy? A systematic review and meta-analysis of the literature. BJOG. 2011;118:790–7.

7. Østensen M. Sexual and reproductive health in rheumatic disease. Nat Rev Rheumatol. 2018;13:485–93.
8. Tosounidou S, Gordon C. Medications in pregnancy and breastfeeding. Best Pract Res Clin Obstet Gynaecol. 2020;64:68–76.
9. Holmes LJ, Yorke JA, Dutton C, et al. Sex and intimacy in people with severe asthma: a qualitative study. BMJ Open Respir Res. 2019;6:e000382.
10. Carlsson-Lalloo E, Berg M, Mellgren Å, et al. Sexuality and childbearing as it is experienced by women living with HIV in Sweden: a lifeworld phenomenological study. Int J Qual Stud Health Well-being. 2018;13:1487760.
11. Reid GJ, Siu SC, McCrindle BW, et al. Sexual behavior and reproductive concerns among adolescents and young adults with congenital heart disease. Int J Cardiol. 2008;125:332–8.
12. Haberer K, Silversides CK. Congenital heart disease and women's health across the life span: focus on reproductive issues. Can J Cardiol. 2019;35:1652–63.

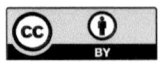

Effects on Sexuality of Medication Used in Pregnancy and Childbirth

19

Erna Beers ⓘ and Annelies Jaeken

This chapter aims to provide an overview of the sexual side effects of the medication used in midwifery and obstetrics. Side effects that frequently tend to be forgotten.

The chapter will also provide practical advice to the midwife to discuss the possible sexual side effects and deal with those effects.

19.1 How Pregnancy Affects the Effects of Medication

Pregnant women are excluded from clinical drug trials, mainly because of the risk of harm to the unborn child. As a result, knowledge about the effectiveness and safety of medication during pregnancy is limited.

During pregnancy, but preferably already when the woman or couple desires a pregnancy, it is necessary to compare the risk of aggravation or recurrence of a medical condition for the unborn against the risks of prescribing medication during pregnancy.

19.1.1 A Few Words on Pharmacokinetics and Pharmacodynamics

Some knowledge of pharmacokinetics or pharmacodynamics helps understand the side effects of medication. Although they seem complex and abstract processes, PK and PD can be explained quite easily.

The original version of the chapter has been revised. A correction to this chapter can be found at https://doi.org/10.1007/978-3-031-18432-1_31

E. Beers (✉)
Pharmacosexology, SUNSCKS, Hilversum, The Netherlands

A. Jaeken
PXL University College of Applied Arts and Sciences, Healthcare Department, Midwifery, Hasselt, Belgium

© The Author(s) 2023, corrected publication 2024
S. Geuens et al. (eds.), *Midwifery and Sexuality*,
https://doi.org/10.1007/978-3-031-18432-1_19

Pharmacokinetics (PK) is about the journey of a medicine through the body, from intake to excretion. After all, if a drug does not reach its target organ or tissue, it will not be effective.

A drug first enters the body, usually through the mouth and gastrointestinal tract or the anus. Furthermore, a drug may enter the body through the lungs, skin, vaginal mucosa, or an intravenous, intramuscular, or subcutaneous injection.

After that, the drug is absorbed into the blood circulation, thereby passing to the liver. Certain enzymes in the liver make drugs more water-soluble (hydrophilic) in order to excrete them via the urine or the faeces. This process is called metabolism.

The drug then is distributed throughout the body. It depends on the characteristics of the drug whether it prefers to spread in a 'watery' environment (the plasma and muscles; i.e. hydrophilic) or in a 'fatty' environment (tissue fat, bone marrow, and brain tissue; i.e. lipophilic). Also, if drugs are bound to proteins in the plasma, they are not capable of leaving the plasma.

Some of these processes change during pregnancy, as we will explain in the next paragraph.

Pharmacodynamics (PD) is about the drug's effect on the body. So, on the one hand, PD is about the therapeutic effect or the effectiveness of the drug. On the other hand, it concerns the unwanted effects or side effects. The effectiveness and side effects are inextricably linked, as most side effects result from the drug's pharmacological effect.

For a drug to have an effect, it must reach a target, mostly a receptor, through which a cascade of consequences leads to the therapeutic effect. However, drugs do not 'know' where to go. The drug merely spreads through the body based on blood circulation and its preference for watery or fatty tissue. As a result, the drug also reaches and triggers receptors in other organs. That is, in short, the mechanism by which side effects occur: the drug affects other receptors than just the target receptor. Consequently, sexual side effects might develop regardless of the medication used.

19.1.2 The Changes in PK and PD During Pregnancy

As midwives are most aware, pregnancy is associated with profound changes in the anatomy and physiology of the body, which affects PK and PD. For example, cardiac output increases in pregnancy. As a result, the blood flow through the liver, kidneys, and lungs increases. Consequently, the time decreases in which medication is metabolised and eliminated.

In addition, the blood plasma volume, the total amount of the 'watery environment', and the 'fatty environment' increase. Hence, hydrophilic drugs will have a lower plasma concentration. Besides, eliminating lipophilic drugs takes more time because they reside in an increased volume of fatty tissue and not in the blood plasma.

The binding of drugs to plasma proteins decreases during pregnancy, which means that a higher amount of the drug can bind to the target and affect whether therapeutic or unwanted.

The activity of the enzymes in the liver that metabolise several drugs change during pregnancy. Some enzymes become more active, while the activity of other enzymes decreases.

In the postpartum period, there is a substantial decrease in sex hormone levels, decreased plasma volume, and normalisation of liver enzyme activity and glomerular filtration rate (*GFR*, renal clearance).

All these PK changes affect the PD. On the one hand, a higher portion of the drug is free to reach the target. On the other hand, the drug might be eliminated faster than before pregnancy. The drug might also be metabolised quicker or slower than before pregnancy.

In conclusion, PK and PD change significantly during pregnancy. However, what it means in daily practice is hardly investigated. Therefore, the midwife's watchful eye is of crucial importance.

19.1.3 What It Means in Daily Practice

In daily practice, there is a clear distinction. Some medication was already taken before pregnancy or will be taken throughout and after pregnancy. On the other hand, there is medication taken only during pregnancy.

A woman who took a specific dosage of medicine before pregnancy might have to change the dosage during pregnancy. Dosage adjustment of medication continued after parturition is also paramount to avoid toxicity or ineffectiveness, depending on whether the woman used a higher or a lower dose during pregnancy. Examples of medication that need dosage adjustments during pregnancy are L-thyroxine, antiepileptic drugs and lithium, most frequently monitored by the prescribing medical specialist.

Dosage instructions are mostly described in the manuals for HCPs. Otherwise, one can consult the summary of the drug's product characteristics (SmPC). This SmPC can be found in the national registers of approved medication or on the European Medicines Agency (EMA) website. An overview of European registers can be found here.[1] The register of the EMA can be found here.[2]

- Please be aware that the general dosage recommendations, as stated in the SmPC or the manuals, might be either too low for a pregnant woman, or too high.

19.2 How Medication Affects Sexuality

As you can read in almost every chapter in this book, sexual responsiveness results from a complex interplay of biological, psychological, and social factors. This also means that sexual side effects of medication, which are in essence biological, can lead to secondary psychological and even social/relational issues.[3] Subsequently, these secondary issues may cause a deterioration of the sexual side effects or a continuation of sexual problems after the medication has been stopped.

---

[1] https://www.ema.europa.eu/en/medicines/national-registers-authorised-medicines

[2] https://www.ema.europa.eu/en/medicines

[3] For a more detailed explanation of this, see Chap. 1 on the BioPsychoSocial Model.

On the other hand, some medication may also improve sexual function, as shown in Table 19.1.

This book will focus on sexual side effects during pregnancy, childbirth and postpartum. In general, sexual issues that women most frequently report are alterations in sexual desire and arousability, in the amount of lubrication (with low lubrication potentially resulting in pain during or after penetration), and altered orgasm capacity.[4]

19.3 Medication in Detail

Pregnant women are, as said before, excluded from clinical medication trials. Therefore, the knowledge of side effects in pregnant women is scarce. Sexual side effects are not very well studied either. Furthermore, most medication prescribed during pregnancy is given for a short period. As a result, it was a complex task to provide an overview of sexual side effects associated with medication prescribed during pregnancy. Nonetheless, the list in Table 19.1 can be used as a guide.

The list intends to be as complete as possible for the safety and well-being of the woman. Hence, our purpose is neither to encourage nor to discourage prescribing the mentioned medication. Besides, we do not give judgement on the need for the medication or possible alternative therapies.

The list contains generic names since brand names differ per country. Only possible sexual side effects are mentioned. For the purpose of this book, we do not include teratogenic side effects.

---

[4] For a more detailed overview of sexual problems, see Chap. 3 on 'How sex works'.

Table 19.1 Potential sexual effects of medication prescribed before, during or after pregnancy

Medication group	Medication	Potential effects on sexuality during pregnancy
Vitamins	Vitamin D	No sexual side effects are described in scientific literature. Adverse effects on the sexual functions of the pregnant woman are unlikely Vitamin D positively influences gonadal hormone synthesis. Both desire, arousal, and orgasm may improve by vitamin D, and vaginal pain may diminish [1, 2]
	Folic acid	No sexual side effects are described in scientific literature. Adverse effects of folic acid are unlikely Theoretically, improved arousal might occur in pregnant women using folic acid. This assumption is based on a positive effect of folic acid therapy described in men with erectile dysfunction [3]
Analgetics	Butylscopolamine	No sexual side effects are described in scientific literature. Based on the mechanism of action, vaginal dryness and diminished arousability might occur during prolonged treatment

Table 19.1 (continued)

Medication group	Medication	Potential effects on sexuality during pregnancy
	Phloroglucinol	No sexual side effects are described in scientific literature. The mechanism of action is not well defined [4]. Therefore, no indication can be provided on the odds of causing sexual side effects
	Paracetamol/ acetaminophen	No sexual side effects are described in scientific literature. Adverse effects on the sexual functions of the pregnant woman are unlikely
	Pethidine	Opioids, like pethidine, are associated with a dose-dependent decline in sexual function due to a decrease in testosterone levels [5]. Women report a decline in arousal and, as a result, in lubrication [6]. Odds for sexual dysfunctions increase with treatment duration. Since pethidine is usually administered during a short period, sexual side effects are not very likely to occur
	Nitrous oxide gas	Positive sexual effects of analgesic nitrous oxide have been long reported anecdotally. Small scientific studies describe an objective decline in arousal since nitrous oxide is an opioid [7]. However, subjective arousal may occur due to increased sexual phantasies [8]. This effect is of short duration due to the wearing out of the gas
	Remifentanil	Opioids, like remifentanil, are associated with a dose-dependent decline in sexual function due to a decrease in testosterone levels [5]. Women report a decline in arousal and, as a result, in lubrication [6]. Odds for sexual dysfunctions increase with treatment duration. Since remifentanil is usually administered during a short period, sexual side effects are not very likely to occur
	Epidural morphine	Opioids, like morphine, are associated with a dose-dependent decline in sexual function due to a decrease in testosterone levels [5]. Women report a decline in arousal and, as a result, in lubrication [6]. Odds for sexual dysfunctions increase with treatment duration. Since epidural morphine is usually administered during a short period, sexual side effects are not very likely to occur
	Ketoprofen	Nonsteroidal anti-inflammatory drugs (NSAIDs) might be associated with erectile dysfunction in men [9]. The odds of sexual side effects (arousal) in pregnant women are low since the treatment duration is short
	Acetylsalicylic acid (aspirin®)	No sexual side effects are described in scientific literature. However, aspirin might increase vascular functions associated with objective arousal
Antibiotics		No sexual side effects are described in scientific literature. Adverse effects of antibiotics on the sexual functions of the pregnant woman are unlikely
Anticoagulant	Heparin	No sexual side effects are described in scientific literature. Adverse effects of anticoagulants on the sexual functions of the pregnant woman are unlikely

(continued)

Table 19.1 (continued)

Medication group	Medication	Potential effects on sexuality during pregnancy
Antidepressants	Selective serotonin reuptake inhibitors (*SSRIs*)	Sexual dysfunctions are common side effects of SSRIs. However, the indication itself is also associated with sexual dysfunction [10]. In pregnant women, it is expected that sexual side effects might occur as often as in non-pregnant women. Desire, arousal, lubrication, and orgasm may all be impaired. In scientific research, women most frequently report a decline in arousal, whereas in clinical practice (in the Netherlands), women most frequently report problems experiencing orgasms [11]
	Serotonin noradrenaline reuptake inhibitors (*SNRIs*)	Sexual dysfunctions are common side effects of SNRIs. However, the indication itself is also associated with sexual dysfunction [10]. In pregnant women, it is expected that sexual side effects might occur as often as in non-pregnant women. Desire, arousal, lubrication, and orgasm may all be impaired. In particular, orgasm might be delayed or absent [12]
	Tricyclic antidepressants (*TCAs*)	Sexual dysfunctions are common side effects of TCAs, most due to affinity for cholinergic, histaminergic, and adrenergic receptors [12]. However, the indication itself is also associated with sexual dysfunction [10]. In pregnant women, it is expected that sexual side effects might occur as often as in non-pregnant women. Desire, arousal, lubrication, and orgasm may all be impaired. Odds might be somewhat lower compared to SSRIs
Antiemetics		No scientific literature is available. However, because of the antiemetics' central dopamine antagonist property, they can be a potent stimulant of prolactin release. This might result in impaired desire and arousal
Beta-blockers	Labetalol	In healthy female volunteers, labetalol appeared to reduce vaginal lubrication [13]. Such effects can also be expected during pregnancy
Miscellaneous	Bisacodylum	No scientific literature is available. Based on its mechanism of action, sexual side effects are not expected
	Miconazole	No scientific literature is available. However, sexual activities during treatment are discouraged, since miconazole is administered through vaginal application. Local irritation of the vaginal mucosa might occur, leading to pain or contact bleeding during intercourse
	Progesterone	High progesterone levels negatively influence sexual desire in women, with a delay of 1–2 days [14]
	Thyroxine	Nearly 50% of women with hypothyroidism experience sexual dysfunctions (impairments in desire, arousal/lubrication, orgasm, satisfaction, and pain during intercourse) [15]. Thyroxine treatment has been shown to resolve such issues. If not, adding liothyronine can ameliorate the sexual issues [16]. However, higher-than-normal levels of thyroxine may cause vaginal dryness, resulting in pain during intercourse

Table 19.1 (continued)

Medication group	Medication	Potential effects on sexuality during pregnancy
	Topical steroids	No scientific literature is available on topical steroids and sexual side effects. However, chronic systemic treatment with steroids decreases testosterone levels in men [17]. This can also be expected to occur in women during pregnancy. Reduced testosterone levels result in impairment in desire and arousal. Topical steroids may have systemic effects if administered for several days and on severely affected skin or a large surface
	Calcium	No scientific literature is available on calcium supplement intake and sexual side effects. However, in patients with hypercalcemia due to hyperparathyroidism, sexual dysfunctions are reported [18]. Theoretically, pregnant women with higher-than-normal calcium levels could experience sexual impairments, but it is not very likely
	Iron	Iron deficiency anaemia is associated with sexual dysfunctions. Suppletion of iron improves sexual functions in females [19, 20]. However, iron overload impairs sexual function due to decreased luteinising hormone (LH) production—i.e. hypogonadotropic hypogonadism, which, in turn, could affect the pregnancy [21]. Therefore, iron overload should be avoided
	Human intravenous immunoglobulin	There are no data on human intravenous immunoglobulin and sexual side effects in scientific literature [22]. No sexual impairment is to be expected
	Insulin	No scientific literature is available on sexual side effects associated with the use of insulin. The lack of studies might be the result of diabetes itself being a significant risk factor for sexual impairment. Based on its mechanism of action, it is not to be expected that insulin might cause sexual side effects in pregnant women
Antacids	Aluminium-magnesium hydroxide carbonate	No scientific literature is available on this antacid and its sexual side effects. Based on its mechanism of action, it is not to be expected that aluminium-magnesium hydroxide carbonate might cause sexual side effects in pregnant women
	Magnesium sulphate	No scientific literature is available on magnesium sulphate and sexual side effects. Based on its mechanism of action, it is not to be expected that it might cause sexual side effects in pregnant women
	Prostaglandin	Prostaglandin E1 as a topical agent applied to the clitoris increases the peak systolic blood flow in the clitoris [23]. This could lead to a feeling of sexual arousal. When applied to the cervix, it is not expected that such effects will occur
	Oxytocin	Increased sexual arousal and, as a result, lubrication have been reported anecdotally after incidental nasal application of oxytocin [24]. It is also known that breastfeeding, leading to an oxytocin peak, can lead to sexual arousal. However, in clinical studies with nasal application of oxytocin, no facilitatory effect of oxytocin on sexual functioning could be confirmed [25–27]. In conclusion, sexual feelings might occur during this stage of pregnancy but are not very likely

(continued)

Table 19.1 (continued)

Medication group	Medication	Potential effects on sexuality during pregnancy
	Betamethasone	No scientific literature is available on antenatal glucocorticoid therapy and sexual side effects. Based on its mechanism of action, sexual side effects might occur in pregnant women due to lower free testosterone levels as a side effect of chronic oral glucocorticoid therapy [28]. If glucocorticoid therapy is given for a short time, then no sexual side effects are expected
	Atosiban	No scientific literature is available on atosiban and its sexual side effects. Based on its mechanism of action, it is not to be expected that it will cause sexual side effects in pregnant women
	Nifedipine	The scientific literature on nifedipine and sexual side effects describes problems with ejaculation in men [29]. Reduced sexual desire has been described in women during treatment with calcium channel blockers [30]

19.4 How to Deal with Suspected Sexual Side Effects

19.4.1 When to Suspect a Sexual Side Effect

Determining whether an undesired symptom is an adverse drug reaction (*ADR*) is difficult. The reported symptom could be caused by the medication, by the underlying indication for which the drug has been prescribed, or by other factors which might be unrelated. In the case of sexual symptoms, psychological or social factors may play a role or even be the causal factor of a sexual undesired symptom.

An Illustrative Case

A 38-year old married woman receives antidepressant medication for a depressive disorder. After 2 months, she reports a slight improvement in her depressive symptoms. As side effects, she states that her weight has increased from 63 to 68 kg and that she cannot reach orgasm during sex with her husband. This is new to her.

Although lack of orgasm is a well-known side effect of antidepressants, other factors should be considered. First, the underlying disease could play a role, as depression is most frequently associated with declining sexual satisfaction. Second, the weight increase might result in lower self-esteem in the woman or a decline in her husband's sexual appetite. Both might lead to a reduction in sexual satisfaction. Third, the partner might be over-focused on his wife having orgasms, resulting in pressure on the woman.

Table 19.2 WHO-UMC causality categories (https://www.who.int/medicines/areas/quality_safety/safety_efficacy/WHOcausality_assessment.pdf)

Causality term	Assessment criteria[a]
Certain	• Event or laboratory test abnormality, with plausible time relationship to drug intake • Cannot be explained by disease or other drugs • Response to withdrawal plausible (pharmacologically, pathologically) • Event definitive pharmacologically or phenomenologically (i.e. an objective and specific medical disorder or a recognised pharmacological phenomenon) • Rechallenge satisfactory, if necessary
Probable/likely	• Event or laboratory test abnormality, with reasonable time relationship to drug intake • Unlikely to be attributed to disease or other drugs • Response to withdrawal clinically reasonable • Rechallenge not required
Possible	• Event or laboratory test abnormality, with reasonable time relationship to drug intake • Could also be explained by disease or other drugs • Information on drug withdrawal may be lacking or unclear
Unlikely	• Event or laboratory test abnormality, with a time to drug intake that makes a relationship improbable (but not impossible) • Disease or other drugs provide plausible explanations
Conditional/unclassified	• Event or laboratory test abnormality • More data for proper assessment needed, or • Additional data under examination
Unassessable/unclassifiable	• Report suggesting an adverse reaction • Cannot be judged because the information is insufficient or contradictory • Data cannot be supplemented or verified

[a]All points should be reasonably complied with

In daily practice, establishing a causal relationship is merely based on clinical judgement. However, this assessment depends on the knowledge and experience of the HCP. To overcome this issue, several causality assessment tools have been developed. A systematic and validated method for the appraisal of the probability of an ADR is the Naranjo score. Answering ten questions leads to a probability score of an ADR. However, the Naranjo score is more time-consuming than the World Health Organization-Uppsala Monitoring Center (WHO-UMC) criteria [31]. Therefore, the latter is shown in Table 19.2. The WHO-UMC has written a comprehensible text on using the criteria, which can be found via this link.

19.4.2 How to Inquire After Sexual Side Effects?

General reccommendations with regard to talking about sex are discussed in other chapters. Therefore, this paragraph will focus only on the inquiry into the sexual side effects of medication.

Consider talking about side effects in general and sexual side effects as your responsibility since you are a medical professional who will talk about sexuality and sexual side effects more frequently than the woman sitting in your office. Naturally, it might not be easy, but gradually you will become more comfortable.

Before starting, it might help to tell the patient that many people, both patients and HCPs, find sexuality a bit difficult topic to talk openly about, but you consider it too important to avoid the subject. Then you ask for permission or make a general statement. Here are some examples the authors frequently use:

'Many people using antidepressants experience sexual difficulties. Does that also apply to you?'

'Many people with these medications have an increase or a decrease in sex drive. Others experience no difference. May I ask how it applies to you?'

'Sexual complaints are often reported with this medication. Do you mind if we talk about that?'

'Some people report an improvement in their sexual functioning; others a deterioration. Since starting your medication, have you noticed a change in your sexual functioning?'

After receiving an answer, consider it your duty to inquire as detailed as necessary to understand the exact problem. In addition, consider other factors in order to assess a causal relation with the medication. Next, explain your thoughts or conclusions. Do that also when you do not know what to do. Most women will feel relieved having talked about their concerns.[5]

19.4.3 How to Manage Sexual Side Effects

Most side effects are not severe and only need explanation. This holds for sexual side effects as well, and even more for medication prescribed during a short period.

When the woman is suffering from sexual side effects, and an explanation is insufficient, dose reduction might be an option. Since dose reduction usually implies a reduction in the therapeutic effect, it is important to consider whether the woman needs the therapeutic effect for her own well-being or for her unborn child.

> **Another Illustrative Case**
>
> A pregnant woman had epilepsy, including grand mal seizures. That is successfully treated with levetiracetam (an antiepileptic drug). The patient reports a decline in desire, arousal, lubrication and orgasm since the start of the medication. She wishes to switch the medication or lower the dose because she suffers from stress due to the side effects.
>
> In this case, one should consider the following strategy. First, although levetiracetam may improve sexual function, patients may experience a decline [32]. Second, the woman experiences stress due to the sexual side effects. This stress will have a certain influence on the unborn child. Third, dose reduction increases the risk of a return of the seizures, which can be supposed

---

[5] For more information on how to talk about sexuality with clients, see Chap. 26 on "Talking Sex".

to be a more significant threat to the woman and her unborn child. Therefore, a dose reduction or cessation of the antiepileptic medication might be considered inappropriate.

Again, it is important to state that even if dose reduction or cessation of the medication is appropriate, the sexual problems might continue. In that case, the causal relation with the medication might be questioned, or the problems might have evolved into secondary psychological or relational issues.

Most of the time, the cessation of medication due to sexual side effects will not be very common in midwifery since the medication will only be given during a (very) short period. In any case, always follow the tapering (i.e. dose reduction) and cessation advice of the medication guidelines.

When prescribing medication, the midwife has to inform the pregnant woman of possible side effects. This chapter provided support for adequate information about sexual side effects.

19.5 Conclusion

In conclusion, the medication used before and during pregnancy and in the perinatal period may affect sexuality. The role of the midwife in discussing sexual side effects is most valuable, given their role as a 'spider' in the medical 'web' of the pregnant woman. Even if a midwife does not have prescribing rights, inquiring after sexual side effects is essential. With the knowledge provided in this chapter, the midwife can undertake a judgement of the causality of sexual changes. And when sexual side effects are present, referral to the prescribing physician is recommended. And of course, referral to a sexologist is also preferable, especially if psychological or social (relationship) factors play a role.

References

1. Jalali-Chimeh F, Gholamrezaei A, Vafa M, et al. Effect of vitamin D therapy on sexual function in women with sexual dysfunction and vitamin D deficiency: a randomised, double-blind, placebo controlled clinical trial. J Urol. 2019;201(5):987–93. https://doi.org/10.1016/j.juro.2018.10.019.
2. Krysiak R, Szwajkosz A, Marek B, et al. The effect of vitamin D supplementation on sexual functioning and depressive symptoms in young women with low vitamin D status. Endokrynol Pol. 2018;69(2):168–74. https://doi.org/10.5603/EP.a2018.0013.
3. Elshahid ARM, Shahein IM, Mohammed YF, et al. Folic acid supplementation improves erectile function in patients with idiopathic vasculogenic erectile dysfunction by lowering peripheral and penile homocysteine plasma levels: a case-control study. Andrology. 2020;8(1):148–53. https://doi.org/10.1111/andr.12672.
4. ANSM (Agence national de sécurité du médicament et des produits de santé). Résumé des caractéristiques du produit—Phloroglucinol/trimethylphloroglucinol. [Online] 2022 [cited 2022 Jan 31]. http://agence-prd.ansm.sante.fr/php/ecodex/frames.php?specid=60294485&typedoc=R&ref=R0373253.htm.

5. Rubinstein AL, Carpenter DM, Minkoff JR. Hypogonadism in men with chronic pain linked to the use of long-acting rather than short-acting opioids. Clin J Pain. 2013;29(10):840–5. https://doi.org/10.1097/AJP.0b013e31827c7b5d.

6. Ajo R, Segura A, Inda MM, et al. Opioids increase sexual dysfunction in patients with non-cancer pain. J Sex Med. 2016;13(9):1377–86. https://doi.org/10.1016/j.jsxm.2016.07.003.

7. Gillman MA. Assessment of the effects of analgesic concentrations of nitrous oxide on human sexual response. Int J Neurosci. 1988;43(1-2):27–33. https://doi.org/10.3109/00207458808985777.

8. Gillman MA, Lichtigfeld FJ. The effects of nitrous oxide and naloxone on orgasm in human females: a preliminary report. J Sex Res. 1983;19(1):49–57. https://doi.org/10.1080/00224498309551168.

9. Shiri R, Koskimäki J, Häkkinen J, et al. Effect of nonsteroidal anti-inflammatory drug use on the incidence of erectile dysfunction. J Urol. 2006;175(5):1812–5. https://doi.org/10.1016/S0022-5347(05)01000-1; discussion 1815-6.

10. Jing E, Straw-Wilson K. Sexual dysfunction in selective serotonin reuptake inhibitors (SSRIs) and potential solutions: a narrative literature review. Ment Health Clin. 2016;6(4):191–6. https://doi.org/10.9740/mhc.2016.07.191.

11. Serretti A, Chiesa A. Treatment-emergent sexual dysfunction related to antidepressants: a meta-analysis. J Clin Psychopharmacol. 2009;29(3):259–66. https://doi.org/10.1097/JCP.0b013e3181a5233f.

12. Higgins A, Nash M, Lynch AM. Antidepressant-associated sexual dysfunction: impact, effects, and treatment. Drug Healthc Patient Saf. 2010;2:141–50. https://doi.org/10.2147/DHPS.S7634. Epub 2010 Sep 9.

13. Duncan L, Bateman DN. Sexual function in women. Do antihypertensive drugs have an impact? Drug Saf. 1993;8(3):225–34. https://doi.org/10.2165/00002018-199308030-00004.

14. Roney JR, Simmons ZL. Hormonal predictors of sexual motivation in natural menstrual cycles. Horm Behav. 2013;63(4):636–45. https://doi.org/10.1016/j.yhbeh.2013.02.013.

15. Gabrielson AT, Sartor RA, Hellstrom WJG. The impact of thyroid disease on sexual dysfunction in men and women. Sex Med Rev. 2019;7(1):57–70. https://doi.org/10.1016/j.sxmr.2018.05.002. Epub 2018 Jul 26.

16. Krysiak R, Szkróbka W, Okopień B. Sexual function and depressive symptoms in young women with hypothyroidism receiving levothyroxine/liothyronine combination therapy: a pilot study. Curr Med Res Opin. 2018;34(9):1579–86. https://doi.org/10.1080/03007995.2018.1448771.

17. MacAdams MR, White RH, Chipps BE. Reduction of serum testosterone levels during chronic glucocorticoid therapy. Ann Intern Med. 1986;104(5):648–51. https://doi.org/10.7326/0003-4819-104-5-648.

18. Norman J. Sexual dysfunction and loss of sexual desire due to hyperparathyroidism [Online]. 2013. https://www.parathyroid.com/blog/sexual-dysfunction-sex-problems-hyperparathyroidism. Accessed 31 Jan 2022.

19. Gulmez H, Akin Y, Savas M, et al. Impact of iron supplementation on sexual dysfunction of women with iron deficiency anemia in short term: a preliminary study. J Sex Med. 2014;11(4):1042–6. https://doi.org/10.1111/jsm.12454.

20. Nikzad Z, Iravani M, Abedi P, et al. The relationship between iron deficiency anemia and sexual function and satisfaction among reproductive-aged Iranian women. PLoS One. 2018;13(12):e0208485. https://doi.org/10.1371/journal.pone.0208485.

21. Gabrielsen JS, Lamb DJ, Lipshultz LI. Iron and a man's reproductive health: the good, the bad, and the ugly. Curr Urol Rep. 2018;19(8):60. https://doi.org/10.1007/s11934-018-0808-x.

22. Orbach H, Katz U, Sherer Y, et al. Intravenous immunoglobulin: adverse effects and safe administration. Clin Rev Allergy Immunol. 2005;29(3):173–84. https://doi.org/10.1385/CRIAI:29:3:173.

23. Dirim A, Goren MR, Peskircioglu L. The effect of topical synthetic prostaglandin E1 (misoprostol) on clitoral hemodynamics. J Sex Med. 2011;8(3):800–5. https://doi.org/10.1111/j.1743-6109.2010.02096.x.

24. Anderson-Hunt M, Dennerstein L. Increased female sexual response after oxytocin. BMJ. 1994;309(6959):929. https://doi.org/10.1136/bmj.309.6959.929.
25. Kruger THC, Deiter F, Zhang Y, et al. Effects of intranasal oxytocin administration on sexual functions in healthy women: a laboratory paradigm. J Clin Psychopharmacol. 2018;38(3):239–42. https://doi.org/10.1097/JCP.0000000000000863.
26. Melis MR, Argiolas A. Oxytocin, erectile function and sexual behavior: last discoveries and possible advances. Int J Mol Sci. 2021;22(19):10376. https://doi.org/10.3390/ijms221910376.
27. Muin DA, Wolzt M, Marculescu R, et al. Effect of long-term intranasal oxytocin on sexual dysfunction in premenopausal and postmenopausal women: a randomised trial. Fertil Steril. 2015;104(3):715–23.e4. https://doi.org/10.1016/j.fertnstert.2015.06.010.
28. Björk Y, Smith Knutsson E, Ankarberg-Lindgren C, et al. Androgens in women after allogeneic hematopoietic cell transplantation: impact of chronic GvHD and glucocorticoid therapy. Bone Marrow Transplant. 2017;52(3):431–7. https://doi.org/10.1038/bmt.2016.268.
29. Suzuki H, Tominaga T, Kumagai H, et al. Effects of first-line antihypertensive agents on sexual function and sex hormones. J Hypertens Suppl. 1988;6(4):S649–51. https://doi.org/10.1097/00004872-198812040-00204.
30. Goldberg JP, Crenshaw TL. ACE inhibitors and calcium channel blockers. In: Goldberg JP, Crenshaw TL, editors. Sexual pharmacology. New York: Norton Professional Books; 1996. p. 239–50.
31. Belhekar MN, Taur SR, Munshi RP. A study of agreement between the naranjo algorithm and WHO-UMC criteria for causality assessment of adverse drug reactions. Indian J Pharm. 2014;46(1):117–20. https://doi.org/10.4103/0253-7613.125192.
32. Yang Y, Wang X. Sexual dysfunction related to antiepileptic drugs in patients with epilepsy. Expert Opin Drug Saf. 2016;15(1):31–42. https://doi.org/10.1517/14740338.2016.1112376.

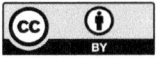

Part IV

Introduction to Module 4: 'Special Topics'

Woet L. Gianotten, Sam Geuens, and Ana Polona Mivšek

In midwifery training courses, the student will gradually expand the areas of knowledge and expertise. One starts with the normal processes before the less familiar and more demanding areas are addressed. This book has followed the same logic.

In Module 2, we first addressed the various sexual aspects of the physiological course before addressing in Module 3 the sexual aspects when physical diseases and other conditions disturb that process of prenatal, intranatal and postnatal period. The midwife usually goes through a comparable learning curve. At the beginning of the training, the average student will learn custom cases, after which gradually, the less common cases will appear in the training process: women from a different culture, with a different sexual orientation, women who have been sexually abused or who have been circumcised.

Because sexuality can be rather different in the life of these women, we have included separate chapters for each of those areas.

The module will start with two chapters on topics that we cannot put under the caption 'different midwifery practice cases'. The first one will deal with the sexual aspects of contraception, the other with the experiences of a male partner.

We advise readers, especially midwifery students, who use this book as a textbook, to start with Chap. 26 on how to communicate about sexuality, which is an essential skill needed to put the information of Module 4 to good use in clinical practice.

Chapter 20: Contraception and Sexuality

In some countries, midwives have become responsible for part of general contraceptive care. That is different from many other countries where contraception is not a part of the midwife's scope of practice. They might counsel only about contraception with respect to intervals between pregnancies. For healthy motherhood and good parenthood, the young mother should not become pregnant within a year and a half after childbirth. So counselling or even prescribing contraception, as an integral part of good postpartum care, falls under the midwife's responsibility.

Whatever contraceptive method we consider, every method has advantages and disadvantages, whether physical, emotional, relational, or sexual.

This chapter will address the sexual consequences of various contraceptive methods. It will provide up-to-date information on the advantages and disadvantages of each method regarding sexuality. In the context of this book, contraception during postpartum and breastfeeding will get extra attention.

The chapter will include information on emergency contraception and the situation when contraception fails.

Chapter 21: Sexual Aspects of Pregnancy and the Postpartum in Non-Mainstream Orientation

In some parts of the world, one can barely imagine that a woman could have a sexual relationship with another woman. However, in other countries, same-sex marriage has become accepted and legalized.

As a logical part of that social and legal development, lesbian couples can decide on pregnancy and motherhood. This chapter will deal with relevant aspects of sexuality in lesbian couples who have decided to start a family with their own children.

The chapter will pay attention to the phase of decision, conception, and beyond. It will also provide recommendations on how to give good care to the lesbian couple, especially concerning sexuality. Those lessons are relevant for everyone, especially for HCPs in cultures where people have not yet developed a greater degree of acceptance (and respect) for lesbian women.

Chapter 22: Male Experience(s)

In the Western world, the man's role in pregnancy has long appeared somewhat limited. After the joint activity of creating the pregnancy, the man barely got attention till the birth, and even then, he was often portrayed as nervously smoking in the waiting room. Nowadays, that has become very different in many parts of the world, with men participating in antenatal classes, birth, and parenting courses.

This chapter will address various aspects of the male partner, which will go beyond only his role during the birth or his role as a father-to-be. It will also look into the psychological and existential changes he faces throughout pregnancy, childbirth, and postpartum. The chapter will also discuss the physical (and even hormonal) changes that can happen to him. All these processes can affect his sexuality.

It will elaborate on the man's sexual life during and after this life-changing experience. One reason to pay good attention to this area is that in postpartum, the difference between the man's and the woman's sexuality can become a hot topic and even a serious couple problem.

The other reason to address this area is that, in many places, midwifery is a nearly exclusively female profession that hence almost exclusively deals with women's issues. However, for good, family-focused care, the midwife needs some understanding of the male's view. This chapter offers some specific information on such 'male perspective'.

Chapter 23: Relevant (Sexual) Aspects of Cultural Differences

One cannot properly address sexuality in midwifery without also paying attention to culture, one of the most important elements influencing the sexual lives of people. Factors like traditionalism, religion, polygamy, machismo, and feminism influence sexuality and also cultural ideas about motherhood and sex roles.

Cultural differences do not only exist by merit of geographical distance since cultures get intermingled. There are differences between our own home and 'next-door'. Due to economic migration, political refugees, and global traffic, our neighbourhoods and patient populations have become multicultured and multicoloured.

Even midwifery as an organized profession and a field of study has significant cultural differences between one country and another. While in some countries, the midwife can guide childbirth independently at home, other countries prohibit this by law. While in some countries, the midwife provides postpartum contraception, in other countries, they don't. This cultural context also affects the practice that midwives provide.

Since this is an English language book, one could conclude that the focus will be more or less on Western maternity care. It will certainly have a European touch as most authors work in Europe. At least one of the advantages of Western and Northwestern Europe is a more open and pragmatic discussion of sexual topics. While sexuality is essential everywhere, we are aware that a basic need for health and luxury must be fulfilled before it seems relevant to tackle some of the problematic aspects of sexuality. Therefore, we believe this book will be of value to midwives working in middle and high-income countries or environments worldwide [1]. On the other hand, much of the information will also be handy for urban midwives in middle and low-income countries.

Chapter 24: Sexual Effects of Trauma Experience on Pregnancy and Labour

No woman who becomes pregnant is a tabula rasa ('a blank slate'). She carries memories and experiences from her past—usually a mixture of positive and negative ones. However, those experiences and memories are mainly negative or very negative for some women. Incidentally, the list of traumatic experiences does include not only incest and rape but also other forms of family violence, emotional deprivation, war traumas, and bullying.

To provide good care, the midwife/HCP should be aware that those negative experiences can strongly influence how the woman reacts to various direct forms of physical contact. As a consequence of those negative experiences, some women can respond differently to the pregnancy, the birth, and sometimes even to their newborn baby. That can happen consciously and somewhat unconsciously based on deep-down memories of the traumatic experience. A history of forced vaginal penetration can later make a vaginal examination a traumatic experience. A history of sexual abuse involving the breasts can later make breastfeeding a frightening experience.

This chapter will elaborate on the sexual consequences and other consequences of traumatic experiences and practical implications, including how the midwife/HCP should or should not behave when caring for women with a traumatic past.

Chapter 25: Relevant Aspects of Female Genital Mutilation

FGM is also named female genital cutting or female circumcision. In 2016, UNICEF estimated that, across the globe, 200 million women and girls had undergone this procedure. It is practised mainly in some 30 countries in Africa and the Middle East, and from those countries, many women and girls migrated to countries in Europe and other parts of the world.

The physical damage and consequences of FGM depend on the extent of the procedure and on the medical and hygienic conditions during the event. On the one hand, these women deserve proper care regarding their medical and obstetrical side effects. This chapter will address some of the expected urological, gynaecological, and obstetrical consequences for the midwife who meets women with FGM through-out pregnancy, childbirth, and postpartum. On the other hand, this chapter will include some of the variety of psychological, sexual, and social impacts of FGM.

It can be somewhat confusing for the midwife who doesn't work (or doesn't yet work) in a multicultural setting when confronted with women after FGM. So the chapter will elaborate on 'How to approach the woman after FGM in a respectful and caring manner'.

Reference
1. Rosling H, Rosling O, Rosling-Rönnlund A. Factfulness; ten reasons why we are wrong about the World and why things are better than you think. Sceptre. 2018.

Contraception and Sexuality

20

Johannes Bitzer [ORCID]

20.1 Introduction

Contraception separates sexuality from reproduction, thus allowing women and men to express and live their sexuality (more or less) free of the fear of unintended pregnancies. Not wanting to get pregnant is based on a myriad of reasons which have to do with life circumstances and life plans.

Thus, contraception is an essential contribution to sexual and reproductive health, both before becoming pregnant and after the pregnancy. Unplanned pregnancies can confront the woman and her partner with a difficult decision regarding termination or continuation. Both options pose medical and psychosocial risks to the woman's health and the child's health in case of continuation. Proper contraception allows reliable planning and preparation for a pregnancy in a reproductive life plan.

For the woman's optimal reproductive and sexual health, contraception after childbirth deserves the same respect and attention. Another pregnancy soon after childbirth increases the risk of pregnancy complications, reduces the vital period of breastfeeding, and endangers family stability and child development. A pregnancy within 18 months increases premature rupture of membranes and placenta previa compared with becoming pregnant after 18–36 months [1].

Therefore, the midwife has a crucial role in contraceptive counselling and care before pregnancy and postpartum.

This chapter will start with general information about contraceptive counselling, followed by an overview of contraception and sexuality. The different contraceptive methods will be reviewed for their possible positive or negative impact on sexuality, followed by specific aspects of postpartum counselling. Since any method can fail,

J. Bitzer (✉)
Department of Obstetrics and Gynecology, University Hospital Basel, Basel, Switzerland
e-mail: johannes.bitzer@usb.ch

© The Author(s) 2023
S. Geuens et al. (eds.), *Midwifery and Sexuality*,
https://doi.org/10.1007/978-3-031-18432-1_20

the chapter will address two backup possibilities, including emergency contraception and abortion. Finally, the elements and practice of sexual counselling in contraception will be explained.

20.2 Contraceptive Methods

Just as a reminder, Fig. 20.1 gives a pictorial overview of the most common contraception methods and their reliability (redrawn from: https://www.optionsforsexualhealth.org/facts/birth-control/).

Contraceptive methods can be associated with health risks.

The WHO regularly updates the scientific evidence regarding these risks in the Medical Eligibility Criteria [2]. These criteria describe the risks for the most important clinical conditions for all available methods. The risk classification comprises four categories.

Category 1: A condition for which there is no restriction on the use of the contraceptive method.

Categories 2 and 3: A condition where one can weigh the advantages and risks of using the contraceptive method.

Category 4: A condition representing an unacceptable health risk for a given contraceptive method.

Fig. 20.1 The reliability of contraception

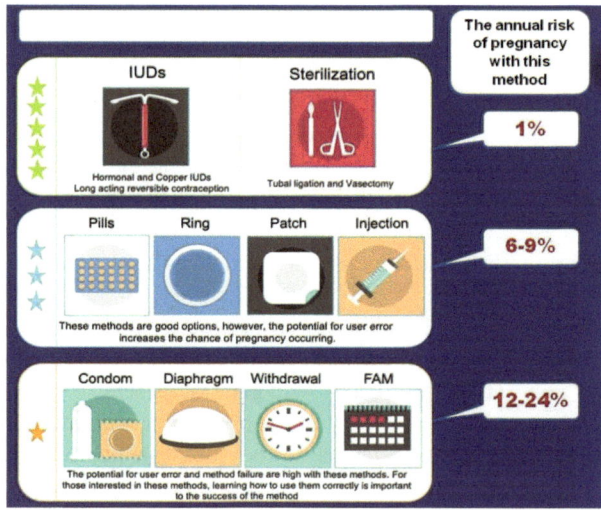

20.3 Contraception and Sexual Function

Although contraception plays a significant positive role in women's sexual and reproductive health, many studies indicate that women and men may experience both positive and negative consequences of contraception on their sexual well-being and sexual function.

How is this possible?

There are several levels or dimensions on which contraceptive methods can interact with the sexuality of the woman (or man) and the couple.

Separating reproduction from sexuality, although being the objective of contraception and although intended to create freedom, can on an emotional level also be experienced as a deprivation of a profound potency or detract from the essential meaning of the sexual encounter

(a) Contraceptive methods can interfere with *the physiology and neurobiology of the sexual response.*

   The physiology of the sexual response is under the influence of a complex interaction of three hormones: oestrogens, testosterone, and progesterone.

   Estrogens make the brain receptive to the influence of testosterone, and they are essential for the integrity of the vaginal mucosa.

   Testosterone (and other androgen hormones) are needed for sexual desire and influence the frequency of sexual thoughts, sexual fantasies, and nocturnal genital responses. With significant interindividual differences, androgens increase the sensitivity of brains and genitals to sexual stimulation (arousability or 'being horny') [3].

   Progesterone's role in sexuality is not yet well understood. It may have an indirect effect via a reduction of anxiety and stress. But that is still under investigation.

   These hormones exert their effects via the interaction with different neurotransmitters like serotonin, noradrenaline, and acetylcholine, in that way allowing a large variety of responses depending on the receptors in the target cells of the brain.

   Hormonal contraceptives influence these physiological processes resulting in changes that may go unnoticed but may also have obvious consequences. The results of those changes can facilitate but also inhibit the sexual response mechanisms.

(b) Contraceptive methods can both have a negative and a positive *impact on the general physical and mental well-being.*

(c) Contraceptive methods can *directly impact the relationship and the sexual encounter.*

(d) Contraceptive methods can have a 'social image' that may influence sexual well-being (an example, anxiety regarding risks may harm sexual arousal).

The impact of all these factors can be further modified and influenced by pre-existing sexual health conditions or pre-existing sexual problems.

20.3.1 Combined Hormonal Contraceptive (CHC)

20.3.1.1 Separating Sexuality and Reproduction

The contraceptive pill ('the pill') has two features that can affect inwardly ambivalent women about this separation. One is the high efficacy which makes the separation so effective, thus activating the ambivalence. The other is controlling this effect by the user's adherence or non-adherence.

Ambivalence can thus manifest itself in sexual 'dysfunction' or compliance difficulties.

20.3.1.2 Impact on the Physiology and Endocrine Regulation

Combined hormonal contraceptives contain oestrogens and progestogens. The progestogens are the primary ovulation-inhibiting substance. Since, during hormonal contraception, the ovaries do not produce enough (endogenous) oestrogens, artificial oestrogens are added ('replaced').

Combined hormonal contraceptives can interact with sexual physiology on several levels:

(a) They reduce the fluctuation of ovarian hormones through the cycle and block ovulation.
(b) They increase to different degrees SHBG,[1] reducing the free testosterone levels. SHBG is a globulin in the bloodstream that tightly binds to testosterone and oestradiol, by which they lose their bioavailability. Then, the body can use only the tiny part that stays bioavailable.
(c) They partly replace the natural hormones and change the sum of estrogenic and progestogenic actions.

We must realise that most women do not become aware that these changes are physical or mental symptoms because the female body is 'used' to hormonal fluctuations and changes in hormonal concentration (like menstrual cycle and pregnancy).

In part of the women, these changes may have the following effects:

- Not enough oestrogen action: irregular blood loss. Some women can get vaginal dryness.
- That is not the same as lacking lubrication (insufficient lubrication during sexuality usually means insufficient sexual stimulation).
- *Too much oestrogen action: increased SHBG → reduced free testosterone level with subsequent lowered desire and arousability.* Those anti-androgenic effects of oestrogen may or may not be counteracted by the more or less androgenic potency of the progestogen used.
- *Not enough testosterone action: lowered desire and arousability.*
- *Too much testosterone action: skin and hair problems.*

---

[1] SHBG = Sex hormone-binding globulin, a protein in the bloodstream.

- *Too little progestogen:*?
- *Too much progestogen: antiestrogenic effect.*

20.3.1.3   Impact on General Well-Being
Combined hormonal contraceptives can have positive or negative effects on general well-being, which indirectly can influence sexual well-being.

Possible positive effects of CHC are:

- Reduction of heavy menstrual bleeding and dysmenorrhea.
- Reduction of cycle-related complaints like PMS (premenstrual syndrome) and PMDD (premenstrual dysphoric disorder) mainly when used in a long-cycle-manner (i.e. continue taking pills for several cycles or till a breakthrough bleeding).
- Improvement of hyperandrogenic skin and hair disorders (acne, hirsutism) with a positive impact on body image.

Possible adverse effects of CHC are:

- Irregular bleeding,
- subjective weight gain,
- irritability,
- mood instability,
- skin symptoms.

20.3.1.4   Impact on the Relationship
CHC can help partners enjoy sexuality without fear of pregnancy and the consequences of unintended pregnancies on the relationship.

However, one partner, especially the woman, can view the responsibility for using contraception as 'unjust', expecting that the other partner should take over the responsibility. The woman may feel forced into taking hormones which may change her personal view on the tolerability of the method, and the sexual encounter.

20.3.1.5   The Role of the Social Image
As mentioned before, the woman can, on the one hand, perceive combined hormonal contraceptives as welcome tools of female emancipation. On the other hand, she can perceive them as 'big pharma' manipulation tools that will depend on the information in the media and the lack of proper reproductive health education (including pictures and stories). The threats and dangers of taking the pill are extensively spread in some countries, whereas the beneficial effects do not receive attention ('Only bad news is good news!'). It is, for instance, seldomly mentioned that having used CHC for some years will substantially reduce the incidence of colorectal cancer and even strongly reduce the incidence of ovarian cancer and endometrial cancer [4].

20.3.2 Progestogen-Only Contraceptives

Progestogen contraceptives include progestogen-only pills, LNG-IUDs, LNG implants, and long-acting progestogen injections (medroxyprogesterone = Depo-Provera®).

20.3.2.1 Separating Sexuality and Reproduction

The impact on the separation between sexuality and reproduction is the same as described above for CHC. When it comes to the long-acting methods like LNG-IUDs and LNG implants, the fact that the method needs a medical professional for insertion and removal may increase the feeling of loss of control, which can negatively impact the inner perception of the method and the emotional reaction to it (being a foreign body which is not under control like ingesting a pill).

20.3.2.2 Physiology of the Sexual Response

Progestogen-only contraceptives effectively inhibit ovulation.

The main differences in comparison with CHC are the following:

(a) There is no increase in SHGB and thus no reduction of free testosterone. In observational studies, progestogen-only users do not observe the loss of interest or desire as seen in users of combined hormonal contraceptives.
(b) There is a reduction of oestrogen supply, with different degrees in different methods.
    That depends on the dose of the progestogen applied. The highest progestogen exposure is in the users of Depot progestogen injections. A rather negative impact could be the reduction in the thickness of the vaginal wall and a reduction in blood flow during arousal. But there are no studies yet proving this.

20.3.2.3 Impact of Progestogens on General Well-Being

Possible positive effects:

• They can improve well-being by reducing dysmenorrhea and heavy menstrual bleeding,
• In some women, they may mitigate pre-existing premenstrual syndrome (PMS).

Possible negative effects:

• Irregular bleeding,
• Unwanted amenorrhoea,
• Acne,
• Weight gain (especially with Depo-Provera®).

The impact on the relationship can be the same as with combined hormonal contraceptives.

The role of the social image depends very much on whether the progestogen-only contraceptives are perceived as 'hormones like in the pill' (bad news) or as to how dose preparations without thrombotic risks (good news).

Another aspect of the social image concerns news about depression, mainly in adolescents.

20.3.3 Copper IUD

The copper IUD is an effective contraceptive method with a good safety profile.

There is no impact on the physiology of the sexual response.

An indirect negative impact would be on those women who have heavy menstrual bleeding or pain during or between menstruations.

When the threads are cut too short, they can cause pain to the penetrating penis.

The psychological impact of a very effective method outside the woman's control may also have an indirect negative effect on the 'inner representation' of the method, which she could theoretically experience as less pleasurable sexuality.

There are, however, no studies proving such an association.

20.3.4 Local Barrier Methods (Condom, Cervical Cap, Female Condom)

Both male condoms and female condoms protect against unwanted pregnancies and many STIs when properly used. Therefore, they are crucial preventive instruments in Sexual and Reproductive Health Care.

This aspect can be very motivating regarding the use of the male condom. Partners can experience using condoms as an expression of shared responsibility, which then can improve their sexual experience.

On the other hand, condom use demands an interruption of the sexual interaction at the time when both partners are sexually aroused. Whereas some couples experience that interruption as a loss of arousal, in others, it will be a boost in their sexual arousal. For some men, the condom means less sensation and less pleasure at penetration and intravaginal movements. For some women, it will mean unpleasant feelings or dyspareunia. Without a condom, the foreskin of the uncircumcised penis will retract during penetration, gradually unfolding the glans, diminishing the risk of dyspareunia. Finally, there may be a negative impact on the enjoyment of the sexual encounter due to insecurity and fears regarding pregnancy.

Especially after alcohol or an intense orgasm, both can fall asleep before leaving the vagina, with the risk of losing erection and semen seeping into the vagina.

Table 20.1 Method satisfaction, overall sexual satisfaction, and negative mood changes concerning different current and past contraceptive methods in a population-based survey [5]

Method	N=	Satisfaction with Method	Overall Sexual Satisfaction	Negative Mood Changes
Oral contraceptives	1.303	68%	44%	16%
Condom	996	30%	11%	23%
IUD	342	59%	30%	
FABM	428	43%	28%	30%
Female sterilisation	139	92%	57%	

20.3.5 Fertility Awareness-Based Methods (FABMs or FAMs)

Fertility awareness methods have no impact on the physiology or anatomy or the sexual response, nor do they have adverse side effects which may impact sexuality besides the insecurity and fears regarding a possible failure in preventing pregnancy (see condom above).

They may positively impact the sexual experience because women using FABM are usually very interested in learning more about their bodies and their body responses. They feel empowered, and by developing security and a positive feeling towards their body, their sexual response will be more welcome and enjoyable.

20.3.6 Overall Effects of Various Contraceptives

A German population-based survey among 1.466 current and past female users of different contraceptive methods looked at satisfaction with the method, overall sexual satisfaction, and negative mood changes [5]. (see Table 20.1). The overall effects of contraceptive use on various aspects of sexuality are positive.

20.4   Contraception after Childbirth

The best time to start discussing contraception is during the pregnancy for several reasons. With all its emotions, the immediate postpartum period is frequently not ideal to think and decide quietly.

For those couples who have reached their desired family size, it is valuable to discuss sterilisation already during the pregnancy. Vasectomy can be performed during the pregnancy. Tube ligation can be done during a caesarean section or in the first 7 days postpartum.

The last trimester of pregnancy is also an excellent time to discuss child-spacing. Usually, it is recommended to wait 18–24 months before getting pregnant again (but less than 5 years) to diminish pregnancy complications and health problems [6].

Postpartum contraception requires special knowledge of how suitable a method is. Whether and how the woman is breastfeeding is a relevant factor.

Table 20.2 When to safely start the various family planning methods in relation to childbirth?

Family planning method	(Nearly) Fully breastfeeding	Partially breastfeeding	Not breastfeeding
Lactational amenorrhoea method	Immediately	Not applicable	
Progesterone releasing Vaginal ring	4–9 weeks postpartum	If breastfeeding ≥4/day, start at 4–9 weeks postpartum	Not applicable
Progestin-only injectable	6 weeks postpartum	6 weeks postpartum	Immediately
Combined oral pills (CHC) Combined patch Combined vaginal ring Monthly injectables	6 months postpartum	6 weeks postpartum	21 days postpartum
Male sterilisation (vasectomy)	Immediately or during the partner's pregnancy		
Female sterilisation	Within 7 days; or during the caesarean section; Or from 6 weeks postpartum		
Male or female condoms	Immediately		
Spermicides	Immediately		
Copper IUD/ LNG-IUD	Within 48 h; or from 4 weeks postpartum		
Diaphragm	Can be fitted from 6 weeks postpartum		
Fertility awareness methods	For symptom-based methods: Start when normal secretion has returned For calendar-based methods: Start after three regular menstrual cycles For breastfeeding women, one can start later		

Since early times, LAM (lactation amenorrhoea method) has been the common child-spacing method. As long as the woman practices exclusive breastfeeding, the risk of becoming pregnant stays in the first 6 months below 1–2%. The ovulation risk is lowest with a higher frequency of breastfeeds, with a longer duration of each feed, and with the inclusion of night feeds.

Table 20.2 shows the earliest time that a woman can start a family planning method after childbirth.

Particular factors to be considered in postpartum contraceptive counselling.

Several studies have shown that the postpartum period is accompanied by an increased risk for sexual problems in both partners. Here are some of the contributing factors.

Prolactin is increased in breastfeeding women, and this hormone is known to reduce sexual desire.

During breastfeeding, oestrogen levels are low, which may contribute to thinning of the vaginal mucosa (increasing the risk of all-day vaginal dryness and itching), and testosterone levels are also low, causing diminished desire and arousability.

The psychosocial transition from a dyad to a triad may lead to emotional distress and insecurity about roles, expectations, and difficulties to adapt to the new interpersonal situation.

All these factors should be considered when women complain about negative changes in their sexual life during the postpartum period.

During the postpartum period, it is recommended to counsel women also about emergency contraception.

20.5   In Case of Failure?

Proper contraceptive care has to be accompanied by solutions if things go wrong.

On the one hand, when the woman/couple realises that sex (with ejaculation) took place without adequate contraceptive protection, there should be the possibility of emergency contraception. Examples of unprotected intercourse (UPI) are a torn condom, a forgotten pill, or non-consensual sex.

On the other hand, when the woman discovers to have conceived, there should be the backup possibility of safe induced abortion. Those backup possibilities are relevant for women's empowerment and will positively influence sexual health. That is the care reality in those countries where the laws do not restrict abortion.

20.5.1 Emergency Contraception

Emergency contraception is indicated when a woman or couple has had unprotected intercourse (UPI) independent of the menstrual cycle. In some countries, oral emergency contraception is also called the morning-after pill. There are several methods with different reliability, here mentioned in decreasing reliability (Copper IUD > Ulipristal > oral levonorgestrel > Yuzpe regimen) [7].

20.5.1.1   Copper IUD
The copper IUD is the most effective emergency contraception method, with the additional advantage that the woman can continue using the copper IUD as a long-acting contraceptive method.

20.5.1.2   Ulipristal 30 mg
Ulipristal is effective up to 120 h after UPI and seems to be more effective than LNG

- Ulipristal does not affect an existing pregnancy and is not associated with congenital abnormalities for 1 week after the use of Ulipristal.
- Breastfeeding women should express and discard the breastmilk.

Contraindications: severe asthma; severe hepatic impairment; using liver-enzyme-inducing drugs.

Side effects: nausea, breast tenderness, dizziness, fatigue, gastrointestinal discomfort, headaches, menstrual cycle irregularities, mood alteration, myalgia, nausea, and pelvic pain are side effects that may occur but are rare. After Ulipristal, the woman should wait for 5 days before starting suitable hormonal contraception to avoid reducing its effect by the progestogens from oral contraceptives.

20.5.1.3 Levonorgestrel (LNG) Oral 1.5 mg

LNG is licensed for use up to 72 h after UPI. After that period, it is unlicensed, with established efficacy of up to 120 h but less than Ulipristal. LNG 1.5 mg does not affect existing pregnancies.

20.5.1.4 Yuzpe Regimen

Within 72 h, the woman takes several of the usual CHC pills. One can use this less reliable method when other emergency methods are unavailable.

20.5.2 Abortion

Women/girls with an unintended pregnancy can decide to continue or terminate the pregnancy. Some of those who continue the pregnancy will get an unwanted baby, which is neither good for the mother, nor the child. When living in those parts of the world where laws restrict abortion, there is the risk of (self-induced or other) unsafe abortion, with severe consequences to her life, health, and well-being.

Where abortion has become legal, two kinds of safe induced abortion are available: aspiration ('surgical abortion') and medication ('medical abortion'). Both are very safe, with a complication rate far lower than the complication rate of ongoing pregnancies. Neither of these methods influences future fertility unless there is a very rare complication.

Surgical abortion takes place in a clinic or hospital. Most of the procedures occur by vacuum suction, with the blood loss being less than normal menstruation.

Medication abortion takes several days. Mifepristone, a progesterone-receptor antagonist, stops the pregnancy, after which (2 days later) misoprostol, a prostaglandin analogue, is given to empty the uterus. The blood loss tends to be more than in a monthly period.

The WHO provides detailed information on: medical management of abortion [8].

Psychological factors, religion, and society's attitudes strongly influence the emotional and sexual consequences of induced abortion. After international studies on abortion outcomes, there is a strong consensus that relief is the dominant feeling in the immediate and short-term aftermath and that the incidence of severe negative responses is low [9]. A year after the abortion, most women viewed the sequels as a process of growth and maturation. However, grief and guilt were also found, especially in women with a religious upbringing. The minimal research on sexuality after induced abortion neither gives consistent positive nor consistent negative consequences [10].

20.6 Sexual Counselling in the Context of Contraception

Based on the above-described possible positive and negative effects of contraceptive methods on sexual function, it will be evident that sexual counselling must be tailored to the individual patient when a problem arises. It is helpful to structure the counselling process into different steps

1. Encourage the patient to talk about the problems, for instance, by introducing the issue of sexual health. *'Contraception shall help you enjoy sex without any fear of unintended pregnancy. For the large majority of women, contraceptives positively affect their sexual life. Nonetheless, some women may feel changes in their desire or arousal or other aspects of their sexual life, and then it is important to talk about it and see what we can do!'*.
2. Describe the worries as problems with desire, arousal, orgasm, pain, or satisfaction and find a common language with the patient to make the dialogue comfortable for her.
3. Ask about pre-existing sexual function and take *a sexual history* (how was sexuality lived before, what has changed, what was positive?).
   (a) It may be that this is the first time that the patient is encouraged to talk about sexuality and that there are longstanding problems that she never talked about, like early abuse, violence, et cetera.
   (b) Other factors like job, stress, partner, and anxiety about the method's side effects may contribute to the problem.
   If these method-independent factors seem important, keep them in mind for further counselling and help.
4. Assess whether method-typical changes could contribute to the problem (see above for possible adverse effects on physiology and anatomy).
5. Look for a solution:
   (a) If method-specific changes are present, look for possible solutions like changing the method, decreasing or increasing the oestrogen component, using natural oestrogen, et cetera.
   (b) Symptomatic treatment of side effects.
6. Arrange a follow-up consultation to check for improvement. If other contributing factors (see above) are important, provide individual or couple sexual counselling.

The midwife should be aware that contraceptive counselling may be the first and only opportunity to track down sexual problems, even if these problems are not directly related to the method.

Healthcare professionals should use this opportunity.

References

1. Brunner Huber LR, Smith K, Sha W, Vick T. Interbirth interval and pregnancy complications and outcomes: findings from the pregnancy risk assessment monitoring system. J Midwifery Womens Health. 2018;63:436–45.
2. WHO 2015: https://apps.who.int/iris/bitstream/handle/10665/172915/WHO_RHR_15.07_eng.pdf;jsessionid=E7E56AFD0B1C7B6428FC03822747B44B?sequence=1.
3. Bancroft J. Sexual effects of androgens in women: some theoretical considerations. Fertil Steril. 2002;77(Suppl 4):S55–9.
4. Bahamondes L, Valeria Bahamondes M, Shulman LP. Non-contraceptive benefits of hormonal and intrauterine reversible contraceptive methods. Hum Reprod Update. 2015;21:640–51.
5. Oddens BJ. Women's satisfaction with birth control: a population survey of physical and psychological effects of oral contraceptives, intrauterine devices, condoms, natural family planning, and sterilisation among 1466 women. Contraception. 1999;59:277–86.
6. Damessi YM. L'espacement des naissances: une pratique simple mais d'un avantage certain Birth spacing: a simple practice with a definite advantage. Fam Dev. 1992;63:10–4.
7. NHS https://www.nhs.uk/conditions/contraception/emergency-contraception/
8. WHO. 2018 Medical management of abortion. Geneva: World Health Organization; 2018. https://apps.who.int/iris/bitstream/handle/10665/278968/9789241550406-eng.pdf?ua=1
9. Kero A, Lalos A. Ambivalence—a logical response to legal abortion: a prospective study among women and men. J Psychosom Obstet Gynaecol. 2000;21:81–91.
10. Bradshaw Z, Slade P. The effects of induced abortion on emotional experiences and relationships: a critical review of the literature. Clin Psychol Rev. 2003;23:929–58.

Further Reading

Family Planning; a global handbook for providers. 2018, Updated 3rd ed.
Under the World Health Organisation Department of Reproductive Health and Research umbrella.
    Free copies are available 'for providers in developing countries'.
Via orders@jhuccp.org (add your name, complete mailing address, and telephone number).
Or via http://www.fphandbook.org/orderform

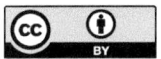

Sexual Aspects of Pregnancy and the Postpartum in Non-Mainstream Orientation

21

Astrid Ditte Højgaard ⓘ and Bente Dahl ⓘ

21.1 Introduction

In some parts of the world, society accepts women having sexual relations with other women and perceives same-sex marriages and legal rights for lesbian couples as a normal variation. Then, assisted reproduction and pregnancy are apparent consequences.

This chapter will deal with relevant aspects of sexuality in lesbian couples deciding to have children. regardless of sexual orientation, some women want (biological) children, and some do not. Healthcare providers (hcps) should realise that women of sexual minorities may also have reproductive wishes [1]. the chapter wraps up with recommendations on how to give good care to the lesbian couple during pregnancy and beyond.

21.2 Prevalence of Lesbianism and Professional Acceptance

When assessing the prevalence of homosexual women, it is important to distinguish between sexual behaviour (with whom I have sex), erotic attraction (with whom I want to have sex), self-identification (sexual orientation defined by oneself), affective preference (romantic preference), and social identification (social labelling).

Like earlier estimations from other countries, in a recent Danish national survey with >62.000 randomly selected adult respondents, 0.6% of all women identified as

A. D. Højgaard (✉)
Sexological Centre, Aalborg University Hospital, Aalborg, Denmark
e-mail: a.hoejgaard@rn.dk

B. Dahl
Faculty of Health and Social Sciences, University of South-Eastern Norway, Kongsberg, Norway

© The Author(s) 2023
S. Geuens et al. (eds.), *Midwifery and Sexuality*,
https://doi.org/10.1007/978-3-031-18432-1_21

lesbian, and 2.6% as bisexual. A proportion of 8% had had sex with another woman, 3% felt a strong attraction towards women, and 27% did ever feel attracted to a woman [2].

In a study of Commonwealth and American lesbian women who had suffered a pregnancy loss, 27% reported experiences of heterosexism, homophobia, or prejudice from HCPs, and another 8.6% were unsure about this [3]. Midwifery and other HCP-curricula must pay extra attention to a non-biased approach and care of non-heterosexual patients.

21.3 The Prevalence of Lesbian Motherhood

It is common that lesbian and bisexual females have been pregnant [4]. Thus, 37% of women of these minorities have ever delivered a child [5], with more pregnancies in bisexual than in lesbian women. It is difficult to determine the number of children growing up in 'rainbow families'.[1] From the very detailed social registers in Denmark, one may estimate (Table 21.1) that at least 0.2% of all children have two parents of the same gender that are registered or married–but many same-sex couples never get married or registered as partners. Furthermore, some single women are lesbian, which adds to the underestimation of the number of rainbow families. Many models of rainbow families are difficult to read from demographic statistics, such as a single lesbian mother with children with a gay couple.

Table 21.1 Family statistics, Denmark (DK statistics) [6]

Number of children according to family structure (2020)		
Single men	36.076	4.6%
Single women	151.367	19.5%
Different-sex married or cohabiting couple	588.789	75.7%
Same-sex married or registered couple	1.541	0.2%

[1] A 'rainbow family' is a family with same-sex parents or a transgender parent.

21.4   Marital and Reproductive Rights

There is a great variety of judicial frameworks concerning marital and reproductive rights for lesbian women, including the parental and adoptive rights for co-mothers/partners. Whereas same-sex marriage and reproductive rights for lesbian women are legally recognised in many countries, other countries still consider same-sex relationships illegal or even punishable by death.

In 1989, Denmark was the first country to allow same-sex civil partnership. Twelve years later, the Netherlands was the first country to institute same-sex marriage. Today, same-sex marriage is legal in many countries (or states) on the Globe. In several countries, legal access to assisted fertilisation, adoption rights, and parental rights have been changed or introduced along with the same-sex marriage law. The legislation on homosexuality ranges from the death penalty to equal rights throughout the world—see Fig. 21.1 for an overview of the situation in December 2020 [7].

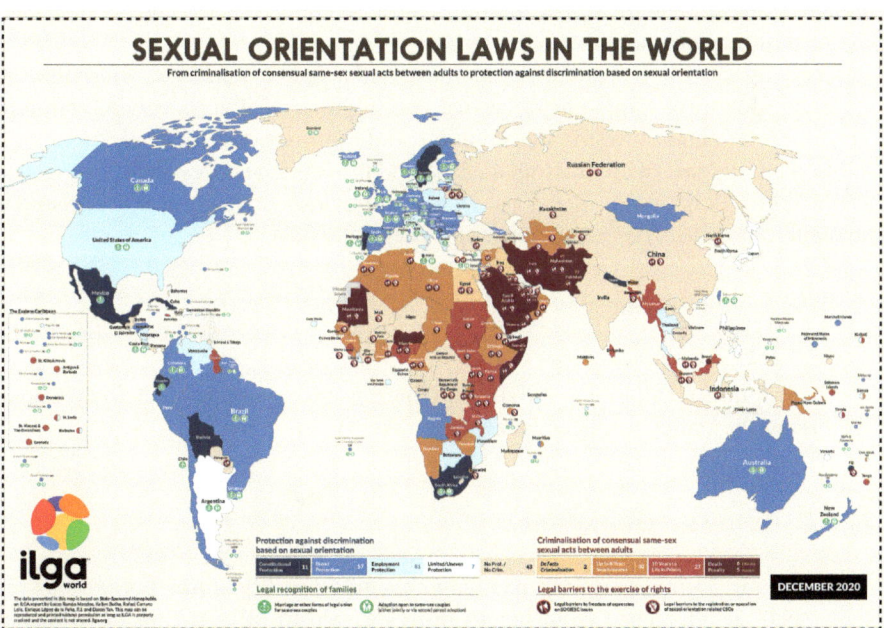

Fig. 21.1 Global legislation regarding homosexuality. (Reproduced from ilga.org)

21.5   The Decision to Have a Child

Just as some heterosexual couples dearly want children and others do not, the same goes for lesbian couples. Whereas in the heterosexual woman or couple, conception cannot happen 'accidentally', for the lesbian woman, it has to be a deliberate decision, and additional steps are needed to achieve a pregnancy.

Fertility clinics offer intrauterine insemination (IUI) to lesbian women in many affluent countries. This method ensures safety regarding screening for various STDs. Most sperm banks also perform donor screening to minimise the risk of major inherited diseases (like cystic fibrosis or spinal muscle atrophy) and other common genetic diseases. Another relevant decision considers using sperm from an anonymous or a known donor (depending on the country's laws).

The methods to conceive depend on the country where the couple lives. In an online Swedish study, 42% used anonymous donor IUI at a clinic, 28% used known donor insemination outside the clinic setting, 7% used IVF with anonymously donated sperm, one had IVF with identified donated sperm, 14% conceived through sexual intercourse with a male partner, and 1% conceived through sexual intercourse with a man who was not her partner [3].

Knowing that many lesbian women have had sexual experiences with men, one might consider proposing a heterosexual one-night stand[2] for conceiving, but most women are reluctant towards this solution. Relevant reasons not to encourage this solution are the risk of contracting an STD and the limited success rate. In countries where sperm donation is illegal but available for lesbian women, the woman can 'explain' a pregnancy as an accident of a one-night stand.

21.5.1 IUI-D

The conception results after IUI-D (Intrauterine insemination with frozen donor sperm) are the same as in heterosexual women [8].

21.5.2 Home Insemination

For achieving a pregnancy, one need not consult a fertility clinic. For various reasons, such as reluctance from health professionals to offer treatment to lesbian women, some women prefer to try home insemination.

If a known donor is fathering the child, the biological father's role afterwards must be considered. In such situations, there is a need of having a contract. See the case story.

---

[2] A one-night-stand is a momentarily one-time sexual contact.

Case Story

Minnie (32) and Lisa (37) have been happily married for 3 years. None of them has been pregnant before. Minnie works as an accountant in a large international firm, and Lisa is a schoolteacher. They live in a lovely suburb and are financially stable. During the last year, they have become increasingly confident that they want to have a baby. As Minnie is the younger one, they decide that she should be the biological mother. Minnie is in doubt about whether her fallopian tubes are open. She contacts her gynaecologist because, at age 18, she had appendicitis causing peritonitis. The gynaecologist reluctantly refers Minnie to have a laparoscopy, as she does not support lesbian motherhood.

Minnie's tubes are open. Due to the unpleasant discussion with the gynaecologist, the couple decides not to be treated by the gynaecologist. They contact Steve, a gay friend, who is willing to be tested for STIs. When all tests are normal, they start home insemination. Since Steve wants to be part of the child's life, the three sign a contract to guarantee this. After three tries, Minnie is pregnant. During the pregnancy, Minnie, Lisa and Steve encounter many opinions from health professionals, some kind, others less so.

During childbirth, Steve and his mother are nervously pacing the waiting room. A beautiful baby boy is born. As Lisa and Minnie are married, Lisa is automatically granted parenthood. That is not so for Steve since a child cannot have three parents in the country where they live. In the years afterwards, Steve takes care of his son every third weekend and during some holidays. The boy refers to him as 'Dad' and to his mothers as Lisa and Minnie.

21.5.3 IVF

Many lesbian women strongly wish to have children, just like many heterosexual sisters, despite judicial obstacles. In some countries, lesbian women can have IVF with donor sperm. Many other countries limit such reproductive freedom by prohibiting IVF for lesbian couples or single mothers (independent of sexual orientation) that has resulted in cross-border reproductive care (CBRC), the extent and consequences of which are hard to assess [9].

A new option is 'shared motherhood' (also called 'Reception of Oocytes from PArtners (ROPA)'; 'interspousal egg donation'; or 'reciprocal IVF'). In this option, one of the mothers goes through ovarian stimulation and ovum pick-up. After fertilisation with donor sperm cells, the embryo is placed in the uterus of the recipient mother, who has been primed with oestrogen and progesterone. Thus, both women are maximally involved in the pregnancy. ROPA is mainly relevant when one of the women has health problems or fertility problems [10]. ROPA has some inborn hazards, such as a high risk for the recipient mother. Egg donation is associated with a higher risk of pregnancy and birth complications, including caesarean section, preterm birth, small-for-gestational age babies, and preeclampsia [11].

21.5.4 When Artificial Reproductive Techniques Fail

In countries where adoption is possible, heterosexual couples might consider adoption if artificial reproductive techniques fail. Same-sex adoption is legal in many countries, but this is not a possibility in other countries. Furthermore, some donor countries restrict adoptions only to heterosexual couples. The authors recommend readers to be aware of the local legislation and its consequences.

21.6 Pregnancy and Childbirth

The pregnancies of lesbian women are more susceptible to low birthweight, premature birth, and even stillbirth [12].

This higher risk of complicated pregnancies, including preeclampsia, is linked to a lack of regular pre-conception exposure to paternal seminal fluid [13] (see also Chap. 5).

21.7 Maternity Care and Midwives' Area of Responsibility

Throughout the world, countries organise maternity care services in different ways. In many countries, registered midwives or nurse-midwives are the main providers of maternity care for low-risk women. Midwives work with the childbearing family to provide support, care and advice during pregnancy, labour, and postpartum, including advice on sexual and reproductive health. The International Code of Ethics for Midwives [14] says that the midwife should offer equal care to all clients, along with evidence-based professional standards.

Overall, good quality maternity care for lesbian women is carried out just as the care for heterosexual women, focusing on health and well-being and preparing for healthy parenthood. Nevertheless, midwives should be aware that some factors related to sexual orientation make dealing with lesbian couples different from the common situation. Examples are heteronormativity in attitude, documents and registration, and the role of the co-mother.

21.7.1 Creating a Safe Environment

The understanding that all human beings are heterosexual, often referred to as heteronormativity, is a social norm in our culture. In a heteronormative setting, the lesbian woman is assumed to be heterosexual until she discloses her sexual orientation to the midwife. The decision to reveal one's sexual orientation may be challenging. Midwives can make women feel welcome and safe by demonstrating awareness about different sexual orientations. An office with a rainbow sticker or a poster with various family constellations signals acceptance and recognition and makes it easier for a lesbian woman or couple to open up. If another woman accompanies a pregnant woman in the antenatal care appointment or at the labour ward, the midwife may politely ask whether the women are partners or friends. Friendly greeting both women can help the couple lower their shoulders.

21.7.2 Paying Attention to Details

When dealing with lesbian women, midwives should pay attention to details more than average. The use of eye contact, inclusive language, and a welcoming smile may signal that she has a positive attitude. For individuals who have experienced stigmatisation, such details may be important signals of being recognised and respected. Lesbian women often experience that it takes some time before midwives find a way to provide tailored care, and most midwives demonstrate uncertainty in the first encounters [15]. Uncertainty is uncomplicated if there is a positive attitude. However, lesbian couples sometimes meet a midwife who seems more interested in the couple's sexual orientation rather than focusing on pregnancy and birth in antenatal consultation. Where professional curiosity about health matters serves an HCP well, satisfying personal curiosities with patients of any gender or orientation is always unprofessional.

21.7.3 Demonstrating Knowledge About Differences

A significant difference between heterosexual couples and lesbian couples planning to start a family is that both women may be able to conceive and give birth to a baby. If both women want to become birth mothers, they sometimes decide to conceive simultaneously, but more often, they take turns becoming pregnant. Midwives should be aware that not all lesbian women want to have a child, or some may want a child but cannot conceive for various reasons, like infertility or age. That may be a challenging subject to bring up when providing antenatal care. Still, the midwife should tactfully address this area as some co-mothers experience jealousy or grief about not being able to conceive and find it difficult to share these feelings with their partner. If that seems too difficult, inviting the co-mother for a 'partner talk' could be a solution.

Although underreported in the literature, we mention the possibility for both women to breastfeed the baby. For co-mothers who have previously nursed a baby, re-lactation is possible. For the co-mother who has not given birth, milk production can be stimulated by hormonal treatment and frequent breast pump use (see Chap. 15, Sect 15.7). Addressing, during the pregnancy, the possibility of breastfeeding for the co-mother and properly guiding that process is a sign of real midwifery professionalism.

21.7.4 Recognising and Including the Co-Mother

In this chapter, we refer to the nonbiological mother as co-mother, nonbirth mother, or social mother.

The fact that, in the lesbian couple, both are a woman may provide a first-hand understanding of pregnancy and labour, especially if the co-mother has previously given birth herself. Still, far from all co-mothers feel comfortable in the labour ward, and a co-mother who has given birth herself may find it challenging to attend her partner's birth because she is well aware of the pain her partner is experiencing.

In many contexts, co-mothers struggle to find a way to be recognised as the baby's legal and social mother. Midwives can demonstrate an understanding that families and parenthood may take different forms by avoiding names that position the co-mother as inferior. Referring to her as 'the other mother' could be experienced as negative or marginalising.

Furthermore, she can include her when providing information and counselling after birth. For midwives, a way of dealing with this situation is to adjust and adapt language and documentation forms to fit the couples' situation, e.g. by using the word 'donor' rather than 'father' when filling out forms and replacing the word 'father' with 'partner' when conducting birth-preparation courses.

21.8 How to Guide a Lesbian Couple on Intimacy and Sexuality

During pregnancy and postpartum, the physical and hormonal changes of lesbian and heterosexual women are alike. However, it is unknown how lesbian couples cope with those changes. Some information on sexuality during pregnancy and postpartum might be relevant (combined with some advice). Many lesbian couples enjoy penetrative sex (see Fig. 21.2).

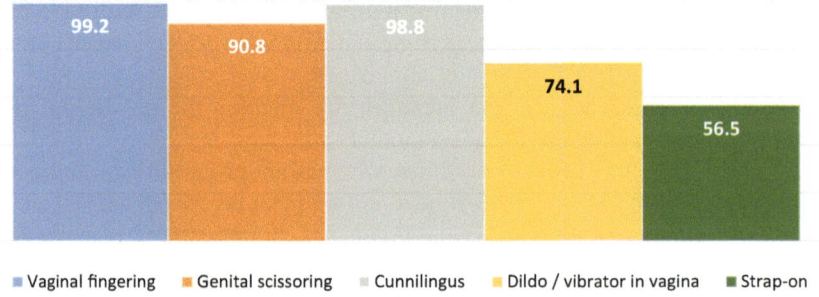

■ Vaginal fingering ■ Genital scissoring ▪ Cunnilingus ▪ Dildo / vibrator in vagina ■ Strap-on

Fig. 21.2 Common Sexual Practices among lesbian women (%). NB Genital scissoring means: genital on genital rubbing or grinding. A strap-on means a dildo attached to the body by a harness [16]

The dildos used for penetration can cause the transmission of various organisms and STIs [16]. Lesbian women have a higher than average incidence of bacterial vaginosis. Since bacterial vaginosis and vaginal infections can cause premature birth and postpartum infections, it is relevant to integrate information on cleaning sex toys before sharing and using barriers (a good reason to inquire about orientation).

If there is postpartum discharge and the cervical orifice is open, any penetrative or vaginal sex should be discouraged, with the addition that all other sexual activities are allowed.

With the newborn child certainly demanding attention, the lesbian mother/couple should be reminded not to forget intimacy, just as in heterosexual couples. With the breasts being important for lesbian sexual pleasure, breastfeeding might be problematic for those mothers who are confused or ashamed when sexually aroused by nipple stimulation. Independent of sexual orientation, 35–50% of nursing mothers experience breastfeeding as erotic ('an incredibly intense physical lust'), and some reach orgasm during breastfeeding. But one-quarter feels guilty because of such sexual arousal [17].

21.9   Offspring of Lesbian Women: Should We Be Concerned?

Although an increasing number of people worldwide express positive attitudes towards homosexual men and lesbian women, people are more reluctant about their reproductive rights and family creation. That reluctance may be related to social norms regarding motherhood and parenting roles [18]. Deviation from the common nuclear family is commonly assumed to increase the risk of children's psychological health [19]. Research does not support this. In families with two female parents, the absence of a male is not associated with child adjustment problems. However, the homophobia in the surrounding society can represent a problem for the children, although most children make average progress through school.

21.10 General Recommendations

Include sexuality and sexual orientation as an issue in all maternity care areas, particularly in midwifery education. Health professionals should bear in mind that not all women are heterosexual—if you do not ask—they probably do not tell. Until you know, use gender-neutral wording.

One can do it easy: After *'Do you have a partner?'*, just ask *'A man or a woman?'*

Or a little more careful: *'I do not know if your partner is a man or a woman, so I want to know if you need me to advice you on contraception?'*

Or: *'Will your partner take part in the birth of your baby? What is the name of your partner?'*

Please pay particular attention to verbal and non-verbal language and ask direct questions to both partners to help them both feel acknowledged as parents. Focus on everyday signs of recognition to counterbalance ambiguous situations and feelings of being invisible or overlooked and recognise both mothers by showing an understanding that there are many ways of parenting and family life.

Be also aware not to focus too much on the sexual orientation of the lesbian woman or couple. Many of their questions and problems are common pregnancy or postpartum issues.

Not all minority women are victimised and oppressed, but many women are in some world regions.

All HCPs should be aware of their own assumptions, attitudes, and cultural bias. Meeting the minority woman/couple with an open mind and heart can be a most rewarding experience.

References

1. Stoffel C, Carpenter E, et al. Family planning for sexual minority women. Semin Reprod Med. 2017;35:460.
2. Frisch M, Moseholm E, Andersson M, et al. Sex in Denmark. Key findings from project sexus. Copenhagen, Denmark: Statens Serum Institute and Aalborg University; 2017.
3. Peel E. Pregnancy loss in lesbian and bisexual women: an online survey of experiences. Hum Reprod. 2010;25:721–7.
4. Moegelin L, Nilsson B, Helström L. Reproductive health in lesbian and bisexual women in Sweden. Acta Obstet Gynecol Scand. 2010;89:205–9.
5. Gates GJ. LGBT parenting in the United States. Los Angeles, CA: Williams Institute, UCLA School of Law; 2013.
6. Denmark Statistics. https://www.dst.dk/en/Statistik/emner/borgere/husstande-familier-og-boern/husstande-og-familier.
7. ILGA World, Mendos LR, Botha K, Lelis RC, de la Peña EL, Savelev I, Tan D. State-sponsored homophobia 2020: global legislation overview update. Geneva: ILGA; 2020. https://ilga.org/sites/default/files/downloads/ENG_ILGA_World_map_sexual_orientation_laws_dec2020.png.
8. Griessler E, Hager M. Changing direction: the struggle of regulating assisted reproductive technology in Austria. Reprod Biomed Soc Online. 2017;3:68–76.
9. Zeiler K, Malmquist A. Lesbian shared biological motherhood: the ethics of IVF with reception of oocytes from partner. Med Health Care Philos. 2014;17:347–55.
10. Fassio F, Attini R, Masturzo B, et al. Risk of preeclampsia and adverse pregnancy outcomes after heterologous egg donation: hypothesising a role for kidney function and comorbidity. J Clin Med. 2019;8:1806.
11. Nordqvist P, Smart S. Relative strangers: family life, genes and donor conception. Houndmills: Palgrave Macmillan; 2014. p. 1–10.
12. Everett BG, Kominiarek MA, Mollborn S, et al. Sexual orientation disparities in pregnancy and infant outcomes. Matern Child Health J. 2019;23:72–81.
13. Saftlas AF, Rubenstein L, Prater K. Cumulative exposure to paternal seminal fluid prior to conception and subsequent risk of preeclampsia. J Reprod Immunol. 2014;101–2:104–10.
14. ICM International Confederation of Midwives. International Code of Ethics for Midwives. (Internet). 2020. https://www.internationalmidwives.org/assets/files/general-files/2019/10/eng-international-code-of-ethics-for-midwives.pdf. Accessed 20 Feb 2020.
15. Spidsberg BD. Vulnerable and strong—lesbian women encountering maternity care. J Adv Nurs. 2007;60:478–86.

16. Schick V, Rosenberger JG, Herbenick D, et al. Sexual behaviour and risk reduction strategies among a multinational sample of women who have sex with women. Sex Transm Infect. 2012;88:407–12.
17. von Sydow K. Sexuality during pregnancy and after childbirth: a metacontent analysis of 59 studies. J Psychosom Res. 1999;47:27–49.
18. Plummer K. Intimate citizenship: private decisions and public dialogues. Seattle, WA: University of Washington Press; 2003. p. 39.
19. Golombok S. Modern families. Cambridge: Cambridge University Press; 2015. p. 32–69.

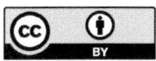

Male Experience(s)

22

Joeri Vermeulen ⓘ, Evelien Luts, and Maaike Fobelets ⓘ

22.1 Introduction

In the Western World, the man's role regarding pregnancy appeared, some decades ago, rather limited. After conception, the man barely got attention till the birth, and then, he was often portrayed as nervously waiting in the hallway. Nowadays, this has changed, with men participating in antenatal classes and parenting education courses in many Western countries, while this still might be different in other parts of the world. Despite wide variation across different contexts, globally identified barriers to men's involvement in pregnancy and childbirth commonly include beliefs that men's participation is unnecessary or that it's inappropriate for them to participate. Besides, men are systematically not (actively) invited to attend services, consultations, etc.

J. Vermeulen (✉)
Department of Health Care, Brussels Centre for Healthcare Innovation, Erasmus Brussels University of Applied Sciences and Arts, Brussels, Belgium

Department of Public Health, Biostatistics and Medical Informatics Research Group, Faculty of Medicine and Pharmacy, Vrije Universiteit Brussel (VUB), Brussels, Belgium
e-mail: joeri.vermeulen@ehb.be

E. Luts
Department of Health Care, Brussels Centre for Healthcare Innovation, Erasmus Brussels University of Applied Sciences and Arts, Brussels, Belgium

Sexologist, Antwerp, Belgium

M. Fobelets
Department of Public Health, Biostatistics and Medical Informatics Research Group, Faculty of Medicine and Pharmacy, Vrije Universiteit Brussel (VUB), Brussels, Belgium

Department of Teacher Education, Vrije Universiteit Brussel (VUB), Brussels, Belgium

This chapter will address various aspects of the male partner's role, beyond just conception and childbirth or his role as a father-to-be. We will also look into the psychological and existential changes that men face before and throughout pregnancy, childbirth, and postpartum. Additionally, the chapter will address the possible physical (and even hormonal) changes that men can experience throughout these specific life events.

We will also elaborate on the man's sexual life. Male partners can feel pressured to impregnate, be scared about the influence of sexual activity in pregnancy, and even fear that sex can cause miscarriage or premature birth. Without being adequately addressed by the midwives and other healthcare professionals (HCPs), these worries will not disappear. Another reason to pay a good amount of attention to this area is that—especially in the postpartum—the difference between the man's and the woman's sexual desire can become a hot topic and even a severe couple problem.

The fact that midwifery is a nearly complete female profession in many places asks for a touch of 'male information'.

22.2 Physical and Hormonal Changes

Transition to parenthood or fatherhood can be a challenging time. For nearly all men, first fatherhood is accompanied by many emotional and physical consequences. Even the gonadal hormones, and their influence on sexuality, change in the course of pregnancy.

Although there is little recognised physiological basis, we should, in this context, mention the Couvade syndrome. This syndrome is a psychosomatic phenomenon affecting male partners mainly during the first and third trimesters of pregnancy and disappearing early in the postpartum period [1]. In first-time expectant fathers, the Couvade syndrome is linked to various physical and psychological changes. Physical symptoms might include changes in appetite, digestion problems, fatigue, nausea, food cravings, weight loss, and weight gain. One of the fathers we interviewed expressed: '*I got lost in unhealthy food cravings and gained weight during my partners' pregnancy*'. Psychological symptoms can be insomnia, mood swings, irritability, and not being interested in usual activities. Since women and men often laugh at the syndrome, many men feel embarrassed admitting they have Couvade syndrome-related symptoms [2]. One interviewed father expressed: '*I think the Couvade syndrome is somehow stigmatising, I would call this "sympathy pregnancy", like in our case, e.g. situations where the partner sympathises with the partners' increased appetite*'. Another father we interviewed stated that these psychological changes in pregnancy are '*Not evident to talk about, but I don't want to burden my partner with this*'.

Some men lose weight during their wife's pregnancy, while some future fathers explain they want to be healthier to set a good example to their children. Yet, more men appear to gain weight during the transition to parenthood, and since men do not undergo the physical demands of pregnancy, the underlying mechanisms are multidimensional [3]. Using a biopsychosocial model to look at sexual health helps us to see how biological and hormonal mechanisms (testosterone and cortisol changes), social and behavioural mechanisms (sleep, physical activity, and diet), and psychological mechanisms (depression and stress) are identified as potentially influencing physical changes in fathers-to-be.

Several hormonal levels change in men. In the preconception phase, some men have hormonal changes. In couples trying to conceive, the men have monthly fluctuations in their testosterone levels [4]. On the other hand, men have lower testosterone and cortisol levels during their partners' pregnancy, and some have higher oestrogen levels [5]. The low testosterone level could explain the diminished sexual interest found in many men at the end of the second trimester. Research indicates that pair-bonding and paternal care are associated with lower male testosterone levels, while searching and acquiring sex partners are associated with higher male testosterone levels [6].

22.3 Male Experiences in the Preconception Phase

When trying to conceive, couples undergo hormonal and psychological changes. In the first months after they stopped using contraception, many men experience more satisfactory and more frequent sexual intercourse. One of the interviewed fathers stated that he found the potential impregnation of his partner exciting and even animal-like. When the man is ambivalent about a possible pregnancy or a child, sexual problems might appear, with sometimes anxiety to ejaculate, low sexual desire, or erectile dysfunction. When conception does not take place, the function of sexuality usually shifts from having fun to 'trying to conceive' [7].

22.4 Male Experiences in Pregnancy

A systematic review of the literature examining sexuality among couples during pregnancy and postpartum demonstrates that the sexual experiences of the male partner have been largely neglected [8]. Most studies of sex during pregnancy and postpartum have focused on women. Moreover, past research mainly focused on vaginal intercourse, while other aspects of sexuality were ignored or not considered [9]. Therefore, we know little about the influence of pregnancy on male sexuality. The consideration of men's emotional, physical, and sexual experience in the perinatal period is limited [9], although the minds of expecting men and young fathers are influenced by various hormonal, physical, emotional, existential, and relational causes [9]. According to the limited studies, becoming a father can greatly impact how sexuality is experienced and expressed [10]. Some men have fears and anxieties about their sexuality during pregnancy and postpartum [11].

While describing various aspects of male partner behaviour, we need to acknowledge that there is much variance among men. Throughout pregnancy and postpartum, sexual activity for individuals is highly variable [9]. Yet, both average sexual interest and coital activity decline slightly in the first trimester of pregnancy, show variable patterns in the second trimester, and decrease sharply in the third trimester. Overall, there is a significant difference in mean scores for sexual activity between females and males. In the PASSION study (Pregnancy and Sexual Relationships Study Involving wOmen and meN), partners reported less frequent intercourse during pregnancy than before pregnancy [12]. Fathers-to-be acknowledge the declined sexual frequency as an important issue between them and their partners. Although some feel guilty to admit they expect more from their partners, while she suffers from many pregnancy-related symptoms. But not only the frequency of intercourse determines sexual satisfaction in expectant fathers. If there is decreased sexual activity in pregnancy, increased affection can often compensate for this [13].

Most men acknowledge that other aspects of sexuality become more important in pregnancy. Male masturbation tends to remain stable throughout the progressing pregnancy and postpartum. For many men, masturbation functions as a backup when intercourse with their partner is not desirable or possible [5]. Some men have problems adapting when their partner's role changes from a sexual partner to a future mother [13]. While some find the pregnant woman's changing body desirable and attractive, others do not. One of our interviewed fathers described sex during pregnancy as disgusting or awkward. Both situations have effects on sexual desire in men. Moreover, men often reported fear of hurting the foetus as one of the main reasons they refrained from having intercourse during pregnancy [14]. Other reasons for men not to have sexual intercourse during pregnancy are concerns about inducing labour [9, 15] and fear of harming their partner [8]. Especially in late pregnancy, men are willing to sacrifice sexuality with their partner for the good of mother and baby. Affection and tenderness through kissing, hugging, and non-genital, non-orgasmic caressing can continue and are highly encouraged, reinforcing the emotional connection between both partners [13].

22.5   Male Experience of Childbirth

Despite the near-universal attendance of fathers at childbirth in affluent Western countries, there is comparatively little research on men's experience of this event. In addition, there is scant focus on men during childbirth education and labour [16].

Most fathers are willing to attend labour and birth yet express feelings of fear and helplessness during the event due to unrealistic expectations, deficiency in antenatal preparation, or lack of midwives' guidance [17]. The most challenging for men is the pain experienced by their partner and being unable to help or alleviate the pain [18]. Some men are confused about their role during childbirth [14]. Men often feel helpless if they do not have a clear role during labour, such as helping their partner cope with contractions through massage techniques. Some expecting fathers do not know where to sit, what to do, and what to say. Some do not recognise their partner because she is in pain like never before. That is why most men find childbirth both wonderful and distressing at the same time. Especially young fathers and those expecting their first baby reported feeling uncomfortable during childbirth more frequently than others [18]. Through their lack of knowledge and perceived control, they struggle to find a role here [19]. Midwifery support, the midwife's presence, and sufficient information about labour progress are important aspects of a father's positive birth experience. When the (male) partner is present during childbirth, the process of birth can be a complex choreography for each party. During childbirth, the midwife's role is important to the father, and respecting his individual needs will enhance a positive birth experience [20]. Meeting the father's needs will result in a calm father-to-be, which will reflect positively on the partner giving birth, whereas a father-to-be that feels lost or stressed might be a factor that could negatively impact the mindset of the partner giving birth.

Fathers describe the moment the baby enters the World as the best experience ever. Directly after childbirth, most fathers experience pride related to fatherhood and love towards their partner and the newborn [21]. Some new fathers experience pride for their partner for what she has accomplished. Many fathers describe the birth as the beginning of fatherhood. Fathers who were present during childbirth reported that their attendance resulted in a closer emotional bond with their partner and newborn [22].

22.6 Male Experiences in the Postpartum

The frequency of most shared sexual activities declines during pregnancy, reaches almost zero in the first 3 months postpartum, and then begins to increase [23]. At 6–12 months after birth, sexual responsiveness is reduced in about 20% of the fathers [9]. Most couples do not practice intercourse for about 2 months after childbirth [9]. A meta-analysis of 59 studies found no significant correlations between birth complications, the severity of birth pain and forceps assistance, and postpartum coital activity, sexual interest, enjoyment, or responsiveness [8]. Though men are concerned about hurting their partner, the first time they have intercourse [13]. Men reported fear of harming and expressed concerns about the healing of her lacerations and stressed that it was important that the woman felt comfortable again before trying to resume sexual intercourse [11]. Additionally, fathers have commented that tiredness and disruptions with the baby and waiting for the six-week postpartum check-up affected sexual activity [9]. Some men experience this as an embargo period they were put on.

In studies on men's sexual experiences during their partners' pregnancy and postpartum, the focus had been predominantly on the frequency of sexuality during that period. Often both partners are dissatisfied with the frequency, the women because it was 'too often' and the men because it was 'too seldom' [9]. In a longitudinal study, at 6 months, 4 years, and 8 years postpartum, the mothers had a lower sexual desire than the fathers on all three occasions of measurement [24]. Most studies confirmed a decrease in sexual activity due to a lack of time and energy [10]. Several men expressed that unfinished tasks and household duties made their partners less interested in having sex. So, negotiating sex in this situation was bound to be unsuccessful [11]. Too significant desire differences may threaten the relationship, sometimes decreasing intimacy and sliding down to emotional and physical detachment.

Many assume that parents do not prioritise the sensual and sexual aspects of their relationship during this intensive period of their life. New fathers focused on the baby and were prepared to postpone sex until both parties were ready for that [11]. After having a child, fathers experience that sexuality becomes tailored according to circumstances [10]. The relationship with one's partner is frequently reported as the most important determinant of sexual satisfaction, with a unique role for mutual closeness [14]. A new form of togetherness can evolve between the partners after having a baby. As in late pregnancy, men can focus on other ways of expressing sexuality and prioritise showing love, affection, and consideration in the postpartum period [10]. The fathers' perceptions of sexual life extended to include all kinds of closeness and touching, deviating from the stereotype of male sexuality [11]. Most of the fathers' satisfaction with their sexuality after having a baby can be related to judging the situation as a transient phenomenon, but some question if the relation and sexual life will ever be the same as before.

The metanalysis of von Sydow (1999) found between 4% and 23% of young fathers have an extramarital affair postpartum [8]. For 15% of the men, the affairs developed before the pregnancy. There are various explanations for these extramarital affairs; the medical advice for prolonged coital abstinence, the need to prove his male independence, or dealing with confusing emotions of becoming a father. When a man is not used to masturbation, his inability to masturbate could also lead to male extramarital sex around childbirth [5]. This might be context or cultur-driven.

Like some of their female partners, some men also experience postpartum depression. Paternal postpartum depression (PPD) within the first postpartum year is estimated to occur in 4–25% of new fathers [25] and can affect sexual health. The definition of PPD used in many studies is that paternal PPD is depression that occurs within the first 12 months postpartum. The highest rates are found at 3–6 months postpartum, while mothers' onset of postpartum depression is generally in the early postpartum period. The most significant risk factor of paternal PPD is postpartum depression in the mother. Some speculate that paternal PPD is related to a decrease in the father's testosterone level. Although the link between low testosterone levels and depression is not clear in the literature, there is a clear link between low testosterone levels and a decline in sexual desire. Research indicates that paternal PPD can also lead to a loss of interest in sex. Education of both parents by childbirth professionals is vital to increase awareness of the condition and decrease stigmas associated with PPD and the combination of PPD and sexual health issues.

22.7   What Can Midwives Do? The Role of Midwives Within a Biopsychosocial Sexology Approach

Medical staff rarely discuss sexual issues with their patients during pregnancy or the postpartum period [8]. In fathers' encounters with perinatal care professionals, they want to be acknowledged and involved as a partner and a parent-to-be. Yet, their experience of maternity care services is as a 'non-patient' and a 'non-visitor'. One of our interviewed fathers stated: '*You are like an informal caregiver, not the patient. I was somewhat involved, but … clearly on the side-line*'. This situates men in an interstitial and undefined place (both emotionally and physically) with the risk that many will feel excluded and fearful [26]. Although men emphasised the need to support their partner and protect their partnership as central to the successful navigation of fatherhood, fathers questioned their entitlement to support, noting that services should be focused on mothers [27].

It seems imperative to provide information to both partners about postpartum sexuality, both during prenatal and postnatal care [10]. HCPs should invite men to share their concerns during pregnancy and offer a chance to voice them [9]. For instance, using the ICE model (see Chap. 26) to address both partners' ideas, concerns, and expectations concerning their sex life as new parents. They need their sexual changes acknowledged and normalised. Midwives and other HCPs need to understand how new fathers look upon their sexual relationship during the transition to parenthood [11] and to take care not to make culturally charged assumptions like men wishing to have more sex and women less.

There is consensus in the literature that discussing sexuality should begin early in pregnancy and that each subsequent prenatal visit should keep the discussion ongoing [11]. Midwives have to develop the skills and acquire the confidence to talk to couples about sexuality during pregnancy and parenthood, assisting the couples in their transition into parenthood. Midwives can inform men, and their pregnant partners that talking about sexuality is a part of their job. We recommend asking men and their pregnant partners for permission to speak about the subject, making them aware that their opinion matters and that they are in control. Midwives can refer to (fictional) couples and situations or existing research to start talking about the subject. Besides addressing sexuality in prenatal visits, the perinatal education classes or workshops should encourage men to discuss sexual changes [13]. We suggest asking dads questions such as: 'how do you experience sexuality during pregnancy?' or 'how do you experience intimacy since you are a father?'

It appears valuable that new fathers meet and exchange experiences. Men need reassurance and information to feel connected to the new family situation [11]. Daddy's classes are now more common in several Western countries. That could be an interesting method for distributing this information [12]. In most cases, 90% of the challenge is information giving, followed by reassurance in normalising their feelings and concerns [13]. Young fathers benefit from better communication skills that include the role of sexuality and sensuality during the transition to parenthood and beyond.

Sharing the right information at the right time will help men and their partners gain new knowledge and bring comfort and reassurance [13]. Midwives must be aware that, after having a child, sexuality can be expressed in many different ways and that it deserves a biopsychosocial approach. Midwives need to be cautious to not only include information about sexual activities [10]. Addressing only sexual function without the aspect of intimacy can be as harmful as not addressing sexuality at all.

In most sexuality studies, participants are white, educated middle class, married, and selected from antenatal classes [15]. Culture-specific trends in sexual activity can explain differences found in research. For instance, Europeans claim more sexual experience than North Americans [23]. The wide cultural variation encompasses sexual taboos before and after birth, lasting for different periods [15]. Additional research is needed to explore the variability between fathers of different cultures and backgrounds. Be also aware of reporting bias with data on men's sexuality, often relying on self-report. This is true for the bulk of research on human sexuality and a reason for interpreting the findings with caution. By concentrating on sexual functioning, activity, and satisfaction, studies of men's postpartum sexuality tend not to use a biopsychosocial approach [10]. Besides, the quantitative nature of most research does not allow to articulate and hear individual experiences [9]. We have to develop sociocultural-sensitive interventions within a tailor-made approach to facilitate a smoother transition to fatherhood [28].

Some health professionals are comfortable talking about sexuality while others avoid the subject [13]. Still, every midwife needs to develop the communication skills necessary to put the subject on the table. Today's HCPs must be aware of the fathers' needs and the impact gender aspects have on their professional support, as counselling or parent classes mostly address women's needs, making it doubtful if the fathers benefit from participation [29]. HCPs need to be aware that midwifery care can only be good care when the couple's sexuality is adequately addressed. Men's sexual and other needs during pregnancy and postpartum deserve more attention.

Acknowledgements The authors wish to thank Nathan, father of a 1.5- and a 3.5-year-old; Alessandro, father of a 2.5-year-old and a newborn baby; Adriaan, stepfather of a 4-year-old and father-to-be; and Dennis, father of children of 4, 7 and 9 years old for sharing their own experiences and their critical appraisal of this chapter.

References

1. Brennan A, Ayers S, Ahmed H, Marshall-Lucette S. A critical review of the Couvade syndrome: the pregnant male. J Reprod Infant Psychol. 2007;25:173–89. https://doi.org/10.1080/02646830701467207.
2. Ganapathy T. Couvade syndrome among 1st time expectant fathers. Muller J Med Sci Res. 2014;5:43. https://doi.org/10.4103/0975-9727.128944.
3. Hirschenhauser K, Frigerio D, Grammer K, Magnusson MS. Monthly patterns of testosterone and behavior in prospective fathers. Horm Behav. 2002;42:172–81. https://doi.org/10.1006/hbeh.2002.1815.

4. Saxbe D, Corner GW, Khaled M, et al. The weight of fatherhood: identifying mechanisms to explain paternal perinatal weight gain. Health Psychol Rev. 2018;12:294–311. https://doi.org/10.1080/17437199.2018.1463166.
5. Gianotten WL. Pregnancy and sexuality. Sex Health. 2007;2:167–96.
6. Pollet TV, Cobey KD, van der Meij L. Testosterone levels are negatively associated with fatherhood in males, but positively related to offspring count in fathers. PLoS One. 2013;8:e60018. https://doi.org/10.1371/journal.pone.0060018.
7. Gaskins AJ, Sundaram R, Louis GMB, Chavarro JE. Predictors of sexual intercourse frequency among couples trying to conceive. J Sex Med. 2018;15:519–28. https://doi.org/10.1016/j.jsxm.2018.02.005.
8. von Sydow K. Sexuality during pregnancy and after childbirth: a metacontent analysis of 59 studies. J Psychosom Res. 1999;47:27–49. https://doi.org/10.1016/S0022-3999(98)00106-8.
9. Williamson M, McVeigh C, Baafi M. An Australian perspective of fatherhood and sexuality. Midwifery. 2008;24:99–107. https://doi.org/10.1016/j.midw.2006.07.010.
10. MacAdam R, Huuva E, Berterö C. Fathers' experiences after having a child: sexuality becomes tailored according to circumstances. Midwifery. 2011;27:e149–55. https://doi.org/10.1016/j.midw.2009.12.007.
11. Olsson A, Robertson E, Björklund A, Nissen E. Fatherhood in focus, sexual activity can wait: new fathers' experience about sexual life after childbirth. Scand J Caring Sci. 2010;24:716–25. https://doi.org/10.1111/j.1471-6712.2009.00768.x.
12. Dwarica DS, Collins GG, Fitzgerald CM, et al. Pregnancy and sexual relationships study involving wOmen and meN (PASSION study). J Sex Med. 2019;16:975–80. https://doi.org/10.1016/j.jsxm.2019.04.014.
13. Polomeno V. Men's sexuality in the perinatal period: what do perinatal educators need to know? Int J Childbirth Educ. 2011;26:35–9.
14. Nakić Radoš S, Soljačić Vraneš H, Šunjić M. Sexuality during pregnancy: what is important for sexual satisfaction in expectant fathers? J Sex Marital Ther. 2015;41:282–93. https://doi.org/10.1080/0092623X.2014.889054.
15. Pacey S. Couples and the first baby: responding to new parents' sexual and relationship problems. Sex Relatsh Ther. 2004;19:223–46. https://doi.org/10.1080/14681990410001715391.
16. Dellmann T. "The best moment of my life": a literature review of fathers' experience of childbirth. Aust Midwifery. 2004;17:20–6. https://doi.org/10.1016/S1448-8272(04)80014-2.
17. Shibli-Kometiani M, Brown AM. Fathers' experiences accompanying labour and birth. Br J Midwifery. 2012;20:339–44. https://doi.org/10.12968/bjom.2012.20.5.339.
18. Vehviläinen-Julkunen K, Liukkonen A. Fathers' experiences of childbirth. Midwifery. 1998;14:10–7. https://doi.org/10.1016/S0266-6138(98)90109-7.
19. Longworth HL, Kingdon CK. Fathers in the birth room: what are they expecting and experiencing? A phenomenological study. Midwifery. 2011;27:588–94. https://doi.org/10.1016/j.midw.2010.06.013.
20. Hildingsson I, Cederlöf L, Widén S. Fathers' birth experience in relation to midwifery care. Women Birth. 2011;24:129–36. https://doi.org/10.1016/j.wombi.2010.12.003.
21. He HG, Vehviläinen-Julkunen K, Qian XF, et al. Fathers' feelings related to their partners' childbirth and views on their presence during labour and childbirth: a descriptive quantitative study. Int J Nurs Pract. 2015;21:71–9. https://doi.org/10.1111/ijn.12339.
22. Dragonas TG. Greek fathers' participation in labour and care of the infant. Scand J Caring Sci. 1992;6:151–9. https://doi.org/10.1111/j.1471-6712.1992.tb00143.x.
23. von Sydow K, Ullmeyer M, Happ N. Sexual activity during pregnancy and after childbirth: results from the sexual preferences questionnaire. J Psychosom Obstet Gynecol. 2001;22:29–40. https://doi.org/10.3109/01674820109049948.
24. Hansson M, Ahlborg T. Quality of the intimate and sexual relationship in first-time parents—a longitudinal study. Sex Reprod Healthc. 2012;3:21–9. https://doi.org/10.1016/j.srhc.2011.10.002.

25. Stadtlander L. Paternal postpartum depression. Int J Childbirth Educ. 2015;30(2):11–3.
26. Steen M, Downe S, Bamford N, Edozien L. Not-patient and not-visitor: a metasynthesis fathers' encounters with pregnancy, birth and maternity care. Midwifery. 2012;28:422–31. https://doi.org/10.1016/j.midw.2011.06.009.
27. Darwin Z, Galdas P, Hinchliff S, et al. Fathers' views and experiences of their own mental health during pregnancy and the first postnatal year: a qualitative interview study of men participating in the UK born and bred in Yorkshire (BaBY) cohort. BMC Pregnancy Childbirth. 2017;17:45. https://doi.org/10.1186/s12884-017-1229-4.
28. Poh HL, Koh SSL, He HG. An integrative review of fathers' experiences during pregnancy and childbirth. Int Nurs Rev. 2014;61:543–54. https://doi.org/10.1111/inr.12137.
29. Premberg Å, Hellström A, Berg M. Experiences of the first year as father. Scand J Caring Sci. 2008;22:56–63. https://doi.org/10.1111/j.1471-6712.2007.00584.x.

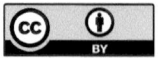

Relevant (Sexual) Aspects of Cultural Differences

Sandrine Atallah ⓘ and Aida Martín Redón ⓘ

> In all cultures, the midwife's place is on the threshold of life, where intense human emotions, fear, hope, longing, triumph, and incredible physical power enable a new human being to emerge. Her vocation is unique. (Sheila Kitzinger)

23.1 Introduction

In order to have a comprehensive biopsychosocial approach to sexuality, it is essential to acknowledge that culture is an inherent part of the person as a unique holistic being. Furthermore, gender roles, male-centred societies, feminism, laws related to sexuality, religious beliefs, and behaviours considered appropriate or not are examples of culturally determined elements that significantly impact the development of a person's sexuality. Therefore, in the midwife's professional practice, the influence of someone's historical and sociocultural context cannot be ignored when addressing this subject.

This chapter aims to clarify some relevant aspects of cultural differences in the field of midwifery and sexuality. This topic is especially important in an era in which multiculturalism, intergenerational differences, and diversity of values, religions, ideals, and traditions coexist throughout the globe.

To this end, we will offer an overview of several sexual elements that can generate controversy and difficulties in the midwife's handling of sexuality, depending on their cultural perspective.

S. Atallah (✉)
Women Health Center, American University of Beirut Medical Center, Beirut, Lebanon

A. M. Redón
Department of Obstetrics and Gynaecology, BovenIJ Hospital, Amsterdam, The Netherlands

© The Author(s) 2023
S. Geuens et al. (eds.), *Midwifery and Sexuality*,
https://doi.org/10.1007/978-3-031-18432-1_23

Furthermore, when talking about this topic, one cannot leave out the influence of the HCP's own culture, which also plays a determining role in the midwife–woman relationship and how the midwife approaches the client's sexual sphere. Therefore, this chapter also intends to reflect on factors such as the midwife's type of education and training, sociocultural context and personal characteristics; in order to raise cultural awareness among HCPs and promote culturally sensitive, safe, and non-discriminatory care.

Nevertheless, we must consider culture as a dynamic and changing element that implies comprehensive individual and temporal diversity within each group. Thus, the existence of cultural identity does not override the importance of considering the personal identity and the woman's autonomy. So, besides cultural scripts, women can make their own decisions and behave based on their own beliefs, values, knowledge, and experiences. Hence, we invite the reader to avoid understanding the contents of this chapter in a deterministic way. We precisely aim to prevent stereotypes, stigmas, and cultural generalisations. We will address structural, socio-economic, and educational aspects and language barriers and acculturation.

Last but not least, we have developed a series of recommendations with some theoretical and practical keys for midwives regarding a culturally sensitive approach to sexuality. These recommendations include a section dedicated to the organisational and structural aspects of the midwifery governing bodies and institutions in order to contribute to reducing barriers in this area. All this aims to promote adequate and non-discriminatory care for every woman in matters of sexuality.

23.2 Female Sexualities

Within the biopsychosocial model, sociocultural factors, psychological and biological factors mould our sexuality, influence how we perceive our sexual self, our sexual behaviours and practices, and even our sexual function [1]. It also influences the clinical practice with our clients. However, HCPs, including midwives, regularly neglect the effect of social and cultural components on sexual health and wellbeing. Considering sociocultural contributors in midwifery is critical as they shape the "dreaded" and embarrassing "sex talk". Culture also partly predetermines if a woman is willing and able to discuss her sexuality with the midwife.

Saying that there are as many female "sexualities" as they are women would not be an exaggeration. Every woman is unique in her sexuality. However, we can determine and be aware of several socio-cultural impacting elements. For example: in many regions of the world, religious beliefs, patriarchy, and family traditions drastically weigh on female sexuality. Conservative values and practices often limit access to sexuality education, restrict women's knowledge of their own bodies, stigmatise female desire and pleasure, and further silence female sexuality because of taboo and shame. In nontraditional parts of the planet, mass media and social media play, in contrast, a major role in how women learn about and view their sexuality. However, we should be aware that access to information does not guarantee accurate sexuality education. Stereotypes and "norms"[1] can also distort women's understanding of sexuality, sexual pleasure, and consent.

For instance, being Western or not, having a high educational level[2] or not, and so on, does not necessarily suggest that a person knows what a clitoris is and how to use it.

Understanding the impact of cultural differences on female sexuality gets even more complex when considering the variety in "acculturation" (the process of incorporating language, values, customs, et cetera after migrating into new surroundings) [2]. In this process, the two main movements are (1) embracing standards, morals, and practices of the destination culture and (2) keeping principles, dogmas, and attitudes of the native/original culture.[3]

Sexuality (just like contraception methods) is an essential aspect of someone's level of acculturation. In other words, in our clinical setting, we cannot assume one's understanding of sexuality and sexual practices, so we simply have to ask.

Despite the infinite diversity of sociocultural factors, several cultural aspects of female sexuality seem universal. Among those is the heteronormative view of women's sexuality that considers penile-vaginal penetration as the only valid form of sex. In this regard, the woman from a conservative culture frequently wants, above all, to protect her "virginity" since her so-called intact hymen symbolises the honour of the family. On her wedding night, the same woman is supposed to surrender herself "completely" to her spouse. Vaginal sex is then not only validating her marriage and changing her social status into a "real" woman, but it is also the only way to "fulfil" and "keep" her husband. Nevertheless, in "liberal" cultures, intercourse is still portrayed as the most fulfilling type of sexual activity.

In both scenarios, guilt and anxiety can accompany failing, by which this topic is seldom discussed in the clinical setting. Even today, women worldwide are often silent about their sexual concerns, as they feel abnormal and too embarrassed to talk about it. Many midwives consider sexual pain, penetration difficulties, and lack of sexual pleasure shameful issues that they do not address. Besides, as exposed later in this chapter, midwives rarely ask about it because of their own discomfort and lack of training skills. And even when inquiring about the client's sexuality and sexual concerns, the midwife might not get an answer because of having a different origin, culture, age, marital status, or gender.

Therefore, all cultures and subcultures influence how we perceive sexuality, its meaning or importance in our lives, what is considered normal and abnormal, and if or with whom we are ready to engage in a conversation about sexuality. Even if sexuality is viewed in a "positive" and empowering way, our view of its different

---

[1] Norms can be related to socioeconomic scripts or a person's subculture, e.g. concerning work, sexual orientation or age.

[2] Even as a midwife.

[3] Information about the challenges of working with sexual and reproductive health of refugee and migrant women is extensively covered in an Australian research report [3].

dimensions[4] is filtered by our cultural biases and sometimes tainted with shame and stigma.

In the next section, we will discuss examples illustrating some of the potential effects of sociocultural factors on female sexuality. Be aware that these illustrations cannot be generalised and should not be used to label or stigmatise people belonging to a particular cultural group.

This chapter does not address female genital mutilation since that topic will get ample attention in Chap. 25.

23.3   Attitudes and Practices

A great example of a sexual and socio-cultural problem is unconsummated marriage (UM), encountered especially among couples from conservative Middle Eastern cultures, accounting for up to 17% of visits to sexual health clinics in certain countries [4]. It is a condition where newly married couples cannot achieve penile-vaginal intercourse for variable periods, despite the desire and frequent attempts. Vaginismus (the involuntary vaginal muscle spasm as a reaction to the fear of some or all types of vaginal penetration) represents three-fourths of the female causes of UM [5]. Likewise, the high prevalence of UM in communities that strictly prohibit premarital sex is attributed to the social and cultural constraints that profoundly pressure the couple. In these conservative societies, the lack of sexuality education, sexual prohibition, misconceptions about sexuality, and unrealistic expectations, contribute to UM and vaginismus. In communities with ample opportunities for premarital coitus and where culture and society do not prohibit such contact, vaginismus is less prevalent. However, any practising midwife might meet women with UM or vaginismus without even knowing. For example, she might be following a pregnant woman who has never had vaginal sex and is afraid of a pelvic exam. One might think that these cases are sporadic and mostly anecdotal. The reality is that some women get pregnant either through outercourse (having sex with ejaculation but without penile-vaginal penetration) or with the help of assisted medical procreation. The same is true for women of different sociocultural origins living in the West and perfectly adapted to their environment, wanting to engage in vaginal sex but dealing with sexual difficulties related to penetration. Western HCPs should not dismiss UM or its distress as"a lack of socio-cultural skills". That might be traumatising for the woman and severely aggravate UM's impact on both partners.

Another strongly culture-specific aspect of sexuality refers to *"wet sex"* versus *"dry sex"* [6]. In Western cultures, vaginal lubrication is a sign of arousal, an essential for pleasurable sex, and needed to prevent dyspareunia. However, in several Sub-Saharan African countries, people believe that dry sex is more enjoyable for the male partner who feels more friction. For the woman, it usually means pain. That, however, might for her be satisfactory because of pleasing her partner. In order to

---

[4] Such as first-time sex, pleasure, pain, contraception, pregnancy, postpartum, aging, sexual practices, and relationship-forms.

achieve dry sex, women use vaginal products to tighten the vagina, reduce its secretions, and even dry it up. Being confronted with such practices might be difficult for the midwife. However, for fulfilling our care mission, it is essential to listen in a non-judgmental way without imposing our own opinions. It can pave the way to sexuality education and enable to, afterwards, correct false beliefs.

Cultures also vary in the importance they attribute to sexual desire. For some, sexual desire is a sign of a loving and healthy relationship, while decreased desire is viewed as a distressing problem that needs treatment. At the same time, other women consider lack of desire as the norm and are not bothered by it [7]. Some people even consider female sexual desire sinful, with sexual practices a conjugal duty limited to vaginal penetration with procreation as the ultimate goal. By mentioning that, we underscore the importance of knowing our client's beliefs before giving any sexual advice.

There are numerous examples of socio-cultural beliefs surrounding sexuality, and one cannot be proficient in all. However, it is crucial to be aware that, due to those beliefs, many women will wait for the midwife to ask about sexuality. Others might not be sexually active in a vaginal way or might not even know how vaginal intercourse is performed. Therefore, the end of this chapter will offer guidelines and recommendations on how the midwife or HCP could become aware of their own cultural blind spots to allow a culture-sensitive approach.

23.4   Cultural Differences among Midwives Concerning Sexuality Approach

We discussed the great cultural diversity in the world and its impact on women's sexualities. But what do we mean when we talk about "midwives"? Do they constitute a homogeneous group of professionals with a neutral and biomedical perspective in all parts of the globe? Definitely not. Indeed, each reader will probably associate the word "midwife" with specific qualities, way of working, socio-economic status, and skills that may differ depending on the person's cultural background.

Even though we expect that midwives accompany women throughout the different stages of their sexual and reproductive life in a respectful and empathetic manner, various factors make their experiences, beliefs, attitudes, and interventions very diverse worldwide. Some of the most significant disparities are the variety of practices they carry out, how they acquire their knowledge and the organisational differences of the profession in each country.

Overall, midwifery education can range from the generational transmission of knowledge among the community's women to university programs in the most prestigious hospitals in large cities. Likewise, professional autonomy and competencies are heterogeneous. In some contexts, midwives accompany women during the first stage of labour. Still, the gynaecologist will be "in charge" of the last part of the second labour stage. In other places, midwives are responsible for the follow-up of healthy pregnancies, independently accompanying childbirth and postpartum, contraceptive advice, sexuality education, gynaecological cancer screening programs, menopause, and ultrasound scans. Another significant difference is the midwife's autonomy to accompany home births. While in some countries, this practice is fully integrated into the system as one more option for women,[5] in others, it is culturally unacceptable and even legally restrained. In the same way, while there are countries where midwives struggle to have their profession recognised and endorsed by legislation, most of them are part of a hierarchical healthcare system. All in all, midwives' skills and knowledge of sexuality and their role in addressing it are highly diverse from one country to another.

At a global level, the International Confederation of Midwives considers knowing the socio-cultural aspects of human sexuality and acting accordingly as an Essential Competency for Midwifery Practice [8].

Also, the WHO [9] includes "Addressing gender and cultural sensitivity" as one of the seven principles that guide the delivery of the "Packages of Interventions for Family Planning, Safe Abortion Care, Maternal, Newborn and Child Health".

However, midwives consider approaching sexuality itself a complicated task, even more so when dealing with women not adapted to the mainstream culture. Frequently, without proper training regarding sexuality and cultural sensitivity, midwives have to rely on their own values, experience, and cultural scripts to address such topics. In this way, they can learn from their practice, successes, and mistakes and via their colleagues. In the long run, this has the potential to enrich professional practice by gaining on-the-ground experience. Nevertheless, without proper training, this relies on the interest and resources of each midwife and often causes avoiding these topics, fear of failure, a tendency to stereotype, a narrow view of sexuality, and uncertainty or rejection towards clients from different cultures.

Understanding fertility, pregnancy, childbirth, postpartum, and breastfeeding as cornerstones of women's sexuality, the cultural elements inherent to each individual midwife, and their biases in this regard will impregnate the practice. So, whether they address this subject explicitly or not, being aware of one's frame of reference and context becomes especially relevant.[6]

We recommend that the institutions that design midwifery curricula ensure appropriate training in these fields. On the one hand, it may provide confidence and skills to practitioners in approaching issues related to sexuality from a cross-cultural perspective. And on the other hand, an ethno-sensitive educational approach can also help blur the racial, ethnic, and status boundaries.[7] Such development can contribute to upgrading the whole midwifery profession (from university-trained to traditional) towards a comprehensive midwifery care model that safeguards women's rights regarding their bodies, their sexuality, and their motherhood.

---

[5] Or indeed the only option in some parts of the world.

[6] It should be noted that there are certain countries where the priority of midwives is to reduce the ratios of maternal and infant morbidity and mortality, having difficulties even to cover their basic needs. Consequently, and without diminishing the importance of sexuality, we are aware that what is written in these lines is not suitable for all realities.

[7] Which may not only have an impact on the relationship with clients, but also divide the midwifery collective.

Let's focus now on the diversity among co-workers. Various studies show that 99% of US midwives and 99.7% of UK midwives are female. Of these, >88% in both countries are white. However, the population they serve is much more diverse and heterogeneous. This fact implies an impoverishment of the cultural competencies in Western midwifery care, related to disadvantages and discrimination for women with non-Western cultural backgrounds. Not only towards clients but also among colleagues [10, 11].

Regarding male midwives, some women prefer to be accompanied by a female practitioner, regardless of the HCP's competencies and skills. Even more so when it comes to discussing sexuality-related issues [12]. This is about an intersection, among others, of the cultural clashes between conceptions of shame or decency, the principles of tradition and/or religion, the ego of the HCP, and the practicalities of the organization of modern medicine. Also, given that women and men are likely to integrate cultural norms differently, the lack of training, as mentioned above, will often mean that the HCP will approach sexuality from her/his personal frame of reference. An additional relevant cue to recommend adequate training in sexuality. Being aware that such cultural clashes can arise, and being taught how to manage them, might help to understand and deal with these issues in a more satisfactory way for both the professional and the woman or couple.

Furthermore, enhancing the cultural diversity of the midwifery workforce may facilitate the rise of cultural humility, remove barriers in this field, and enrich culturally sensitive practice [13–15].

Case Study
Ioana and the contraceptive advice

After the birth of her ninth child, Ioana went to the regular six-week postpartum consultation. In each of her deliveries, she had placental retention, and on several occasions, her life was in grave danger because of it. From the Western view of health care, the right thing for this woman was to make sure she accepted a long-term contraceptive, and so the midwife tried to convince her.

Ioana spoke a language that the midwife was unfamiliar with, but as the clinic was in a very multicultural area, there was a permanent interpreter whose presence was requested in advance. However, Ioana belonged to a cultural group that was not common in the city, and, in the end, they had to communicate through the help of Ioana's friend and the online translator. Anticipating that this consultation would require more time than usual, the midwife had reserved a double timeslot in her schedule, but that was insufficient. By developing all her abilities and creativity, the midwife somehow succeeded in transferring part of the information to Ioana. Nevertheless, Ioana simply said "no" energetically with her head and finger while smiling embarrassingly.

After several "failed" attempts, the midwife referred this case to the hospital team as a last resort.

Despite all efforts, it didn't work.

But how was this possible if she had used all the available material and human resources?

Question to the reader:

What was the midwife missing? Where, why, and how should you have reacted differently?

The following are some relevant aspects to consider when addressing these issues:

- Unawareness and non-research on what family, sex, fertility, abortion, and contraception mean to the woman and her community.
- Cultural, educational, and language barriers.
- Lack of time.
- Unfamiliarity with specific tools for the culturally appropriate translation of health issues.
- Ethnocentric[8] and paternalistic approach.

With this, we believe that addressing sexuality as part of the midwife's practice is essential, but it does not make sense at all if the cultural aspects, which strongly influence people's sexual lives, are not considered.

23.5 Recommendations for a Culture-Sensitive Approach

Paasche-Orlow described the essential principles of culturally competent care [16]:

Principle 1: Acknowledgement of the importance of culture in people's lives.
Principle 2: Respect for cultural differences.
Principle 3: Minimisation of any adverse consequences of cultural differences.

Based on these principles, we will present some recommendations to provide theoretical and practical keys for midwives regarding a culturally sensitive approach to sexuality.

---

[8] Ethnocentric refers to the idea that the elements of one's own culture are the norm, being considered desirable, superior, and extremely important. From an ethnocentric perspective, one's cultural worldview is used as a yardstick to evaluate those who represent otherness. This can imply the assumption that all people should adapt to the predominant cultural model. Otherwise, they may be labeled as primitive, exotic, irrational, or incomprehensible. In addition, an ethnocentric attitude avoids critically perceiving the own culture, constituting a significant barrier towards diversity. Therefore, midwives should be aware that this issue can have consequences on the interaction with the clients [15].

All this is conceived from a positive point of view, understanding differences in this field as a two-way learning opportunity in which cultural exchange enriches the client, the midwife, the midwifery profession, and the population in general. The reader might feel more at home with some recommendations than others, agreeing more or less with them as a professional. Then, we have succeeded with one of our objectives: to make the intersections between culture and sexuality a topic considered by midwives. From here, new ideas, greater awareness, and even the implementation of actions that promote a real and significant change in this regard may appear.

The recommendations aimed at the individual midwife are the following:

1. Recognise the impact of culture on one's own psychosexual development and sexual life and, in that way, become aware of one's own norms and values regarding sexuality.
2. Be aware that each individual, despite shared cultural backgrounds, is unique in sexuality.
3. Normalise and legitimise non-judgmental discussions concerning sexual health in all cultural contexts by systematically recording aspects of people's sexuality in the clinical history.
4. Keep an open mind and a respectful, active listening stance.
5. Avoid determinism and overgeneralisation on cultural grounds.
6. Detect and manage cultural and communication barriers that may hinder the midwife–woman interaction related to sexuality.
7. Be aware of the influences of one's subculture.
8. Recognise discriminatory situations on cultural grounds occurring in the midwife's workplace.
9. Collaborate and establish alliances between sexual and reproductive health service providers and organisations or associations in various communities (outreach work).

However, to expect all midwives to be experts in cross-cultural sexual healthcare is unrealistic and perhaps unnecessary because of the wide individual diversity within groups with the same cultural background. But also because of barriers that depend on governing structures and institutions. For this reason, we have here below included some structural and organisational recommendations:

1. Improve organisational aspects and provide human and material resources to midwives to allocate time for culturally competent sexual health care to women.
2. Include cross-cultural and sexual health awareness in midwifery training.
3. Promote cultural exchanges within the midwifery training program, between midwives in rural areas and those in cities, traditional and professional midwives, and even performing a minor part of the training abroad.

4. Ensure the availability of adequately trained interpreters or suitable tools (such as specific translating software[9]) to accompany women and professionals in sexually related conversations.
5. Aspire to create culturally diverse staff in midwifery teams.
6. Create a specialised cross-cultural-care midwife or committee, guaranteeing the continuity and quality of care for immigrant women and a reference role for colleagues.
7. Create culturally appropriate materials and educational campaigns related to sexuality for immigrant women and make them in different formats available for midwives.[10]
8. Improve equitable access to sexual and reproductive health services for all women, eliminating discrimination based on cultural background, social class, ethnicity, etc.

23.6 Conclusions

In the practice of midwifery, we may consider cultural differences related to sexuality as an opportunity to face new challenges and discover different behaviours in this regard. Thus, certain situations in this field that at first may seem shocking or even incomprehensible can become a learning process for the midwife and even result in an unexpected approach to the users, being able to minimise cultural barriers.

Together we can gradually develop a more global, coherent, women-centred, individualised, and holistic midwifery care concerning sexuality. An approach responsive to all women's needs and concerns, regardless of their cultural background. In other words, a truly biopsychosocial model that embraces cultural pluralism.[11]

---

[9] Examples of specific translating Apps:

CALD Assist, available online at https://www.csiro.au/en/research/health-medical/overcoming-language-barriers-in-healthcare

Talk-to-me, available online at https://play.google.com/store/apps/details?id=com.neverads.talktome&hl=en_US&gl=US

Care to translate, available online at https://caretotranslate.com/

[10] Examples of online materials and resources:

Zanzu, available online at https://www.zanzu.de/en/

Health Translations, available online at https://healthtranslations.vic.gov.au/

Continuum Complete International Encyclopedia of Sexuality, available online at https://kinseyinstitute.org/collections/archival/ccies.php [17].

[11] Also called biopsychosocial-cultural (BPSC) approach.

References

1. Atallah S, Johnson-Agbakwu C, Rosenbaum T, et al. Ethical and sociocultural aspects of sexual function and dysfunction in both sexes. J Sex Med. 2016;13:591–606.
2. Sam DL, Berry JW. Acculturation: when individuals and groups of different cultural backgrounds meet. Perspect Psychol Sci. 2010;5:472–81.
3. Mengesha ZB, Perz J, Dune T, Ussher J. Challenges in the provision of sexual and reproductive health care to refugee and migrant women: a Q methodological study of health professional perspectives. J Immigr Minor Health. 2018;20:307–16.
4. El-Meliegy A. A retrospective study of 418 patients with honeymoon impotence in an andrology clinic in Jeddah, Saudi Arabia. Europ J Sexol. 2004;13:1–4.
5. Badran W, Moamen N, Fahmy I, et al. Etiological factors of unconsummated marriage. Int J Impot Res. 2006;18:458–63.
6. Martin Hilber A, Hull T, Preston-Whytec E, et al. A cross cultural study of vaginal practices and sexuality: implications for sexual health. Soc Sci Med. 2010;70:392–400. https://doi.org/10.1016/j.socscimed.2009.10.023.
7. Woo JST, Brotto LA, Gorzalka BB. The role of sex guilt in the relationship between culture and women's sexual desire. Arch Sex Behav. 2011;40:385–94.
8. International Confederation of Midwives (ICM). Essential competencies for midwifery practice. 2018. https://www.internationalmidwives.org/assets/files/general-files/2018/10/icm-competencies%2D%2D-english-document_final_oct-2018.pdf.
9. WHO. Packages of interventions for family planning, safe abortion care, maternal, newborn and child health. 2010. https://apps.who.int/iris/handle/10665/70428.
10. Wren Serbin J, Donnelly E. The impact of racism and Midwifery's lack of racial diversity: a literature review. J Midwifery Womens Health. 2016;2016(61):694–706.
11. Nursing and Midwifery Council (NMC). Diversity data 2018–2019. 2018. https://www.nmc.org.uk/globalassets/sitedocuments/annual_reports_and_accounts/edi/edi-2018-19-data-tables.pdf.
12. Small R, Roth C, Raval M, et al. Immigrant and non-immigrant women's experiences of maternity care: a systematic and comparative review of studies in five countries. BMC Pregnancy Childbirth. 2014;14:152.
13. Bly KC, Ellis SA, Ritter R, Kantrowitz-Gordon I. A survey of midwives' attitudes toward men in midwifery. J Midwifery Womens Health. 2020;65:199–207.
14. Kennedy HP, Erickson-Owens D, Davis JA. Voices of diversity in midwifery: a qualitative research study. J Midwifery Womens Health. 2006;51:85–90.
15. Ong-Flaherty C. Critical cultural awareness and diversity in nursing: a minority perspective. Nurse Lead. 2015;13:58–62. https://doi.org/10.1016/j.mnl.2015.03.012.
16. Paasche-Orlow M. The ethics of cultural competence. Acad Med. 2004;79:347–50. https://doi.org/10.1097/00001888-200404000-00012.
17. Francoeur RT, Noonan RJ. The continuum complete international encyclopedia of sexuality. New York: Continuum; 2004.

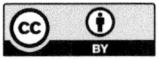

Sexual Effects of Trauma Experience on Pregnancy and Labour

24

Tanja Repič Slavič ⓘ

24.1 Introduction

Sexual abuse can affect various areas of a person's life. One area is motherhood, with related factors like the decision to have a child, getting pregnant, pregnancy experience, delivery, and the postpartum period. In this chapter, we want to present how these areas may be related to the plight of women who have experienced the trauma of sexual abuse. Many aspects of this trauma are comparable to physical and emotional abuse. First, we theoretically explain how memories can affect the present, and then, based on clinical experience with sexually abused clients, we highlight the importance of the facts that should be known to anyone who encounters survivors in their work. Finally, we will add for health care professionals (HCPs) statements of women who shared what would be the most soothing to hear, with examples of specific sentences for HCPs to help promote emotional security and positive experiences.

24.2 Before Pregnancy: Pondering Motherhood and Making the Decision to Have a Child

A decision to have a child is undoubtedly one that calls for the highest degree of responsibility, as when one becomes a parent, one remains a father or mother for the rest of one's life.

Even without a traumatic past, the decision to have a child can awaken various feelings, from excitement, joy, anticipation, and longing to all sorts of fears, doubts, insecurities, and anxieties. These emotional oscillations and adversities can be even

T. R. Slavič (✉)
Marital and Family Therapist at Franciscan Family Institute, University of Ljubljana, Ljubljana, Slovenia

© The Author(s) 2023
S. Geuens et al. (eds.), *Midwifery and Sexuality*,
https://doi.org/10.1007/978-3-031-18432-1_24

more pronounced in women who have experienced sexual abuse. Eventually, they can even lead to re-traumatisation, should memories of sexual abuse be awakened. It is important to emphasise that sexual abuse includes not only sexual violence but also acts that do not involve physical violence and can accompany touching and caressing. The consequences can be similar for sexual abuse that occurs without touch, such as showing pornography, nudity, and masturbation. The main purpose of the perpetrator is sexual arousal, but most of the time, the primary motivation for abuse and sexual gratification is a feeling of dominance, power, control, or even revenge. The victim feels humiliated, ashamed, and guilty because their most intimate boundaries have been violated [1]. Clinical experience shows that victims of physical or psychological violence can experience similar feelings, but in sexual abuse, there tends to be even more disgust and shame. Although the perpetrators are more often men, women are not excluded. When the sexual abuser is a woman, the abuse is often more hidden under the guise of caring for and nurturing the child, and it can leave even deeper wounds.

For the sexually abused woman, even the thoughts about having a child, conceiving, or already being pregnant are often full of distress and questions about whether she will be a good mother or able to protect the child from abuse in a life that is full of suffering, whether she will be able to take care of, play with, emotionally feel, and comfort the child. Sexual activity can also be a problem in the sense that she does not want it, rejects it, and feels repulsion at the very thought of natural conception, so some women opt for alternative forms of fertilisation that do not involve sexual intercourse or even for adoption (Simkin and Klaus, 2004). In clinical practice, abused women often express fears about the child's gender. Some are afraid of having a female child because they project their childhood feelings of helplessness and being abused on their potential daughter [2]. Others fear that a boy growing in their body will awaken memories of the perpetrator, who was also male and that they might not be able to love the boy-child enough [3]. The fear of conceiving and having a child is even worse if the woman has previously experienced one or more abortions or has not been able to conceive, which can raise the worry of being infertile.

On the other hand, many sexually abused women consciously choose rather never to become a mother than expose the child to such a horrible childhood as they have had and are unwilling to take risks. Some even go so far as to consider sterilisation [2].

Important Notes
Never judge. Do not try to convince the woman that, in your opinion, her thoughts or actions are wrong. Let her express her concerns, feelings, and fears and show compassion.

24.3   Pregnancy in a Woman with a History of Sexual Abuse

Pregnancy can be a trigger that may make a woman aware of her experience of sexual abuse for the first time [4]. Even if she does not remember it, her body has memorised this experience and can, during pregnancy, start 'talking' very loudly about that experience. Research shows that, after sexual abuse, pregnant women are more likely to report depression and PTSD symptoms, think more about suicide, have more health problems (high blood pressure, vomiting, pelvic pain, bleeding), and are more likely to be hospitalised [3].

On the other hand, some pregnant women with childhood abuse history can almost wholly disconnect from their bodies, especially from the waist down, to the point that they do not feel the child's movements. That is a defensive dissociation or physical numbness that once served to protect her from the horrors and pains of sexual abuse.

Severe distress can also be caused by the changes in her pregnant body (with the growing belly, and enlarged breasts). Many women feel as if something is wrong, feeling dirty or hurt inside. With unstoppable bodily changes, they often experience a loss of control over what is happening to their body [3].

All of a sudden, the woman's body is more noticeable. As a child, she had to hide every physical sign so that no one would notice that she had been abused. Now, her body has become part of the 'public arena.' People feel they are allowed to comment on it or even touch it [5]. which can activate the memory of sexual abuse. The same goes for more frequent vaginal examinations and procedures that interfere with intimacy because her body is being touched. For instance, the position on the gynaecologist's chair can strongly resemble a sexual abuse situation, with legs apart and the HCP penetrating her vagina with fingers or a clinical instrument. The body has unconsciously memorised the abuse, with sensations that intrusively activate the memory of the trauma, sometimes so disturbing that the woman cannot separate the present from the past. According to clinical practice, the two most common types of responses of women to vaginal examinations are: numbness and freezing because they experience horror and fear and wait for the examination to be over as soon as possible; or they experience ambivalence during these interventions: with on the one hand arousal, and, on the other hand, aversion, disgust, and shame at their bodily responses. Such arousal can be a mixture of physical arousal and explicit sexual arousal. Many women try to avoid vaginal examination because of these problematic effects or visit the gynaecologist or midwife only late in pregnancy.

The HCP must be professional and sensitive, as the woman is even more susceptible to any touch and procedure related to her femininity and her body [6].

If the woman smokes and consumes alcohol or other drugs that she discontinues during pregnancy because she wants to take care of herself and the baby, this can trigger unpredictable stress. These activities often protect her from painful feelings related to sexual abuse and serve to release internal tension. With the loss of these defence mechanisms, repressed memories and emotions can surface, leading to severe anxiety [3].

Clinical experience shows that distress and anxiety are even more intense when an unplanned pregnancy occurs due to unprotected sex or rape. In the case of the former, the woman can experience pregnancy as another abuse or punishment imposed on her by the child's father, society, or God. Thus, they re-experience the feelings of being a victim, helpless, and unable to control their own destiny [3].

As a result, some women choose to terminate the pregnancy, which often brings forth feelings of guilt, either immediately or later, even after several years. In most cases, the man is exempt from decision-making, and she is the only one to choose what to do.

If pregnancy results from rape, it is extra difficult to decide whether or not to keep the child or give up the child for adoption immediately after the birth. In this case, in addition to the trauma of rape, the woman is struggling with an accidental pregnancy, and she questions herself about what to do.

She can quickly see herself as a criminal if she does not accept the child. However, if she accepts the child (due to the pressure of those around her or religious beliefs), the child will remind her all her life of the rape. And she will find it difficult to accept the child or develop a negative attitude towards the child because the progenitor was sexually violent. It was by no means her fault that this had happened to her.

Important Notes
- In the case of **rape** or otherwise unplanned and unintended pregnancy, it is imperative that regardless of the decision whether to keep the child or not, you **do not blame** the abused woman; allow her to say what she feels, what makes her calmer and gives her a sense of security. Avoid WHY-questions, as they always bring about even more guilt than the traumatised person already bears. Many decisions would undoubtedly change if, in such crises, a woman had at least one compassionate, supportive relationship in her life.
- Even if you do not understand the triggers that arouse the memories of abuse, take all her feelings seriously, stay calm, and tell the pregnant woman that she is safe now, that the abuse is just waking up and not happening anymore, and give her the opportunity and a safe space to tell whatever worries and bothers her. The fact that she will be able to speak out loud and be heard when expressing her needs will be reassuring.
- Always ask permission before a vaginal examination.
- Suppose a pregnant woman confides in you her experience of sexual abuse. In that case, it makes sense to refer her to therapy with a sexual abuse specialist before giving birth and work with her and her partner to make a 'safe plan' to ensure that she is as relaxed as possible and that she masters various techniques helpful in childbirth (visualisation, breathing techniques, autogenic training, etc.).

24.4   Labour

A sense of security is a crucial protective factor that contributes to the course of childbirth. If a woman feels safe and can trust, she will find it much easier to cope with the instructions of the HCPs and with what her body tells her. Abused women have learned that losing control means physical and emotional danger, so they feel stronger and safer if they have a structure - if they know what will happen during childbirth, how it approximately will develop, what is normal and what to expect.

This information will help the woman take a break from constant worrying, monitoring, and waiting for what will follow. Those worrying feelings are very much related to abuse, where a person learns that she is 'safer' if she is constantly alert. On the other hand, a sense of being threatened can lead to extreme behaviour—aggression, subordination, rituals, constant crises, etc. Certainly, childbirth is related to a relatively high degree of unpredictability, where the woman faces the uncertainty about when labour will begin, how long it will last, how much it will hurt, how well she will tolerate the pain, how her body will react, if she will suffer injury, or if complications with the child will occur [3].

Since sexual abuse is always also an abuse of power and trust, sexually abused women are very susceptible to this dynamic. That is why she may experience fear of the medical staff because they represent authority, power, and control, reminding her of the people who abused her. As a result, she often doesn't dare to share her worries, discomforts, or disagreements, resulting in feeling insignificant and unseen, precisely what she experienced at the abuse. During vaginal exams, she may thus become completely submissive (or aggressive) due to feelings of threat and fear, but when the situation is over and she feels safe again, anger and sadness may arise [5]. In a good relationship, her partner can offer the best support. But the midwife and the doula (if present) play an additional essential role in the feeling of security, as they accompany the woman for the longest time.

That is why the midwife must know how to create a safe atmosphere while carefully monitoring the woman's reactions. The midwife should be open to a conversation to make the expectant mother feel that abuse is not happening now and that she is safe. More sense of security can be given by the partner or somebody else who knows the fears and feelings of the woman and how to calm her down (since during the abuse, she was alone and nobody protected her and calmed her down). This dual awareness and the ability to distinguish past and present is essential for the expectant mother [7].

Certain body positions, such as lying in bed, can present a problem. Abused women can also be sensitive to words uttered by the staff, as well as painful and escalating contractions, nausea, vomiting, bloody discharge, instinctive responses such as moaning, shaking, grunting, screaming, pelvic dilation, and feeling the baby inside the vagina as they all can awaken the body's memory of sexual abuse. The woman can be upset due to the changes of staff (unpredictability, lost sense of security) and a darkened room (reminiscent of the room that was dark when the perpetrator came to abuse her). She can react in different ways: with excessive fear and panic or by freezing, becoming rigid and numb. The latter—dissociation—enabled her to endure sexual abuse and distance herself from her body and mind.

This reaction (called freezing) often happens to those victims who experienced severe pain during the abuse. Therefore, it is very likely that these women will experience dissociation even during childbirth, float away without feeling physical pain (because they will freeze, the same as during trauma) and thus unconsciously fight the psychological distress, which can significantly prolong and hinder the course of childbirth. In such moments, it is crucial that the woman stays as much as possible 'present' during labour and that the midwife or partner, if he is by her side, 'calls' her back with her name and calming words, reassuring her that she is safe and that she can trust that everything will be fine with her body [7].

Fear of a caesarean section (with general anaesthesia) can also cause fear in a woman, particularly the feeling of losing control over her body. However, general anaesthesia makes it for some women easier to cope with childbirth.

Clinical experience shows that fear can also increase due to the thought of possible injuries (perineum, vagina) and the fact that the child will get dirty because they will come out through the part of her body defiled by the penetration of the perpetrator; the woman can experience immense disgust about her genitals. On the other hand, some women report that childbirth was a positive experience, and they experienced a kind of cleansing—as if the fact that they were able to give birth and that the child came out through the same body part where the abuse 'came in' the childbirth healed this part of the body's memory.

On the outside, the reactions described above may seem exaggerated or inappropriate. Although the cause lies in the past, the reactions are triggered in the present. So, emotions and sensations associated with the abuse that flare up when she is supposed to prepare for the child's arrival can be very stressful. How her partner and the HCPs approach her significantly impacts whether she will feel worthy or re-traumatised.

Important Notes
- For the care of the mother and child, the woman with a history of sexual abuse will be most helped by the presence of the same staff (as few shifts as possible) who provide emotional security. If they know the possible triggers of sexual abuse, they will recognise the woman's reactions when her trauma flares up and, therefore, blocks her, increasing stress and panic.
- If a woman feels it appropriate, she can confide in her experience of sexual abuse. In this case, the staff's response is essential because it can relax the atmosphere or, conversely, cause dissociation. Stress, anxiety, and fear cause the secretion of epinephrine, norepinephrine, and cortisol, hormones that slow down childbirth. Thus, unconscious mechanisms and fears can prevent the progression of the delivery and lead to otherwise preventable surgeries, causing further potential emotional and physical trauma.

- Persons present at birth should listen and take into account the potential needs and wishes of the mother, which may be trivial when observed from the outside, but are very important to her. Allow her to express her worst fears and biggest hopes about childbirth (e.g. absence of students at the delivery, no unnecessary vaginal examinations, only as much nudity as is necessary, and the unacceptability of specific touches and positions, even if they are well-intentioned).
- The key to a sense of security is also that the woman is familiar with the normal course of childbirth, procedures, and interventions and that she has the opportunity to participate in decision-making. She must be assured that her decisions will be respected and taken into account (with the health of the mother and child always coming first). It is wise to talk about all this already during pregnancy.

24.5   After Childbirth: The Beginning of Motherhood

In therapy, it often turns out that things that may seem most self-evident and natural (such as caring for a child, breastfeeding, washing the baby, putting the baby to sleep, soothing the crying baby) can be powerful triggers for an abused woman, additionally increasing tension and anxiety. A child's crying can greatly increase a mother's distress, helplessness, and anxiety because she can be unconsciously reminded of herself crying out loud when a child or calling out in silent cries, begging her closest people to protect her from abuse. On the other hand, embracing and caressing her newborn can be reassuring, as the young mother feels able to soothe her child with her presence, voice, and gazing in the child's eyes and gains hope that she can succeed in giving her love and being a good mother.

For instance, breastfeeding can trigger a memory of abuse in the maternity hospital soon after birth. Breastfeeding is related not only to the mother's body but also very strongly to emotions and experiences. If a sexually abused young mother has an aversion [8] to breastfeeding because it may arouse feelings of abuse and remind her body that someone was disrespectful to it, she should be supported as much as possible and not forced to breastfeed at all costs. Even if her body is fully prepared for breastfeeding, her psyche is not necessarily so, and that is why emotional contraindications should also be considered [6]. Clinical experience shows that this happens more often to women whose breasts have been touched by the perpetrator during abuse, perhaps even commented. As a result, she can feel that her milk is 'dirty' and therefore unconsciously experience a psychological blockage because she doesn't want the child to drink from her 'dirty' breasts in order 'not to 'get the baby dirty'. Sometimes the infant's gender is also related to the feelings accompanying breastfeeding. When the perpetrator was a male, abused mothers tend to be more relaxed with a daughter than with a son. Then a son can cause associations with breastfeeding a male).

The timeslot for breastfeeding can also be an influencing factor. Breastfeeding can be more peaceful during the day than lying in bed at night. A darkened room can create unpleasant associations with the abuse when going to bed as a child. Then, one should look for a more suitable time, place, and conditions without distress.

Nudity alone, remembering nudity, exposure, and insecurity during abuse, may be too much. In many situations in the maternity hospital, the body is exposed in front of others. That occurs in contact with HCPs during medical check-ups, and especially in case of failure to establish proper breastfeeding. Such failure may be enough to awaken the woman's shame, especially if milk production doesn't start properly, which can occur due to all the earlier mentioned distress factors [8].

Motor/vestibular memory of what happened to her breasts during the abuse can awaken. For instance, by being touched by the infant, by herself, and perhaps by a midwife or nurse who wants to help the young mother not yet used to the proper grip. But also by strong, painful sensations in the initial phases of breastfeeding, and she does not know yet whether these are normal. The baby's constant demands and the noticeable pleasure during sucking can cause some mothers to decide not to continue breastfeeding [3].

Clinical experience shows that in extreme cases, some sexually abused women decide, already before childbirth, to bottle-feed their baby because they want to avoid additional stress.

On the other hand, the hardships associated with breastféeding can be the reason for dissociation as a defence mechanism—so the woman does not feel her body and breasts as if they do not exist. In this way, she avoids all feelings and sensations while feeding the baby. For some women, this is the only way to breastfeed at all [8].

Another common challenge can be caring for and bathing the child. The necessary washing of the baby's genitals can awaken the fear that she may somehow violate boundaries. That clearly shows how the mother's abuse is awakening because the perpetrator has violated her boundaries. If the woman is aware of her sexual abuse, then the fear of her abusing the child is a kind of 'protection' that, in most cases, prevents her as a mother from sexually abusing the child. In therapy, some women say that there may be situations where they change, bathe, or breastfeed the baby and feel aroused. Her body tells her that something is happening that is not natural. That can especially happen if she has been sexually abused at the changing table or while bathing and may not even have images in her explicit memory so that she could recall the abuse itself. It is enough that the body remembers the abuse stored in the woman's organic, implicit memory. So if there is arousal or disgust, it is important that the mother learns to control herself, take her time, and evaluate these feelings. In other words, she must set boundaries for herself, know that her abuse is awakening and that her child deserves pure love. If necessary, she also knows how to withdraw, maybe turn to her partner and talk to him about these feelings if she is not yet able to process them independently [9]. But when that does not work, the mother must seek professional help to process these feelings of abuse (disgust, shame).

Important Notes
- HCPs should encourage breastfeeding but never force it or even condemn and blame a woman if she cannot overcome her psychological blockages. The baby is better fed with a bottle and without anxiety than breastfed, absorbing the mother's anxiety with her milk.
- In case the midwife (or lactation consultant) helps the woman or wants to show her how to facilitate breastfeeding with a certain position or grip, she should ask what the woman prefers: to only verbally tell her what to do (i.e. use the hands-off technique) or also use her hands on the mother's breast to show her.
- If the mother's body responds with arousal, disgust, and fear when changing and caring for the baby, this is usually a sign of an unprocessed experience of sexual abuse. Helping her seek professional help is the right thing to do. Otherwise, the fear and guilt can be severe enough for the mother to start avoiding her baby and consequently feeling that she is a bad mother.

24.6 Statements of Abused Women

What They Would Like to Tell the HCP to Get the Most Helpful Responses
1. *"Don't judge me, don't force me verbally if I freeze, start crying, react in a way showing my sadness, shame, and helplessness. Your compassion, calmness, and respect help me feel secure and make it easier to feel that everything will be fine."*
2. *"Don't ask me WHY I'm doing or not doing something because it will only make me feel even more guilty, and it will worsen. Tell me that you are backing me, that I am not alone, that I am 'here and now' and that this is only awakening of some feelings that belong to the past."*
3. *"If I have a sense of control, if I know what's going on or what's going to happen, it's a lot easier for me, so please explain to me earlier what you're going to do. It will be very reassuring to hear that everything happening is normal in certain circumstances."*

In moments of distress when memories of abuse are stirred, some of these sentences are most helpful when uttered by the HCP.

Very important: These words must be spoken slowly and calmly! Before you start talking, say the person's name because it helps disconnect the flow of dissociation, which took her into the past, and recall her back to the present.

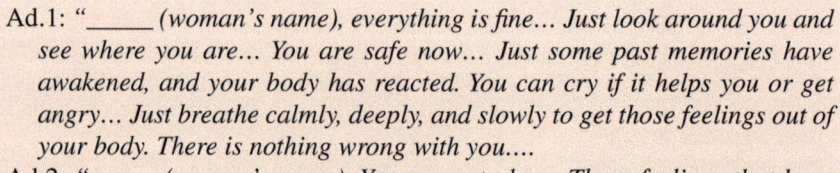

Ad.1: "_____ (woman's name), everything is fine... Just look around you and see where you are... You are safe now... Just some past memories have awakened, and your body has reacted. You can cry if it helps you or get angry... Just breathe calmly, deeply, and slowly to get those feelings out of your body. There is nothing wrong with you....

Ad.2: "_____ (woman's name), You are not alone. These feelings that have flooded your body have awakened and are a thing of the past. It's just the aftershock: the quake is over. Today you are safe, and you can say anything you feel, set a boundary, and have control. I understand. And I feel that it is not easy for you. I'm here with you."

Ad.3: "_____ (woman's name), you are safe. We will explain everything to you as we go, and your responses are perfectly normal, given the circumstances and what you have experienced. Your body is just responding to a traumatic memory of where you couldn't have any control. But here, today, you are in control, and you are not alone. We will do everything in our power to make it easier for you, just tell us; and if something bothers you, you can always set a boundary...".

24.7 Conclusion

A decision to have a child, pregnancy, give birth, and accept motherhood can be a major challenge for a woman who has experienced sexual abuse. These challenges can awaken painful, repressed memories of trauma and leave a woman with a bitter aftertaste, a sense of guilt, incompetence, pain, and betrayal by her own body. Even though she may consciously not remember the abuse, her body remembered it. No matter what comes to the surface, we should never blame a woman for what happened to her. Despite the many triggers that bring new hardships, it is important to point out that, for some abused women, this period can be one of the most positive experiences in their lives, even a 'healing' experience if their partner is understanding and if they are surrounded by professional medical staff who are open to compassion and understanding of their plight. In such safe circumstances, the woman will be able to hear that everything is fine with her, that she is 'normal', that her body is doing something right and can carry a new life, give birth, breastfeed, hug, nurture, and raise her child with love. As a result, she will feel stronger and experience more confidence in her body, her growing child, and her ability to mother.

References

1. Repič Slavič T, Gostečnik C. Relational family therapy as an aid toward resolving the trauma of sexual abuse in childhood in the process of separation in the couple relationship. J Marital Fam Ther. 2017;43:422–34.

2. Reckling AE. Mother-daughter incest: when survivors become mothers. J Trauma Prac. 2004;3:49–71.
3. Simkin P, Klaus P. When survivors give birth: understanding and healing the effects of early sexual abuse on childbearing women. Seattle: Classic Day Publishing; 2004.
4. Lukasse M, Schei B, Vangen S, Øian P. Childhood abuse and common complaints in pregnancy. Birth. 2009;36:190–9.
5. Russell S. Experiences of birth after sexual abuse. Multiple Parts. 2021:18–9.
6. Prescott A. Childhood sexual abuse and the potential impact on maternity. Midwifery Matters. 2002;92:17–29.
7. Tilley J. Sexual assault and flashbacks on the labour ward. Pract Midwife. 2000;3:18–20.
8. Wood K, Van Esterik P. Infant feeding experiences of women who were sexually abused in childhood. Can Fam Physician. 2010;56:136–41.
9. Repič T. Nemi kriki spolne zlorabe in novo upanje (the silent screams of sexual abuse and a new hope). Celje, Slovenia: Celjska Mohorjeva Družba; 2015.

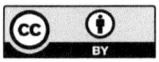

Relevant Aspects of Female Genital Mutilation

25

Suaad Abdulrehman (iD)

25.1 Introduction

Female genital mutilation (FGM), also called female genital cutting (FGM/C) or female circumcision, is a widely practised phenomenon or tradition in many African countries, some countries in the Middle East, and Indonesia. It is defined as 'an intervention on the external female genitalia without medical necessity'.

There is a wide variety in the extent of the intervention, how the intervention takes place, the short and long-term consequences for physical and reproductive health, and the psychological and sexual consequences.

This chapter will give information about FGM so that the HCP can provide optimal guidance to women without compromising their experience or their culture.

The chapter will start with a brief description of the phenomenon with backgrounds and explanations and some figures on prevalence. Then some details of the circumstances and the extent of the procedure will be given, followed successively by the various consequences of FGM: first, the direct results of the intervention, and then the long-term physical, obstetric, psychological, and sexual consequences. The last part will discuss aspects of dealing with clients with FGM.

25.2 A Brief Description of the Phenomenon with Backgrounds and Explanations

The origin of FGM is unclear. In Islamic Africa, it is frequently explained as a religious commitment, assuming that Prophet Mohammed mentioned in one of his Hadiths that *'having undergone Sunna (FGM type 1) is a symbol of cleanliness and purity for a girl'*.

S. Abdulrehman (✉)
Parnassia Groep IPSY/Psyq Almere, Almere, The Netherlands

© The Author(s) 2023
S. Geuens et al. (eds.), *Midwifery and Sexuality*,
https://doi.org/10.1007/978-3-031-18432-1_25

The reality is that FGM is a pre-Christian and pre-Islamic practice.

FGM is deeply rooted in cultural traditions that differ by family, region, and country. Among the arguments to continue with FGM are:

- The clitoris is supposed to be dangerous ('the devil') or hazardous for the man's orgasm.
- A girl without a clitoris is supposed to have no sexual desire, so it is more likely that she will keep her virginity till marriage.
- Without a clitoris, the married woman is neither supposed to have nor show sexual desire. The man should show desire.
- The procedure is regarded as providing beauty, purity, and cleanliness.
- In some countries, circumcision is said to promote fertility and increase male sexual pleasure.
- Circumcision is an initiation rite into womanhood. In some areas, 'not being circumcised' is experienced as being incomplete and lacking social status (or even running the risk of being expelled). Circumcision is then usually considered a 'festive' rite of passage [1].

On the other hand, the WHO very clearly states that FGM violates the human rights of girls and women and that the practice of FGM has no health benefits for them [2]. ICM, the International Confederation of Midwives, recognises and condemns FGM as a harmful practice and a violation of the Human Rights of girls and women [3].

The tradition of FGM reflects the deep-rooted inequality between the sexes and constitutes an extreme form of discrimination against women. It violates a person's rights to health, security, and physical integrity, the right to be free from torture and cruel, inhuman, or degrading treatment.

25.3   Prevalence and Where Can It Be Found

According to UNICEF, more than 200 million women and girls alive today have been cut [4]. They are mainly living in the 30 countries where FGM is commonly practised [4]. The prevalence in those countries varies and is usually given for the 15–49 age group. In part of these countries, the prevalence is decreasing. However, according to UNICEF, the absolute global figures are still growing because of the increasing population.

Egypt is a clear example of that trend. In women aged 15–49 years., the prevalence of FGM decreased from 97% to 70% between 1985 and 2015. The population increase of 85% over this period caused a 35% increase in the absolute amount of FGM.

In a 2013 report by UNICEF, Egypt had the highest absolute number of FGM, whereas Somalia had, with 98%, the highest global prevalence.

Starting in the 1970s, when more migration from Africa and the Middle East got underway, the Western medical world became confronted with women who had FGM. So it gradually became a topic of public discussion.

25.4 Details of the Circumstances and the Extent of the Procedure

FGM is usually performed in childhood. Depending on the different (sub-)cultures, there is much variety in the preferred age. In Yemen, the vast majority occurs in the first week after birth, whereas in Egypt, one quarter occurs at ages 5–9 and 70% at ages 10–14. In the more rural areas of many countries, the procedure was (and regularly still is) traditionally performed without anaesthesia and septic precautions. Frequently, the mother plays a prominent role, e.g. holding her daughter down and keeping her eyes closed.

In many cultures, FGM is a rite of passage and a nearly inescapable major life event, surrounded by festivities. Over many years the girl is, in a way, seduced by various promises. The circumcision is 'the path to make her perfect, with absolute beauty and purity as a woman'.

Despite being aware of the pain, the fear, and the other side effects, they have suffered themselves, most mothers and grandmothers continue to adhere to this tradition.

The extent of the procedure is the basis of the four types of FGM that the WHO distinguishes. Because the clitoris has such an essential role in the FGM arguments and the FGM procedures, it deserves some extra attention. The clitoris is far bigger than the tiny, highly sensitive spot frowned upon in many FGM cultures (see Fig. 25.1). Next to the glans, shaft, and hood (the foreskin), the clitoris has two crura and two spongious bodies that swell when aroused. In none of the FGM procedures, the crura and the spongious bodies are removed. These remaining parts are responsible for the fact that many women, despite FGM, can experience orgasm [5].

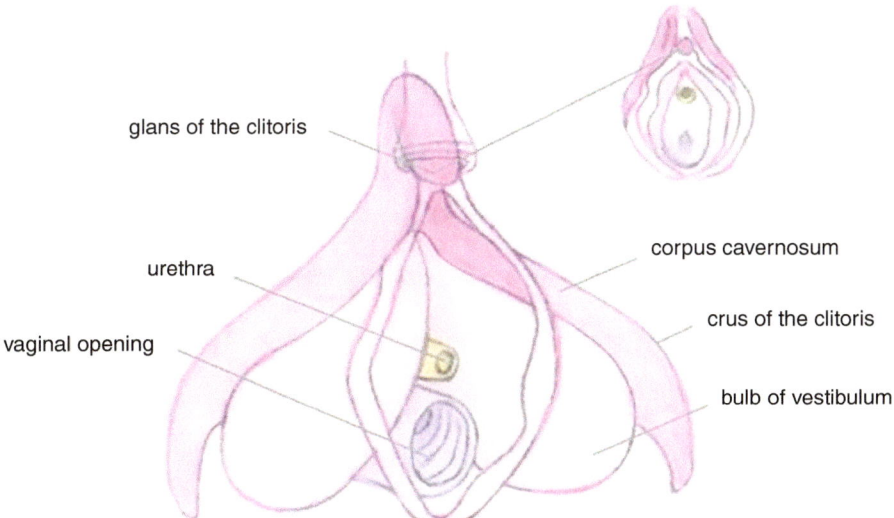

glans of the clitoris

corpus cavernosum

urethra

crus of the clitoris

vaginal opening

bulb of vestibulum

Fig. 25.1 The Clitoris. (Illustration composed by Gabrijela Simetinger and Helena Černej)

25.4.1 The WHO Classification of FGM

Female genital mutilation is classified by the WHO into four major types [2]. See Fig. 25.2.

Type 1: This is the partial or total removal of the clitoral glans (the external and visible part of the clitoris, which is the most sensitive part of the female genitals), and/or the prepuce/clitoral hood (the fold of skin surrounding the clitoral glans).
Type 2: This is the partial or total removal of the clitoral glans and the labia minora (the inner lips), with or without removal of the labia majora (the outer lips).
Type 3: Also known as infibulation, this is the narrowing of the vaginal opening through the creation of a covering seal. The seal is formed by cutting and repositioning the inner lips, or outer lips, sometimes through stitching, with or without removal of the clitoral prepuce/clitoral hood and glans.
Type 4: This includes all other harmful procedures to the female genitalia for non-medical purposes, e.g. pricking, piercing, incising, scraping, and cauterising the genital area.

In the Pharaonic type (Type 3) with infibulation, the small opening for urine and blood is told to be not wider than a grain of rice or the head of a match.

Geographically, there are many differences in the prevalence of the various types. In Somalia and Sudan, close to 98% of girls undergo the Pharaonic type, although, in the last decade, a small percentage of mothers have chosen Sunna (Type 1) for their daughters. In Sunna, the specialised woman takes the clitoris between two fingers and pulls the prepuce very strongly till it tears and starts bleeding (the blood ensures the girl's purity).

Another change is that the procedure is shifting to the medical field. In Egypt, for instance, 60% of girls have undergone the procedure by a physician and 10% by another HCP.

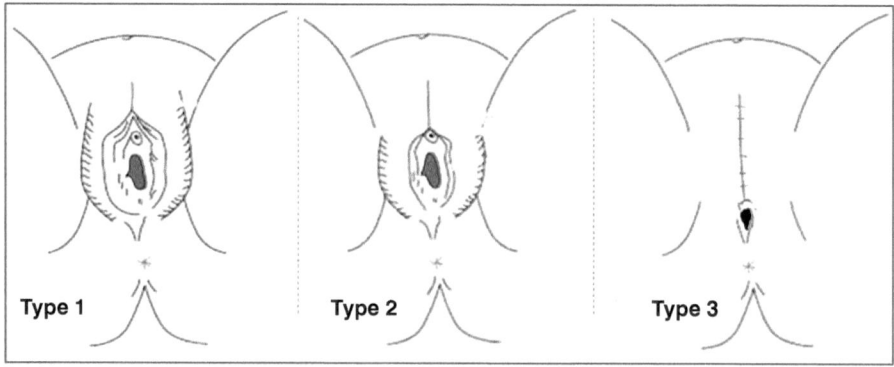

Fig. 25.2 The WHO classification of female genital mutilation. (Redrawn by WL Gianotten)

Instead of relying on geographical prevalence figures, it is better to ask what kind of circumcision the woman has had and by whom.

At the time of marriage, the nearly closed vagina has to be reopened. In Sudan and Southern Somalia, traditional defibulation has to be done by the bridegroom through penile penetration. He has to put sufficient pressure on the infibulation seal, causing it to tear, which is painful for both partners. The time needed for defibulation varies depending on the amount of force and the thickness of the scarred seal. Generally, it is supposed to be accomplished within a week [6].

In other areas, like northern Somalia, the infibulation is cut open by an excisor (circumciser). In both cases, the couple has to continue penetration for several weeks to prevent the vagina from reclosing. This 'maintenance' is painful because of the open wounds, and many women experience this defibulation period as painful as the original infibulation. Infections and bleeding are common [6].

25.5 The Consequences of the Intervention

In the broader sense, FGM is a severe violation of the rights of girls and women, strongly impairing the process of normal development. In the context of this chapter, it can be seen as a complicated and painful process causing damage to physical and mental health and sexuality. The amount of damage depends on many factors.

- The age at which FGM is performed,
- The extent of the procedure and the skills of the person who performs the procedure,
- The practicalities (duration of the operation, hygiene, et cetera),
- The resilience, resistance, and physical power of the girl/woman,
- The balance between emotional support and force,
- Living inside or outside an FGM-endemic society,
- The level of sexuality education and the approach to sexuality.

Many reported data are not very reliable. Partly because of a lack of appropriate comparison groups. And frequently also started from a biased underlying frame of reference [7].

Here a distinction is made between physical ('medical'), reproductive, mental ('emotional'), and sexual consequences.

25.5.1 Physical Disturbances

Among the immediate health complications are:

- Severe pain (especially when performed without anaesthesia).
- Blood loss with haemorrhagic shock.

- Local oedema causing impaired urination and defecation.
- Injury to the urethra, vagina, or rectum.
- Death due to blood loss and infections (including tetanus).

Among the late medical complications are

- Chronic pain from trapped or unprotected nerve endings.
- Dermoid cysts, abscesses, and genital ulcers with superficial loss of tissue.
- Excessive scar formation by keloid. Keloid is extensive scar tissue, common in people with Sub-Saharan African genes.
- Chronic pelvic infections causing chronic backache and pelvic pain.
- Urinary incontinence and dribbling of urine (especially after infibulation), owing to difficulties emptying the bladder and stagnation of urine under the hood of scar tissue. Recurrent urinary tract infections and damage to the kidneys with eventual renal failure.
- Infection with HIV.

25.5.2 Reproductive and Obstetric Disturbances

Especially infibulation, but also the defibulation phase can cause reproductive disturbances.

- Painful menstruation due to the near-complete sealing of the vagina and urethra.
- Endometriosis due to retained menstrual blood.
- Vesicovaginal and rectovaginal fistula (after obstructed labour).
- A narrowed obstetrical birthing channel.
- Perineal tears.
- Postpartum haemorrhage.
- Associated neonatal morbidity.

Whereas traditional defibulation usually creates enough room for sexual penetration, that room is not enough for smooth childbirth. The vaginal outlet can need medical widening during childbirth ('medical defibulation'). In a study from Saudi Arabia, defibulation at birth was performed as a surgical procedure [8]. In that study, the women defibulated at birth had fewer instrumental deliveries and less blood loss (with no differences in the neonatal outcome). The authors concluded that HCPs working with women with FGM type-3 should learn how to perform this medical defibulation [8].

25.5.3 Mental/Emotional Health Issues

The FGM procedure can be an extremely psychotraumatic event depending on various factors. The girls' age at the procedure is a relevant factor. The older the girl, the more likely she will have anxious anticipation, and the more she will be confused (aware that she has to agree without real consenting). During the procedure itself, the pain, the shock, and the amount of physical force by those performing the cutting are relevant elements. That is especially when she feels betrayed (for instance, when the mother forces the girl to surrender). At a later stage, additional damage can develop due to the fear of pain when getting married. And also after marrying due to the pain in the trajectory of defibulation by the husband.

Migrating to a more woman-friendly society without FGM and with apparently more social and sexual freedom creates opportunities for comparison. Whereas in the original culture, 'not being circumcised' can have caused feelings of incompleteness and inferiority, the same feelings can develop after migrating, but now precisely because of having been circumcised [9].

Among the consequences are found:

- Post-traumatic stress disorder (found in 1 in 6 migrant women in the Netherlands) and depression or anxiety (1 in 3) [10].
- Psychiatric and psychosomatic disturbances.
- Lowered self-image, with the feeling of incompleteness and inferiority.
- Chronic irritability, sleep problems, and nightmares.

25.5.4 Sexual Issues

Sexuality after FGM appears an ultimate example of the complex choreography between various bio-psycho-socio-cultural influences. Even with removing the glans, shaft, and hood of the clitoris, there is sufficient remaining erectile clitoral tissue [5]. However, for an orgasm, more is needed than only anatomy. One needs enough and adequate stimulation, which is influenced by the presence and amount of pain, the fear of pain, the erotic support of the partner, and the amount of sexuality-positive education the woman has received.

Infibulation can easily plunge the woman into a vicious circle of pain, fear of pain, low arousal, dry vagina, and high pelvic floor tone. A meta-analysis compared the sexual function of women with and women without FGM. Women with FGM scored worse in all domains (desire, arousal, lubrication, orgasm, satisfaction, and pain) [11]. That can also develop during and in the period after defibulation, resulting in low or no sexual pleasure, potentially leading to relational problems and even divorce.

However, for some other couples, that strenuous defibulation period can also forge a close bond between the partners.

In dealing with FGM, caution appears needed when assessing research questions and results. That was, for instance, clear in Egyptian research [12]. Whereas FGM is supposed/intended to reduce a woman's sexual appetite and increase her chastity, it was not believed to reduce her sexual pleasure. However, sexual pleasure was framed differently by men and women. While (especially younger) men considered sexual satisfaction a cornerstone of marital happiness, women considered themselves sexually satisfied with marital harmony and a satisfactory socio-economic situation.

Acculturation to Western culture can create the request to defibulate, either to get rid of pain or to obtain more sexual pleasure. Proper surgical anatomy reconstruction usually gives patients and husbands high satisfaction [14].

On the other hand, Western HCPs can get confused by women requesting to re-infibulate after childbirth (in other words: narrowing the entrance). Vaginal tightness can be considered a prerequisite for male sexual pleasure and can be intimately linked to infibulation [6].

25.6   Dealing with FGM

In 2015 the global community clearly stated that FGM violates human rights. The Sustainable Development Goals (SDGs) have laid this down under Goal 5. The target is, by the year 2030, to eliminate all harmful practices, such as child marriage, early marriage, forced marriage, and FGM/C,

That has clear consequences for HCPs in countries where FGM is endemic. They should proactively clarify not to agree with these procedures. On the one hand, by participating in public health education about FGM and its harmful consequences. On the other hand, even more important, by not performing these procedures themselves. In several countries, FGM has become strongly medicalised and an important source of income. The International Confederation of Midwives clearly states that midwives should refrain from supporting or participating in any form of the practice at any time and that they have to respect relevant (inter)national codes of ethics [3].

Gynaecological and obstetric HCPs with, in their community, migrants from FGM societies have to be prepared to deal with the consequences of FGM. They have to acquire the skills to defibulate during labour or when women request defibulation to relieve pain or improve their sexual life.[1]

Part of comprehensive care is proper health education for the women of those migrant communities. Having migrated to the Western world is no guarantee that FGM will be abandoned. Up to one-third of North African girls living in Scandinavia were found to be circumcised when visiting their home country [15].

Another aspect of good care is how to deal respectfully with this other reality. Whereas the term mutilation is used in this chapter, using that term with the woman in question can be experienced as offensive and degrading. Then the term circumcision is preferable.

When confronted with FGM, HCPs need to be aware that their response impacts the women. Looks—sometimes spontaneous and unaware—of astonishment or even horror can also damage women's mental health. Many women have felt ashamed of a physical examination and avoided HCPs who did not conceal their astonishment about FGM or how it looked [8].

---

[1] For technical details see: Abdulcadir [13].

References

1. Althaus FA. Female circumcision: rite of passage or violation of rights. Int Fam Plan Perspect. 1997;23:130–3.
2. https://www.who.int/news-room/fact-sheets/detail/female-genital-mutilation.
3. https://www.internationalmidwives.org/assets/files/statement-files/2019/06/eng-fgm-1-letterhead.pdf.
4. https://www.unicef.org/media/files/FGMC_2016_brochure_final_UNICEF_SPREAD.pdf.
5. Catania L, Abdulcadir O, Puppo V, et al. Pleasure and orgasm in women with female genital mutilation/cutting (FGM/C). J Sex Med. 2007;4:1666–78.
6. Johansen REB. Virility, pleasure and female genital mutilation/cutting. A qualitative study of perceptions and experiences of medicalised defibulation among Somali and Sudanese migrants in Norway. Reprod Health. 2017;14:25.
7. Obermeyer CM. The health consequences of female circumcision; science advocacy and standards of evidence. Med Anthropol Q. 2003;17:394–412.
8. Rouzi AA, Berg RC, Al-Wassia H, et al. Labour outcomes with defibulation at delivery in immigrant Somali and Sudanese women with type III female genital mutilation/cutting. Swiss Med Wkly. 2020;150:w20326.
9. Omigbodun O, Bella-Awusah T, Groleau D, et al. Perceptions of the psychological experiences surrounding female genital mutilation/cutting (FGM/C) among the Izzi in Southeast Nigeria. Transcult Psychiatry. 2020;57:212–27.
10. Vloeberghs E, van der Kwaak A, Knipscheer J, et al. Coping and chronic psychosocial consequences of female genital mutilation in the Netherlands. Ethn Health. 2012;17:677–95.
11. Pérez-López FR, Ornat L, López-Baena MT, et al. Association of female genital mutilation and female sexual dysfunction: a systematic review and meta-analysis. Eur J Obstet Gynecol Reprod Biol. 2020;254:236–44.
12. Fahmy A, El-Mouelhy MT, Ragab AR. Female genital mutilation/cutting and issues of sexuality in Egypt. Reprod Health Matters. 2010;18:181–90.
13. Abdulcadir J, Marras S, Catania L, et al. Defibulation: a visual reference and learning tool. J Sex Med. 2018;15:601–11.
14. Nour NM, Michels KB, Bryant AE. Defibulation to treat female genital cutting: effect on symptoms and sexual function. Obstet Gynecol. 2006;108:55–60.
15. Berg RC, Denison E. A tradition in transition: factors perpetuating and hindering the continuance of female genital mutilation/cutting (FGM/C) summarised in a systematic review. Health Care Women Int. 2013;34:837–59.

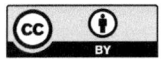

Part V

Introduction to Module 5: Skills and Adaptations

Woet L. Gianotten, Sam Geuens, and Ana Polona Mivšek

All professionals in sexology, sexual health, and sexual medicine have expertise that gradually developed over the years. During their education and years of practice, knowledge and skills were learned, and their attitude was successively refined and shaped according to their professional needs. The needed levels in this triad of knowledge, skills, and attitude will differ for midwives and other maternity care providers. But they too have to pass through a gradual development of expertise.

While the first four modules of this book mainly focused on knowledge, this fifth module will predominantly concentrate on skills, attitude, and teaching.

In healthcare, professionals devote much time to developing manual skills like taking blood pressure, giving injections, auscultation, and vaginal examination. In dealing with sexuality, most skills consist of communication. Activities like taking a sexual history, giving sexuality education, explaining the sexual side effects of an episiotomy, and treating a sexual disturbance all need words and an amount of verbal fluency.

So the first chapter in this module deals with talking sex. Like other skills, one cannot simply learn the skill of talking sex from a book.

The second chapter of this module will focus on the professionals who teach midwives. How should they offer the framework with the necessary sexuality-related midwifery competencies, and how should they implement the triad of sexuality knowledge, skills, and attitude into the midwifery curriculum? Finally, this chapter will also provide concrete strategies for teaching midwives about sexuality, organizing practicals, etc.

The next chapter will concentrate on attitudes. Daily midwifery practice is, on the one side, characterized by pregnant and birthing women with their insecurities and vulnerability. On the other side are the midwife's practicalities and responsibilities and the daily routine of dealing with bodies and pain. This chapter aims to foster awareness among practising midwives and midwifery students about the risks of 'routine care', making us blind to our client's vulnerability, dependency, nakedness, and pain.

The next chapter will address how sexology professionals manage sexual problems. It will explain the skills and toolbox of the psychosexual and sexual medicine professionals in case referral is needed.

The last chapter will look into the future of midwifery. It examines how midwifery can introduce new elements into its field of practice, starting from a sex-positive approach, responding to the cultural taboos and anticipating the gradual changes in society.

Chapter 26: Talking Sexuality

In most Western cultures, people have learned to talk about sexuality reasonably easily, at least at a party or in a pub, with a lot of humour. That, however, is very different from professionally talking about sexuality with patients or clients. For many HCPs, it appears rather difficult to ask about getting lubrication, having a painful orgasm, or loss of desire. It is also difficult to give information on oral sex or intimate masturbation.

This chapter will deal with those communication skills. It presents a specific framework for discussing sex with clients, supplemented by concrete, practical communication examples. The chapter will differentiate between 'talking sexology' (usually in the mutual contact between professionals) and 'talking sex' (what is needed in the communication with clients - the woman or couple).

The chapter follows the broad outline of the 'One to One' model with four stages: proactively raise the issue; encourage the patient to talk for herself; summarize; make an offer. This 'One to One' model is developed by SENSOA, the Flemish Expertise Centre for Sexual Health.

It aims to help HCPs engage more easily and often with the sexuality and intimacy of their patients and enhance the sexual well-being of the community as a whole.

Chapter 27: From Midwifery Competencies on Sexual Wellbeing to Teaching and Training Midwives on Sexuality

This book aims to better integrate the 'sexuality and intimacy' topic in midwifery care.

To achieve that, one has to consider three relevant groups.

On the one hand, there are practising midwives and HCPs who have already finished their basic training. With the current adage of 'life-long learning', we believe that this book offers much valuable and reliable information for private refreshing and further training.

The second group consists of midwives and HCPs in the making. Many schools and university institutions offer midwifery and nursing courses that prepare young people to become the next generation of providers for maternity care and women's healthcare. We hope that this book will contribute to that formation.

The third group consists of the teachers and tutors in midwifery and other healthcare schools.

That group is the main target of this chapter.

Based on the existing midwifery competencies frameworks, it starts with the midwives' role in sexuality and sexual well-being, looks at the adaptations needed in the curriculum, and then moves on to the tutor's skills and capacities. For developing the required expertise, knowledge has to be intertwined with skills and attitude. Such expertise can only be acquired by various forms of 'doing it'. In other words, role-playing, with roles that gradually resemble the daily reality.

The chapter uses KASES, an educational model (knowledge, attitude, skills, emotional attunement, and support) to offer concrete strategies for teaching midwives about sexuality, organizing practicals, etc.

Chapter 28: Various Sexual Consequences of Interventions in Midwifery Practice

Many different elements influence sexuality and intimacy. Whereas some of those elements are entirely outside obstetric care, others are directly related to what happens in the contact with the midwife. This chapter deals with the consequences (the 'sexual side effects') of what the midwife is doing or not doing. It focuses relatively more on behaviour and attitude than on the 'medical or technical' interventions. The chapter will discuss possible sexual implications of the midwife's daily work and of integrating the theme of sexuality with attention to body integrity, boundaries, and respect.

Part of the information is provided as questions for reflective exercises on the professional attitude in daily practice.

This chapter will also include some aspects of personal involvement in the care of the woman and the couple. The midwife is also a person with sexual feelings, and most probably with a sexual life and maybe a sexual relationship. These relevant realities tend to be considered unrelated to their work, but they can influence when the positive and negative aspects of their clients' intimacy and sexuality intensely or repeatedly confront the midwife.

Chapter 29: How Sexual Problems are Managed (by Other Professionals)

This chapter will address how sexology or sexual medicine professionals deal with sexual problems and sexual disturbances. The 'toolbox' of the sexuality professional contains many different elements. Some of them can be developed and used by the midwife. The chapter will describe these elements to clarify what is going on in the sexologist's consultation room so that the midwife can explain what the woman or couple can expect when being referred there.

Based on a detailed case history, the chapter will introduce the various steps of a possible sex therapy treatment programme.

Chapter 30: Midwifery of the Future; A Widening Field of Competences

This book aimed to create more 'sexuality-sensitive midwifery care', which today is often lacking in most places around the world. This last chapter of both the module and the book will try to take midwifery to the next level.

In a broad sense, sexuality-positive midwifery can create space for expanding the domains of women's health.

Why not dream of a change for the better? This chapter will emphasize various motives to look for change. It will delineate some aspects of Swedish midwifery. Sweden is an example of well-developed midwifery care, with a progressive and sexuality-positive approach.

The chapter will then cover various perspectives of sexuality education. Starting with the daily midwifery practice, then on the role of teacher/educator for various groups and thirdly by proactively participating in the society for advocacy and promoting sexual health and rights.

The chapter then reaches for midwifery imagination. Combining social needs and individual dreams can create new job opportunities in the form of midwifery super-specialization.

Talking Sexuality

26

Ruth Borms and Sam Geuens [ORCID]

26.1 Introduction

This chapter offers a concrete, easy-to-use method to introduce the topic of sexuality in your midwifery practice. Based on four easy steps, the midwife, as a healthcare professional (HCP), can start a conversation about sexuality, listen to their client's story, respectfully round up the conversation, and offer possible ways to meet the client's needs. These steps will build on skills you already possess as a midwife. This method is a tool for discussing sexuality, even when you do not yet have experience addressing this topic with your client. Most HCPs will wonder and have questions like: *"Can I bring up sex as a topic of interest? Won't this be too intrusive? What will this woman think of me? How do I introduce sex as a topic? Do I have enough time to address the sexual concerns my client would voice? What if my clients ask me questions on sexuality that I don't (yet) know how to answer?"*

The One-To-One ("1T1") model is based on different (counselling) models; the PLISSIT model [1], Motivational Interviewing [2], ICE client history taking [3], and the biopsychosocial model [4]. The final "1 T1" model (Fig. 26.1) was developed by SENSOA [1] in collaboration with various universities and

---

[1] SENSOA is the Flemish Expertise Centre for Sexual Health and HIV prevention. As part of their focus on enhancing the sexual well-being of the community as a whole, a model was developed to help general practitioners engage more easily and often with their patients on sexuality. This chapter explores the usability of that same model for midwifery practice.

R. Borms (✉)
Sensoa vzw, Antwerp, Belgium & Private Practice, Willebroek, Belgium

S. Geuens (✉)
Department of Healthcare - Midwifery, PXL University College of Applied Arts and Sciences, Hasselt, Belgium

Outpatient Center for Sexual Health, Saint Franciscus Hospital, Heusden-Zolder, Belgium
e-mail: sam.geuens@pxl.be

© The Author(s) 2023
S. Geuens et al. (eds.), *Midwifery and Sexuality*,
https://doi.org/10.1007/978-3-031-18432-1_26

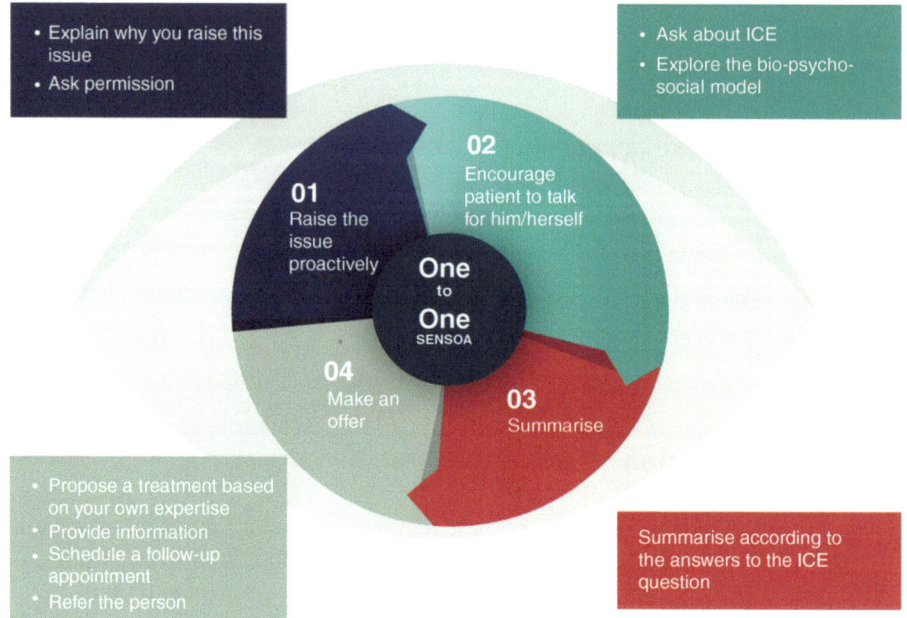

Fig. 26.1 The One-To-One ("1T1") model: Proactively discussing sexual health with clients [5]

professional organisations [5]. This chapter provides a concrete overview of the multiple steps to discuss sexuality with clients proactively. At each stage of the model, it will offer practical advice on how to implement this model in the daily midwifery practice directly.

26.2   Step 1 A: Pro-Actively Put Sex on the Table

This first step offers the HCP a handhold to start a conversation on sexual health topics. Often HCPs hesitate or doubt about proactively discussing sexuality with their clients: *"Is this okay? I don't want to approach this too directly. What will she think of me? Which questions are okay to ask and which are inappropriate? How do I do this in a helping and professional manner?"*

- This step entails nothing more than proactively starting a conversation about sexual health. Women don't often bring up the topic of sexuality themselves. Reasons for this are numerous: feelings of shame and guilt, not knowing if sharing such concerns with the midwife is in line with the midwifery practice, etc. When sexuality is never proactively addressed, sexuality-related worries and troubles will stay hidden, and in addition, we implicitly give the message that sexuality should not be addressed.
- The midwife knows that discussing sexuality can be vital to women's health and well-being. Still, this link is not always clear for all women. That could cause

women to be startled or caught unaware by the midwife raising the topic of sexuality. Two rules can ease this: explain why you want to talk about sex and ask permission.

Out of the blue, "How is your sex life at the moment?" can be a rather intrusive question. Not understanding where that is coming from can raise questions in the woman or couple: *"Why is the midwife asking me about sex? Is there something wrong with me? How am I seen? Why does the midwife want to know these things?"*

While some assertive women might ask these questions, others might feel awkward being put in this position by their midwife and not venting their reactions. One can prevent such reactions by explicitly explaining why one wants to talk about sexuality and linking the question to general health.

Step 1 aims to introduce sexuality as a regular topic of conversation within midwifery practice in a non-intrusive way. It is recommended not to ask direct questions when introducing the theme of sexuality. Getting into details comes in step 2. When you **refer to your midwife's role and explain that looking after people's sexual health is a standard part of midwifery practice**, women and couples can handle the theme easier.

Example *Our job as a midwife is to monitor your general health and well-being, including sexual health. Would it be okay for you to talk about that?*

You can also refer to standard practice or protocol in a midwifery or hospital team. That also depersonalises bringing up sexuality by linking it to one's profession.

Example *"In our team, it is a protocol to talk to all women and couples about sexuality. We know that people don't always bring up questions and concerns about sexuality themselves. Still, we feel it's important to be able to help in this regard when necessary. Would it be okay if we make some time for that now?"*

By explaining that the theme of sexual health is linked directly to your role and function as a midwife, asking about sexuality becomes less personal. This way, you can talk about sexual health positively and more neutrally.

In reality, the midwife will also bring up sexuality when expecting sexual problems. This suspicion can originate from professional instincts but more often because the midwife knows how physical or mental conditions or life events can impact women's sexual well-being. An active childwish, pregnancy, and the postpartum period inevitably will change sexual practice and well-being. So midwives have an objective reason to proactively bring up the topic of sexuality and should always do so. Additional reasons to talk about sexuality with a specific client are, for instance:

- Something you noticed during a physical exam: e.g. muscle tension.
- Something you hear in her story: e.g. experience with sexual abuse.
- Something you read in her file: e.g. history of depression.

The concerns that catch the midwife's attention are often part of the woman's situation or story. Still it remains advisable to introduce sexual health in **a**

depersonalising manner. Like the theme is depersonalised by referring to team protocols or sexual health being "part of the midwife's job" in the examples above, you can depersonalise individual concerns about this specific woman **by referring to your professional knowledge or experience**.

Referring to knowledge means that the midwife states that the concerns she noticed are known possible risk factors negatively impacting sexual health. For instance, saying as a fact: "We know that …". You can also refer to research or professional guidelines. By stating the link between one's concerns and sexual health as a known fact, the midwife again avoids appearing to speak specifically about her current client but rather about women in such positions in general.

Example *Research has shown that hormonal changes during pregnancy impact women's levels of sexual desire and sexual arousability. "They tend to decrease at the beginning of pregnancy, then sometimes increase and again decrease towards the end."*

Other ways to factually introduce the theme of sexuality are: "Fertility problems often confuse a couple's sexual relationship…;" "Young mothers often struggle with sexuality…"; "A pregnancy often induces fear of intercourse in couples…".

The midwife can also depersonalise the topic by referring to her professional experience. By connecting the concerns noticed in this woman with earlier experienced similar situations, you address sexuality less directly. Referring to expertise can always be used, especially when we can't yet refer to research data or protocols.

Example *"Your situation reminds me of other women I've counselled who indicated that young motherhood, with its lack of sleep, impacted their relationship and sex life".*

Some useful phrases are:

– *"Many women who ……. tell me that…."*
– *"Other women with this condition tell me they're also experiencing problems with …"*
– *"Women who I monitor often tell me that …"*
– *"This reminds me of worries other women have shared with me about …".*

Cave In this approach, always **refer to multiple persons**. Talking about one client can be heard as a breach of professional confidentiality between the midwife and the client. That can instil worries about her story being shared with the next woman.

Sometimes there's no concrete reason for the midwife to worry about sexuality, but her professional instincts tell her that this woman might be experiencing sexual problems. When this is the case, the midwife could directly voice her intuitions, but the chance that this will be met with resistance from the women is great.

Case Example Your client has just given birth, and contraception has probably not been addressed yet during pregnancy. Quickly getting pregnant again seems unwise.

You're worrying if she's using contraceptives. You would like to bring up contraception during your next consult.

Directly voicing your concerns: *"I'm worried if you're using contraception as I'm not sure it's a good idea to get pregnant again at this time."* could be met with resistance. The woman can experience that as addressing her reproductive and sexual habits directly and without good reason and as crossing a personal boundary without her permission. Such an approach could provoke insecurities like "what does the midwife think about me? How does she see me? It could even provoke insecurities or anger at what seems to be a judgement of their way of life: "Is this even your business? I don't care what you think I should or should not do. You think I can't handle another child. You just wait. I'll show you".

One can make this line of questions feel less aimed at them as a person by not yet posing questions directly:

Midwife (referring to professional knowledge): *"We know that many women who have recently given birth need time to get their lives back on track, juggling new maternal, social, and financial worries at a trying time with lack of sleep, etc. Because of all this, thinking about contraception can easily be forgotten. Would it be okay with you if we discuss this?"*

An Alternative Phrasing Could Be:

Midwife (referring to professional experience): *"I've counselled multiple women who unwillingly got pregnant again soon after giving birth. Due to the rigours of motherhood, the lack of sleep, etc., they forget about using proper contraception. Many of them had a hard time coping with the pregnancy. You've just given birth yourself. Would it be okay if we discussed contraception and family planning a bit?*

By referring to both knowledge and experience, sexuality is introduced as a theme connected to midwifery care in a non-personal way whilst simultaneously recognising that women might not be alone in experiencing sexual difficulties at this time. Recognising their situation can be a relief when sex is still a theme of shame and guilt. The added implicit message is that talking about sexuality is a normal part of midwifery care and that the woman can call on you when worrying about sexuality.

26.3   Step 1 B: Ask for Permission

After proactively introducing the theme of sexuality on a general level, the midwife will ask permission to further discuss this topic on a personal level. Asking for permission is a technique of motivational counselling that reduces the possible unwillingness to talk on the client's side. It is a potent communication technique, giving the client co-ownership of the conversation, and letting her decide how to proceed.

Some examples: *"Would it be okay for you to discuss this together?"*

"Would it be okay to stay with this topic for a bit?"

"Would it be okay for you if we take some time to discuss this further?"

"Would it be okay if we take some time to talk about it and see how you are experiencing this?"

Asking for permission also means that the clients have the option of refusal; in other words, they could say "No!". When a woman doesn't want this conversation, you offer her a way out of a difficult situation by asking permission. Still, refusing to talk about sexuality is also important information and could be an opportunity to discuss why sex is such a difficult topic.

You can do this fairly simply by asking: "May I ask why you'd rather not talk about it?". Even this way of exploring the issue holds a form of asking for permission. She can still indicate she does not want to go into it any further. Sometimes clients raise questions about professional confidentiality at this point. In such cases, some information about how to handle professional confidentiality can suffice to put the client at ease to open a conversation.

Overview Step 1: Table 26.1

Step 1 summary: Proactively putting sex on the table
• Introduce sexuality as a conversational topic on a general level, and depersonalise your introduction
– Refer to your profession or team protocol
– Refer to the professional knowledge: "We know that... Research shows that..."
– Refer to professional experience: "Other clients tell me that..." "Other people suffering from... also experience..." (plural)
• Ask permission to continue the conversation on a personal level

26.4 Step 2: Have the Client Tell Her Own Story

With permission to continue, the conversation moves to step 2. This step aims to get to know this client's unique situation and experiences concerning sexuality. So, ending step 1 with permission to continue is essential.

What follows is a framework for stimulating the client to tell her story. The midwife's change towards a genuine not-knowing stance and active listening position is more important than which questions to ask. Take in as much as possible of the client's story without making assumptions about her experiences, thoughts, feelings, etc. That might sound evident, but it isn't always as easy. Trained to help people, we HCPs often translate that into taking action, giving advice, sharing tips and tricks, and even getting actively involved to facilitate change. HCPs often forget that active listening should start from a not-knowing stance. Seeing the woman as the expert on her own story, her life, and her problems is essential for creating positive change.

The fact that listening helps isn't because it solves the client's problems, but it can relieve the client from excessive emotional burdens (feelings of shame, guilt, loneliness, etc.). Think about the woman who can finally share her frustrations about not getting pregnant for months on end without having to fear judgement. Such a conversation won't directly facilitate pregnancy but feeling that one can share in a safe environment enables the client to unburden herself, which is already helpful. Ironically HCPs often refrain from talking about sexuality because they don't have readymade advice or answers to offer and thus feel they can't "help" in this respect.

The reasoning behind this step can be found in the PLISSIT Model. Annon, formulating that model in 1976, emphasised the importance of permission-giving: making clear to the client that it's okay to talk about sexuality with you [1]. Feeling one can finally share their sexual burdens or concerns is helping because it creates recognition of those worries and has a potential normalising effect. In 2007, Taylor & Davis further stressed the importance of the impact of permission-giving on creating change through communication. Their EX-PLISSIT model put asking for permission as central to every level of the PLISSIT model, rather than seeing it as just the start of the process [6]. In the Ex-Plissit model, the HCP asks for permission when informing about sexuality, when offering helpful suggestions to the client, and when engaging in intensive therapy. This constant process of asking and receiving permission, along with a continuous form of self-evaluation and reflection on how the process is going, ensures that clients feel at ease talking about a "difficult" topic, such as their sexuality.

For many women, sexual life is taboo, with feelings of shame and guilt mostly kept to themselves. By actively listening from a not-knowing stance, the midwife stands next to the client, a woman with a unique situation and history. How does she experience her situation? What are her primary concerns? Based on what information does she make decisions regarding her sexual health and well-being? Does she require additional information? Does she need help? In short, on top of the helping effect of just listening and not judging, this step provides an opportunity to understand the client's situation, concerns, and feelings so the midwife can formulate an appropriate intervention based on the client's story in step 4.

The core of step 2 is adopting the not knowing stance. The goal is to recognise the client as the expert on her own story. That will enable her to tell her unique story to the fullest. As stipulated before, many HCPs refrain from talking about sexuality because they feel they lack knowledge in this area. Typically, a less professional background in sexology makes it easier to adopt a not-knowing stance when talking about sex with clients. For instance, if you don't know about sexuality in a different cultural setting, you can genuinely ask:

Examples *"Could you tell me how you see this as a Muslima? How do your culture and your religion view sexuality? How do you deal with that in your personal life?"*

Or: "How do you experience thinking about having children with a female partner? How do you feel about your partner getting pregnant?"

The more knowledge and experience one has gathered, the faster one makes assumptions based on recognisable aspects of the client's story. It is a pitfall to unconsciously view these assumptions as being the client's reality, without asking if your assumptions are correct.

Example Working at a hospital's fertility clinic and meeting a couple trying to conceive, the midwife asks: '*Do you have sex when your chances of conception are highest each month?*'. Often couples answer: "*Yes!*". The midwife then writes down the answer on her intake sheet without knowing if the couple understands enough about the menstrual cycle and the fertile window.

Adopting a not-knowing stance is easier if one remembers that each woman has a unique personality, history, sexual history, and sex life. Precisely the uniqueness of her story is what the midwife needs to offer adequate help in step 4.

Once you have learned to adopt the not-knowing stance, you still have to know which questions to ask and how to ask them to make the woman tell her unique story. Step 1 had a general point of concern on bringing about a conversation on sexuality in a less direct manner, ending in the woman's permission to continue talking about sexuality. Step 2 starts with exploring if the general concern linked to sexuality is experienced similarly by her.

Example "*Do you recognise this? How do you experience this?*
Is this causing problems for you too? In what way? ..."

Step 2 focuses on exploring the woman's unique perspective. Adopting a not-knowing stance, the HCP can stimulate the woman to tell her story with different frameworks. Within the "1 T1"-model, we propose to use the ICE framework or the BioPsychoSocial model.

The ICE technique is the first framework for exploring the client's sexual story [3]. ICE stands for Ideas, Concerns, and Expectations. The midwife inquires about what the woman worries about (– Concerns -), if she has any idea how this came to be (– Ideas -), and what she expects of you as a HCP with regards to these concerns (– Expectations -). These questions help focus the conversation on the woman's unique story, experiences, and needs. This line of questioning also contributes to developing a better HCP–client relationship, with the woman telling her story and the HCP understanding her experiences [3].

Ideas: This question explores the woman's views on how her sex life has become as it is now. How does she feel about her current situation? By actively inquiring about this, the HCP will often get information that otherwise could have been excluded from the conversation. It also enables the HCP to identify a lack of or even wrong information or knowledge from the woman's side that the HCP can attempt to correct in step 4.

Example "*What do you think is the cause of this? Do you have any ideas as to what this is related to? ... *".

Concerns: Asking about the client's concerns is relevant because HCPs presume to know what women in this situation need or want. That can lead to an unsatisfied client when the treatment does not focus on her primary concerns. For example, a woman with dyspareunia might not focus on less pain, but on regaining intimacy, like kissing and sitting together. If we presume the pain is the current primary focus, our treatment plan might be ineffective because the woman might not be motivated to address the pain at this point.

The woman's concerns may be different or more severe than the HCP imagines. Or the woman might arrange her priorities differently than the HCP saw in previous women. By actively asking about the woman's concerns, the HCP breaks free of any preconceptions and adopts a genuine not-knowing stance. Asking about her concerns and asking about her priority of concerns will give the HCP a more accurate picture of the woman's needs. In that way, the HCP can propose a tailor-made intervention in step 4.

Example *"About what are you most worried?" "What is the most important thing you hope could change?"*

Expectations: Asking about expectations gives the HCP an idea of how the woman wants to see change occur. Trying to formulate this positively by asking about hope, she can again help tailor an intervention in step 4. Asking about her expectations towards you, as her HCP, will enable meeting the woman's needs more accurately and assessing if her expectations are realistic. Such a line of questioning makes the client feel heard and creates a connection that makes it easier to correct unrealistic expectations if they would arise.

Examples *"How do you expect this to evolve in the future?" "What do you expect will happen if nothing changes?" "What do you hope to reach?" "How do you hope this can change in the future?" "What do you hope and expect me to do as a midwife?"*

Additionally, it can be very worthwhile to ask the woman about her Ideas, Concerns, and Expectations related to sexuality and her sexual life. What are her ideas about having sex after giving birth? Does she expect to resume vaginal intercourse quickly? Does she expect it to be the same or different, or maybe painful? Is she concerned about how her partner will experience this period or what her partner will expect of her?

The BioPsychoSocial or BPS model forms the second usable framework [4]. This model approaches sexual health, just as general health, as the product of a delicate balance between a person's biological or physical, psychological, and social self [4]. Again starting from a not-knowing stance, the midwife explores possible imbalances in the woman's physical, psychological, or social/relational well-being. Such a line of questioning facilitates a broader picture of the woman's possible distress or hindrances. That does not mean the HCP must formulate an intervention for each dimension. Interdisciplinary referrals often are necessary.

Biological or physical impact: *"Does this cause any physical hindrances? Are you experiencing pain anywhere? Do you feel that this also impacts your body? In what manner?"*

Psychological or mental impact: *"How are you dealing with this? What does this do to you as a person? What thoughts or feelings does this bring to the surface? How do you cope with this?"*

Social or relational impact: *"How is your partner handling this? Does this affect the relationship with your partner? Can you find support in your social* *circle? How does your family respond to this? How is this viewed in your cultural/ religious community?"*

It's equally important that our view of the woman's reality is not too problem-focused. The midwife can prevent this by inquiring which aspects of the woman's sexual life are (or are still) okay or even good. A good starting point could be questions like "What's still going well sexually?" "What makes you sexually content?" "What still makes you happy sexually?"

26.4.1 How, Where, and With Whom to Have the Sex Talk?

Compiling two lists of proper and improper midwife questions about sexuality is absurd. One can train oneself to reflect critically on what to ask clients by adhering to a simple rule of thumb: What is my intent? Why am I asking this question? We should not ask sexual questions out of personal interest or curiosity. Sexuality questions unrelated to improving the woman's or couple's health are inappropriate. Asking about sexuality needs to start from the professional intent to monitor and enhance her or their sexual health.

Example The woman you're monitoring is now in the third trimester. Curiously asking if her orgasms feel different (tonic instead of clonic) is not the primary concern about her sexual health. A correct starting question about sexual health could be:" How do you feel about your sexual life during this final phase of the pregnancy? Is this something you would like to talk about?"

HCPs regularly use non-health-related themes as connection catalysts to develop a good working alliance with the client. However, to build a trusting relationship, we better not choose sexuality since that is, for many people, still a taboo subject, evoking feelings of insecurity, shame, and even guilt. There are plenty of other positively connotated themes to use.

Since the topic can also be complex for the midwife, it might be good to ask where and with whom sexuality should be discussed.

Sexuality is a part of our individual lives and part of our connected lives. As an individual, we have sexual ideas and feelings. Our bodies respond uniquely to sexual stimulation, and we have our private sexual life (for instance, fantasies or masturbation). That changes when we look at sex as part of our connected life with its interpersonal dynamics. Sexuality is integral to the dyadic relationship between both partners in a couple. Even in a sexual encounter with a "one-time" partner, sexuality is part of the interplay between those two people. Realising this emphasises the need to inquire about the context in which the woman experiences her sexuality. Solo or partnered? Within or outside a committed relationship? With a man, women or non cisgendered other? We cannot view the sexuality of a woman in a committed relationship as independent from her partner's sexuality. So, if possible, it will benefit to (also) talk about sexuality with both partners present. However, for some women, talking about sex with their partner present is more complicated than a one-on-one conversation with the midwife. That might be due to sexual problems, relational problems, feelings of shame or guilt, sexual abuse, etc. So, again, don't force the sexuality theme onto the client but start the conversation in a non-personal manner and by asking the client's permission. Sometimes a woman might first prefer a one-on-one conversation with the midwife, drawing strength from that conversation to, later on, talk about sex with her partner present. Starting by asking the woman's preference on "how and with whom to talk about sex" can be helpful:

Example *"I'd like to address sexuality. Would you prefer that now, or would you like to postpone that till next time when your partner is also present?"*

Even without being present, the partner's perspective can actively be incorporated into the conversation. For instance, by asking: *"What does he do?"* *"Do you know his ideas about your current sex life?"* etc.

Some example questions might be:

"You've told me that now that you're actively trying to conceive, you sometimes feel like having sex is a burden rather than a joy. How do you think your partner is experiencing this?"

"You told me you prefer waiting after the birth until you feel completely ready for intercourse again. What ideas do you think your partner has on this?"

While the answers on her partner's sexual experiences might seem second-hand and sometimes not correct, asking about the absent partner will at least trigger the client to consider how her partner is experiencing their current sexual relationship.

The context. Almost all clients prefer to discuss sexuality without being overheard by other people. That sometimes seems impossible to do. We might only be separated from the next woman by a hospital curtain. Many women are admitted to an open ward. Such a lack of privacy might hinder clients from talking about sexuality. When the woman is hesitant, actively remarking on these difficulties might benefit the conversation and the connection with her.

Examples *"It is my midwife's job to monitor your general health and well-being, including sexual health. Would it be okay for you to talk about that?"*

When the woman hesitates to answer and remains silent: *"Many people feel more comfortable talking about sexuality in a more private setting. Is it okay for you if we pick up this topic at another time?"*

Or: *"Many people feel more comfortable talking about sexuality in a more private setting. Would you feel more comfortable talking about this in a more private place?"*

Of course, the physical reality of our work accommodation can hinder us. Midwives can deal with such situations creatively. Some clients might prefer to write their questions down, get a written answer, etc. Discussing sex while walking through the hospital together might feel more comfortable than in their room, where other women or staff are eavesdropping.

Overview Step 2: Table 26.2

Structure	What	How	Example
Beginning	Explore the woman's sexual situation and sexual habits	Inquire about the link between general worries (step1) and the woman's sexual life	Do you recognise this? Are you experiencing similar problems? How are you experiencing this?
Middle	Explore the woman's experiences	ICE–questions:	
		– *Ideas*: What are the woman's ideas on this?	*"What do you think is causing this?"*
		– *Concerns*: What are the woman's concerns?	"About what are you most concerned?"
		– *Expectations:* What are the woman's expectations?	*"What do you expect to happen…?"*
		Biopsychosocial	
		– *Biological:* What is the physical impact?	*"What does this do with your body? Are you experiencing physical discomfort?"*
		– *Psychological*: What is the psychological or mental impact?	*"How do you cope with this? How do you feel about this?"*
		– *Social*: What is the relational or social impact?	*"How does this affect your relationship and your social circle?"*
End	Explore what is sexually still good, functioning well, etc		What's still going well sexually? About which sexual aspects are you content? What still makes you happy sexually?

Step 2 summary

- HCP's perspective when connecting to clients: Active listening, starting from a not-knowing stance
- Goal: Getting to know this woman's unique situation, exploring her ideas and knowledge about sexuality, and assessing her primary needs concerning sexuality
- Explore:
    The current situation, experience?
    ICE: Inquire about her ideas, concerns (prioritise), and expectations
    Bio-psycho-social: Explore the impact on the woman's physical, mental, social, and relational well-being
    Inquire about positive, well-working aspects of the woman's sexual life

26.5   Step 3: Summarise

This third step is relatively short but of great importance. It forms the bridge between the woman's story and the midwife's attempt to respectfully round up the conversation, moving towards formulating an offer of assistance.

Respectfully rounding up a session is essential, even more so with the touchy subject of sexuality. As most people seldom talk (to HCPs) about sexuality, ending such a conversation with care can be done by the simple but powerful basic communication skill that stems from motivational interviewing [2]: **summarising.**

With a good conversation summary, the woman will understand that you attentively listened to her story. It structures her story and provides a way to emphasise certain of its aspects. Besides, it enables you to retake control over the conversation, easily change the direction of the conversation if needed, or just round it up respectfully.

The midwife attempts to capture the essence of the woman's unique story, which is her lived reality. Summarising should be based on the answers given by the woman on the ICE or BPS questions. Then check if you have correctly summarised by asking: *"Did I get that right?"*. Using closed questions gives the conversation control back to the midwife if necessary.

Example *"Okay. If I understand it correctly, since the treatment for your endometriosis, you have less sexual desire. That isn't bothering you much, but it hurts when you have intercourse with your husband. You worry about how your partner experiences this situation. Did I get that right?"*

Step 3 summary
- Summarise:
  Repeat the essence of the answers to the ICE questions; or
  Repeat the essence of the answers to the BPS questions
- Check: *"Did I get it right?"*
- In case the partner is absent: *"Do you think your partner will agree, or do you think he would change or add something?*
- Types of summarising:
  Summarising = Respectfully rounding up the conversation whilst making the client feel heard
  Summarising = Giving back the client's story in a more structured way
  Summarising = Retaking control of the conversation

26.6   Step 4: Make an Offer

With this final step, the circle is made whole. After summarising, the woman hears that the midwife has been paying attention. Still, the question of how to move forward remains unanswered. In case an intervention is needed or desired by the woman, the HCP offers the possibility of an intervention tailored to this unique woman's specific story and expectations.

HCPs should realise that having addressed sexual concerns or problems is sometimes enough. It can also be enough for the time being since creating change might need a long process. Besides, some conversations will not contain concrete interventions, providing already the required intervention.

The midwife can propose various interventions when the woman needs or desires concrete interventions. Examples are a treatment within the midwife's expertise, tailored psychoeducational information, a subsequent appointment for in-debt handling of the woman's story, or referring to a colleague with more expertise.

26.6.1 A Treatment Proposal, Based on the Midwife's Expertise

If your conversation with the woman clarifies that she is worried about aspects of her sexual life, and if you, as a midwife, can present a solution in the form of treatment, this can be part of step 4. For example, you are prescribing a contraceptive during the postpartum period (e.g. one that does not negatively impact the woman's sexual desire and arousability). In many situations, adequate psychoeducation or targeted interdisciplinary referrals are necessary to handle sexual difficulties successfully.

26.6.2 Giving Information

Once they feel their story has been heard, many women and couples benefit from adequate psychoeducation. Information such as how specific pathologies (e.g. mastitis or hyperemesis) or situations (e.g. young motherhood) can impact sexuality often normalises what women are experiencing. Such a normalising effect diminishes negative emotions surrounding the problem, thus helping the woman achieve positive change. That does not mean that HCPs should have all the necessary information ready in their minds. Guiding people towards accurate books or online information is sometimes enough to alleviate a problem. It's a challenge for many people to find online understandable and trustworthy sexuality information. Actively exploring the woman's ideas on sexuality in step 2 can indicate if she lacks specific sexual knowledge or holds wrong beliefs on aspects of sexual functioning. Then try correcting the erroneous beliefs as they can be part of what's causing the sexual difficulties. Sometimes this can be enough for women to make the rest of the necessary positive change happen themselves. The midwife should be aware of reliable sources of information in the woman's language. A very reliable, multilingual online source is the webpage www.zanzu.be.

Zanzu has been developed by Sensoa, the Flemish Expertise Centre of Sexual Health and HIV. It has information on sexual health, reproduction, sexual problems, and family planning.[2] It is a good point of reference for HCPs all over the globe.

---

[2] Among the topics are: the male & female body, sexual pleasure, having sex, virginity, hygiene, the sexual body, contraception, getting pregnant, being pregnant, sex during and after pregnancy, unwanted pregnancy, giving birth, young parenthood, STIs, HIV, vaginal infections, condom use, sexual problems, romantic relationships, talking about sex, couple problems, and intimate violence.

Symbols and drawings on the website facilitate navigation and understanding of the information. The information is available in 14 languages[3] and can be played as audio files spoken by native speakers. Zanzu can be used during a session with the woman listening to accurate sexual health information, whilst you can, in your HCP language, strictly follow what the woman hears. Such an experience can strongly impact the relationship with the woman, especially when confronted with cultural and language differences.

26.6.3 Planning a Follow-Up Appointment

When women talk about their sexual concerns for the first time, it could very well be possible that they cannot tell their whole story in step 2, especially given the time constraints that can be in place in different healthcare settings. Planning a follow-up conversation to explore the woman's story can be a valuable intervention. Talking about concerns and worries and feel listened to is essential for any treatment process.

26.6.4 Make an Offer for an Interdisciplinary Referral

Some sexual problems require treatment beyond the scope of the skills and knowledge of the midwife. Perhaps the woman or the couple needs sexological or psychotherapeutic treatment. Treatment by a clinical sexologist, psychosexologist, or psychotherapist trained in sex therapy should always be tailored to the sexual difficulties of the unique woman, her needs and her hopes. Such treatment deserves a biopsychosocial approach and a "couple approach". Sometimes a referral to other medically trained professionals is needed, such as the gynaecologist, urologist, endocrinologist, or pelvic floor therapist, to treat or rule out possible physical causes for the sexual disturbances. Midwives should develop a network of professionals from various disciplines with practical knowledge of treating sexual problems. To successfully treat the more complex sexual troubles, we all require interdisciplinary collaboration, with mutual fine-tuning and open communication between the various professionals.

26.7   Conclusion

As long as sexuality remains taboo, women, couples, midwives, and other HCPs might find this a complex topic to tackle in the conversation. The "1T1" model makes the task of "talking sex" easier by providing a clear framework for the midwife. This model neither requires much working knowledge on sexual health, nor uses up much time. By giving multiple examples within each stage of the

---

[3]Albanian, Arabic, Bulgarian, Dutch, English, Farsi, French, German, Polish, Portuguese, Romanian, Russian, Spanish, and Turkish

model—raising the issue proactively, encouraging the women to tell their story, summarising, making an offer—on how to phrase questions to get the conversation going and how to keep it going, we hope that more HCPs will talk sex and that the woman, the couple, and the HCP will stay behind feeling that this was after all "just another part of the conversation".

References

1. Annon JS. The PLISSIT model: a proposed conceptual scheme for the behavioral treatment of sexual problems. J Sex Educ Ther. 1976;2:1–15.
2. Miller WR, Rollnick S. Motivational interviewing: preparing people for change. 2nd ed. New York: Guilford Press; 2002.
3. Silverman J, Kurtz S, Draper J. Skills for communicating with patients. 3rd ed. Boca Raton, FL: CRC; 2013.
4. Engel GL. The need for a new medical model: a challenge for biomedicine. Science. 1977;196(4286):129–36.
5. Borms R, Vermeire K. Spreken is goud: Seksuele gezondheid bespreekbaar maken met de Onder 4 Ogen methode. Ontwikkeling en implementatie bij huisartsen in Vlaanderen. T v Seksuologie. 2020;44:155–61.
6. Taylor B. Davis S using the extended PLISSIT model to address sexual healthcare needs. Nurs Stand. 2006;21:35–40.

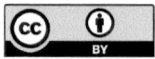

From Midwifery Competencies on Sexual Wellbeing to Teaching and Training Midwives on Sexuality

27

Sam Geuens [ID] and Joeri Vermeulen [ID]

27.1 Midwives' Role Concerning Sexuality and Sexual Well-Being

Midwives are acknowledged, all over the world, as having an important role in sexual counselling and sexual health issues. The International Confederation of Midwives (ICM) and the World Health Organization (WHO) recognise that counselling and education on sexuality and reproductive health are among the tasks of midwives [1, 2]. Since the first *State of the World's Midwifery report* in 2011, evidence indicates that midwives are essential care providers at multiple health system levels. In addition to maternity care, they provide a wide range of clinical interventions and contribute to broader health goals, such as addressing sexual and reproductive rights, promoting self-care interventions and empowering women and adolescent girls [3].

They contribute to SDG 3 (Sustainable Development Goals), including universal access to sexual and reproductive health services, family planning, information, education, and the integration of reproductive health, and SDG 5 aims, to achieve gender equality and empowerment of women and girls. Various sources indicate that sexual education by midwives during pregnancy and postpartum can improve the couple's sexual well-being. An essential element of this midwife's vital role in sexual health is the skill to adequately initiate the conversation on sexuality and

S. Geuens (✉)
Department of Healthcare - Midwifery, PXL University College of Applied Arts and Sciences, Hasselt, Belgium

Outpatient Center for Sexual Health, Saint Franciscus Hospital, Heusden-Zolder, Belgium
e-mail: sam.geuens@pxl.be

J. Vermeulen
Department of Public Health, Free University of Brussel (VUB), Brussels, Belgium

Midwifery Department, Erasmus Brussels University of Applied Sciences and Arts, Brussels, Belgium intimacy based on the necessary knowledge about sexual health and well-being. However, the sad reality is that, within midwifery teaching and practice, this only happens in a small part of the more affluent countries.

While sexual counselling requires a positive and respectful approach to sexuality and sexual relationships [4], personal or societal attitudes towards sexuality may affect the implementation of sexual counselling services [5]. In some countries, sex education[1] is integrated into schools, universities, and media. In other countries, it is far less available or non-existent, or its content is unsatisfactory [6]. When sex education is taboo in a community, the implementation of sexual counselling in health care will be hampered [5]. In addition, the cultural and gender reference points of the maternity care professional may influence the approach towards the couple in counselling [4]. A recent study in Sweden found that midwives' insecurity regarding sexuality was even more remarkable in patients who deviated from the heterosexual norm or had a different cultural background [7]. These insights present significant challenges for midwifery education worldwide.

The ICM Essential Competencies for Midwifery Practice outlines the minimum knowledge, skills, and professional behaviours required by a newly graduated midwife when entering midwifery practice [8]. Regarding sexuality and sexual well-being, the knowledge and skills include anatomy and physiology related to reproduction and sexual development, guidance about sexual and reproductive health, and information about safe sex. Newly graduated midwives are expected to be competent to assess sexual and reproductive health needs comprehensively [8]. Given the extent to which the ICM gives attention to sexuality-related competencies for midwives and the virtual absence of sexuality subjects in many midwifery schools' curricula, one can wonder if midwifery schools today are fully aware of the ICM's stance on sexual health and well-being.

A UK study indicated that midwifery students lacked knowledge or had difficulty translating theoretical knowledge into practical clinical situations regarding postpartum contraception and sexual health advice [9]. A Bulgarian study on teaching midwifery students in contraceptive counselling revealed that interactive work methods and cooperation with a regional family planning centre were critical for skills acquisition in this area [10].

A Turkish study on midwifery students' attitudes towards sexual counselling indicated that their attitude on sexuality was positive, but they were not always comfortable providing counselling, especially to particular groups of women [5]. Another Turkish study showed that midwifery students' attitudes towards sexuality, contraceptive methods, and abortion were strongly influenced by social-value judgements. Many students believed that a girl should be a virgin when marrying, that abortion was morally wrong, and that only married couples should receive information on contraceptive methods [11].

---

[1] We use the term 'sex education', because that is the common term for various forms of education on sexuality. It should not be read as 'education on having sex' or as 'education on how to have sex'.

In a UK study, final-year midwifery students reported a lack of confidence in their knowledge regarding contraception and sexual health, despite considering this part of their professional role. They stated that more practice-based educational methods would increase their confidence [12].

It seems clear that midwifery education must integrate knowledge, skills, and attitude-building regarding sexuality and sexual health into their teaching curriculum. This chapter aims to help midwifery schools ensure that their student midwives enter the workplace with the necessary knowledge and skills, combined with the right attitude, concerning sexuality and sexual health. Then they can proactively integrate these essential topics into the care they provide in the context of pregnancy, postpartum, and young parenthood.

27.2 Implications for Midwifery Education

As described above, international professional organisations have strong arguments to equip students with the knowledge and skills to address sexuality, though not all educational institutions follow the recommendations. Midwifery curricula must implement sexuality and sexual well-being-related aspects defined by the ICM and the EU Directive and emphasise the topic. One could state that *'making midwives experts in sexual or reproductive health issues'* is essential to achieving midwifery's full scope and potential.

The midwifery curriculum requires a model in which theoretical knowledge is reinforced practically, with practice-based scenarios and with the tutor as a role model [12]. As the role of mentors appears to be very important in helping students gain confidence in sexual counselling and sexual health, we will start by elaborating on their function and profile within the scope of this chapter.

27.3 Integrating Sexuality and Sexual Health into your curriculum

To educate midwives with adequate skills and knowledge regarding sexuality and sexual well-being, a midwifery school must tackle two significant tasks. The first task is content related: scanning the existing curriculum for courses that already touch upon sexuality (for a concrete scanning tool, see Table 27.1 Midwifery & Sexuality Curriculum Scanning Tool, based on the chapters of this book). It's seldom the case that midwifery schools have to start from scratch. Carefully scanning the existing curriculum and thus identifying the work already done can make implementing knowledge and skills on sexuality and sexual well-being less daunting. Once the school has identified its current state of affairs, it can fill in the theoretical and practical gaps, making room for those courses needed to make its student midwives experts in sexual health and sexual counselling. The framework and content of this book might serve as a guide through this process of curriculum optimisation.

Table 27.1 Midwifery & Sexuality curriculum scanning tool

Midwifery & Sexuality curriculum scanning tool	Content available in 'Sexuality and Midwifery' chapters	Theory covered in current curriculum	Skills covered in current curriculum
Basic knowledge and terminology with regards to sexuality	1		
Sexual anatomy of the male and female	2		
Sexual functioning	3		
Sexual problems (including dysfunctions)	3		
Health benefits of sexual expression	4		
Talking sexuality	26 and 29		
Sexual counselling	26 and 29		
Sexual aspects of getting pregnant	5		
Physiology: Sexual impact of pregnancy	6		
Physiology: Sexual impact of labour and childbirth	7		
Physiology: Sexuality during the postpartum and young parenthood	8		
Physiology: The sexual impact of breastfeeding	9		
Physiology: The sexual function of the pelvic floor	10		
Pathology: The sexual impact of fertility problems and treatments	11		
Pathology: The sexual impact of high risk pregnancy	12		
Pathology: The sexual impact of labour-induced trauma	13		
Pathology: Sexuality during problematic postpartum or young parenthood situations	14		
Pathology: The sexual impact of problematic lactation	15		
Pathology: The sexual impact of pelvic floor problems	16		
Pathology: The sexual impact of mental health problems (preconceptional, prenatal, and postnatal)	17		
Pathology: The sexual impact of other physical disturbances	18		
The sexual impact of medication & drugs used in daily midwifery practice	19		
The sexual impact of contraception	20		
Sexuality and sexual Well-being in all sexual orientations and identities (preconceptional, prenatal, and postnatal)	21		

Table 27.1 (continued)

Midwifery & Sexuality curriculum scanning tool	Content available in 'Sexuality and Midwifery' chapters	Theory covered in current curriculum	Skills covered in current curriculum
Male experience(s) with regards to sexuality (preconceptional, prenatal, and postnatal)	22		
The impact of culture on sexual Well-being (preconceptional, prenatal, and postnatal)	23		
The impact of trauma experience on sexual Well-being (preconceptional, prenatal, and postnatal)	24		
The sexual consequences of female genital mutilation	25		
The sexual consequences of daily midwifery practice	28		
How sexual problems are managed by other health care professionals	29		

During this exercise, the midwifery school should remember the general rule put forward by the 2021 ICM Standard for Midwifery Education that a good *'midwifery curriculum includes both theory and practice elements in clinical settings'* [13]. This rule also applies to midwifery knowledge and skills in the area of sexuality and sexual well-being.

27.4 Matching the Tutor to the Courses

Once the curriculum has been adapted to include the needed themes, a second task is identifying tutors. On the one hand, they should have the skills and knowledge needed to educate about sexuality in a way that applies to midwifery and, on the other hand, possess the individual traits for successfully educating about that area.

It's a given that the experienced midwifery tutors who integrate sexuality in their own work are the best to teach these subjects. Furthermore, more so than for the other course material in midwifery, we believe that how the tutor covers the topic of sexuality will inevitably serve as a role model for dealing with sexuality. A key component of effective learning and effective practice regarding sexuality is a relaxed but still professional attitude about all matters concerning sex. Only the midwifery tutor who can address a couple's sexual habits equally comfortable as addressing a woman's eating pattern will be able to teach students the communication skills needed to start a conversation about sex. Such a *'teaching by example'* attitude can instil in the future midwife the belief that sex is a normal aspect of the human condition, equally important as other basic functions such as nutrition and rest. Still, even for the midwifery tutor, 'practice creates perfection'. One does not yet have to be 100% comfortable to start teaching about sex, given that one recognises one's current level of expertise and is not afraid to communicate it to colleagues and students alike.

Regarding teaching sexuality, the midwifery tutor is never just educating on knowledge or skills but also on how to position oneself towards sexuality as an everyday part of life. Secondly, the tutor best suited to teach midwifery students about sexuality does not necessarily have to be a midwife. Where the first choice should be a midwife with additional training and experience regarding sexuality, such midwives might not always be at hand. Just as midwives in practice provide the best care when working multi- or even transdisciplinary, one can argue that the best midwifery teaching comes from multi- or transdisciplinary[2] working midwifery faculties. In the words of the ICM: "Individuals from other disciplines who teach in the midwifery programme are qualified to teach in that area" [13].

Transdisciplinary midwifery teaching can be ideal for training sexuality-sensitive and competent midwives. That means that the midwifery faculty can, for instance, choose to take on board a non-midwife clinical sexologist experienced in working with women and couples in the various stages of reproduction, to teach on these specific topics. In this way, the school moves towards multidisciplinary midwifery teaching. Such a sexologist-midwifery tutor can influence the standard midwifery courses to include attention to sexuality and sexual well-being and the midwife-midwifery tutors can foster greater knowledge and understanding of midwifery in their non-midwife colleagues.

Building on this vision, one can imagine that bringing such a lived and experienced form of multi- and interdisciplinarity to midwifery students' practical courses by actively having midwifery students engage with gynaecology residents, sexology students and pelvic floor therapy students would further their formation as practice-experts in the field of sexual health and sex counselling [14, 15]. Finally, the midwifery tutor best suited to teach about sexuality should have experience in 'teaching' sexuality. Teaching sexuality has to go beyond just giving psychoeducation to midwifery clients. Here we refer to experience with actually teaching other professionals, not necessarily midwives, about sexuality and sexual well-being. Ideally, this teaching experience also entails teaching practical skills, e.g. talking about sexuality and also knowledge about sexuality and sexual well-being [13].

In summary, the ideal scenario for a midwifery school is to expand the midwifery faculty with one or more HCPs trained and experienced both as midwives and sexologists. Preferably this midwife-sexologist is already proficient in teaching sexuality to HCPs.

---

[2] For the purpose of this chapter, multidisciplinary collaboration is seen as individuals from different fields of practice working together, within the boundaries of their respective disciplines, to care for a single client, striving towards holistic care by continuous intervention. Transdisciplinary collaboration is seen as health care professionals from different fields of practice working together to care for a single client, with professionals sometimes going beyond the classic boundaries of their own discipline to strive towards holistic care.

27.5   On the Practice of Teaching Student Midwives About Sexuality

Once a midwifery school has made room in its curriculum for sexual health and sexual well-being and has identified a suitable tutor to teach sex or attracted a new colleague with the needed skillset to do so, it just comes down to teaching student midwives about sex. What should go on in the classrooms and training rooms? What are the most effective educational ways to form midwives who are not only knowledgeable about sex but also proficient in talking about sex with clients and can actively integrate sexual health and well-being into their care?

Considering the most effective way to obtain learning goals, an important question is how to match the pedagogical method to the desired learning outcomes. The KASES model, developed by Sensoa, the Flemish Expertise Centre for Sexual Health and HIV, is designed to give a simple overview of matching desired outcomes to the most suited pedagogical methods [16].

KASES is an acronym for Knowledge, Attitudes, Skills, Emotions, and Support. Each learning outcome has its own methods best suited to work towards it.

- Knowledge increase is best achieved through what one could call more traditional forms of education such as research work, academic reading, content exercises, and lectures.
- Fostering attitude-change works better through group work, group discussions, writing, and presenting dissertations.
- Skills are best acquired by combining modelling, role-play exercises, and authentic learning scenarios.
- Emotional attunement and insight are best achieved through performing or watching interviews, testimonials and storytelling.
- Every student, like every client, needs to feel supported for any positive change to occur. Support is best provided by positive feedback scenarios, group and one-to-one coaching, awareness about all possible support services, etc.

The midwifery tutor developing educational materials for midwifery students can then elaborate on which learning outcomes are connected to which part of the course. To achieve learning outcomes related to sexuality and sexual well-being, midwives need competencies with a mixture of knowledge-building, attitude formation, skill-building and emotional attunement. The emphasis is most heavily on knowledge and skills building for obvious reasons.

Globally, midwifery tutors know how to bring new information to students so that they understand it and can incorporate it into their midwifery knowledge. This chapter will not go into detail about how to compose and style lectures on sexuality and well-being. Still, midwifery tutors could do well to be aware that even when just lecturing on sexuality, they are in a perfect position to foster attitude building. One of the most important parts of attitude building regarding sexuality is the lived-through idea that sex is just another part of life, a basic need that obviously can have a major positive or negative impact on people's general health and well-being. Such a sense of sex is central to our human condition. Approaching it as plain as sleep and nutrition is the needed basis for building skills to talk about sex with clients effectively. So even when giving a theoretical lecture on, e.g. sexually transmitted infections or sexual anatomy, one actively influences the students' attitude towards sex. In a sense, the tutor is reshaping a professional way of talking about sexuality, which is the first step into acquiring skills.

Achieving skills requires a combination of modelling, role-play exercises and authentic learning scenarios. Modelling is not enough to foster the skills needed to talk with clients in a relaxed, neutral way about sex. When the tutor shows how to do a sexual anamnesis in front of a group of students, this can only ever be a first step towards the desired outcomes regarding skill-building. To learn how to talk about sex, one actually has to be in the position of the professional. Students need to go through the process of searching for the words to use that suit them, the right tone and posture to take on, etc., when talking about sex with their clients. One can only achieve that by personal exercise.

Where a practical course can start with a theoretical intro, possibly followed by an example by the tutor, classes on sexuality related skills need to move into self exercises quickly. Students must experience taking on this role and having the conversation themselves. Still, putting oneself in the position of the HCP talking about sex can feel somewhat unsafe for students because of the cultural load attached to the topic, possibly combined with the fact that their fellow students are watching them. Going back to the KASES model, the tutor needs to foster support. One way of doing this is by actively installing a positively focused feedback system before the start of role-playing. When the student talking in the role of the HCP can hear the tutor instruct the other students to only pay attention to what their colleague 'does right' during the exercise, this goes a long way to installing enough safety for students to try to talk about sex during role-playing actively. The tutor can instil an even greater feeling of support by declaring that the role-playing student can ask for a 'time-out' at any moment during the exercise to receive input and guidance from the group. At each time-out or at the end of the exercise, the tutor can start by first having the other students give all the positive feedback they've written down for their colleagues, before providing suggestions on how to do it even better. This way, students can feel empowered by one another through these sometimes challenging exercises instead of feeling judged on their performance. Such a combined focus on knowledge, attitude, skills, and support maximises the learning output.

Once the tutor has learned how to install enough safety for the students to try to talk sex during exercises actively, practicals are best organised within a learning curve, aiming for the most authentic learning possibilities in a classroom setting. One can first ask students to practice in small groups, just talking about sexuality-related topics in general. Then one can show examples of how HCPs talk about sexuality with their clients in various settings and conversations (e.g. anamnesis, psychoeducation, problem-solving, therapy). Examples can be pre-recorded and projected, or the tutor can give a live demonstration. At this point, tutors should realise that every student has to develop a personal style of engaging with clients. To prevent students from mimicking the example, providing demonstrations of different professionals/tutors talking with clients can be very helpful. The next step for the students is role-playing in small groups, alternatingly taking the HCP and client roles. Then practicals can move on to group exercises, with students taking the roles of the client and the HCP conducting a conversation for the entire group. If the tutor can install enough safety in the group to allow recording of the exercise, students can benefit greatly from the opportunity of watching themselves work at a later point and reflecting on how to improve their skills. The last step before practising these skills during internships is bringing in simulation clients, strangers to the students, to take on the role of the client during exercises in practicals. The tutor, at this stage, has to decide to work with simulation clients who either take on the client role, drawing on personal experiences as clients, or perform a role written for this exercise by the tutor. We suggest tutors select simulation patients who are sufficiently flexible and emotionally stable to allow them to draw on their own experiences of wanting to conceive, being pregnant, giving birth or caring for a newborn. When possible, it is a great advantage to have HCPs as simulation patients, for they are often familiar with these types of practicals and have experience in giving feedback to students. The ideal simulation patients for midwifery practicals on talking sex are midwives who are mothers (or fathers). Communicating with these 'real women' or 'real couples' pushes students to take their skills in talking about sex to the level required during internships.

27.6 Conclusion

Future midwives need to be aware of the diversities within human sexuality, understand the factors that influence views and norms about sexuality and gain insight into their own values and assumptions about sexuality [4]. Qualified midwives may need additional education and support from sexual and reproductive health services. Further education in sexology for midwives appears to significantly impact their skills and readiness to address sexual issues in their daily work. Stronger and interprofessional collaborations with clinical settings and government systems are required to solve the current challenges to midwifery [13]. We emphasise that multi- and transdisciplinary healthcare teams are the future models of health care, also concerning sexuality and sexual well-being. Therefore, it's worth considering synchronising sexology and midwifery educational and practising teams providing appropriate maternity care for couples and so educate and maintain professional experts geared towards the sexual health and well-being of women and families worldwide.

The wise words of a midwife from the United Kingdom sum it up nicely: *'I encourage midwives to speak to managers and primary care links to discuss the value of acknowledging families' sexual and reproductive health needs within local maternity service provision — with a sense of optimism that in future, maternity service providers and midwives will make sexual health a public health priority'* [14].

References

1. International Confederation of Midwives. International Definition of the Midwife (Revised and adopted at Toronto Council meeting, 2017). 2017. https://www.internationalmidwives.org/assets/files/definitions-files/2018/06/eng-definition_of_the_midwife-2017.pdf.
2. World Health Organization. The role of primary healthcare providers in sexual and reproductive health: results from an intercountry survey. 2011.
3. UNFPA, WHO, ICM. The state of the World's midwifery 2021. 2021. https://www.unfpa.org/sites/default/files/pub-pdf/21-038-UNFPA-SoWMy2021-Report-ENv4302.pdf.
4. Olsson A. Sexual life after childbirth and aspects of midwives´ counselling at the postnatal check-up. Sweden: Institutionen för kliniska vetenskaper, Danderyds sjukhus/Department of Clinical Sciences, Danderyd Hospital; 2009.
5. Ören B, Zengin N, Yazıcı S, Akıncı A. Attitudes, beliefs and comfort levels of midwifery students regarding sexual counselling in Turkey. Midwifery. 2018;56:152–7.
6. Tabatabaie A. Constructing the ideal Muslim sexual subject: problematics of school-based sex education in Iran. Sex Educ. 2015;15:204–16.
7. Percat A, Elmerstig E. "We should be experts, but we're not": sexual counselling at the antenatal care clinic. Sex Reprod Healthc. 2017;14:85–90.
8. International Confederation of Midwives. Essential competencies for midwifery practice 2019. The Hague: ICM; 2019. https://www.internationalmidwives.org/assets/files/general-files/2019/02/icm-competencies_english_final_jan-2019-update_final-web_v1.0.pdf.
9. Walker S, Davis G. Views of final-year student midwives on giving postpartum contraception and sexual health advice. J Fam Plann Reprod Health Care. 2014;40:312.
10. Marinova J, Parashkevova B. Skills acquisition in the area of contraceptive counseling: approaches and challenges in training students in midwife. Trakia J Sci. 2014;12:371–5.
11. Ege E, Akin B, Altuntuğ K. Opinions of midwifery students on adolescent sexuality and reproductive health in Turkey. Soc Behav Personal Int J. 2008;36:965–72.
12. Walker SH, Davis G. Knowledge and reported confidence of final year midwifery students regarding giving advice on contraception and sexual health. Midwifery. 2014;30:e169–76.
13. Barger MK, Hackley B, Bharj KK, et al. Knowledge and use of the ICM global standards for midwifery education. Midwifery. 2019;79:102534.
14. Crisp E. Do we acknowledge families' sexual and reproductive health needs within maternity services? A practising midwife's reflection. MIDIRS Midwifery Digest. 2018;28(2):1–4.
15. Vermeulen J, Vivilaki VG. A value-based philosophy debate on academic midwifery education in Europe. Eur J Midwifery. 2021;5:51–3.
16. Degryse B, Frans E, Peeters K, et al. Relational & sexual education. Textbook for secundary education (relationele en seksuele vorming). Handbook voor secundair onderwijs. Antwerp: Garant/Sensoa; 2011.

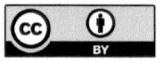

Various Sexual Consequences of Interventions in Midwifery Practice

28

Woet L. Gianotten ⓘ, Ana Polona Mivšek ⓘ, and Sam Geuens ⓘ

> I've learned that people forget what you said, people will forget what you did, but people will never forget how you made them feel.
> (Maya Angelou (African American poet, 1928–2014))

28.1 Introduction

This chapter addresses the sexual aftermath of what happened in the process that took place between the midwife and the woman or the couple. It does not focus on the direct physical consequence of an intervention but on the psychological, relational, and possible sexual implications of the midwife's approach and the surrounding context. Here are two examples:

1. The chapter does not deal with episiotomy causing dyspareunia, but it will deal with the emotional and sexual consequences of how the midwife introduces that episiotomy, communicates about the repair, and explains potential effects.

W. L. Gianotten (✉)
Department of Gynaecology and Obstetrics, Erasmus University Medical Center, Rotterdam, The Netherlands

A. Polona Mivšek
Faculty of Health Studies, University of Ljubljana, Ljubljana, Slovenia
e-mail: polona.mivsek@zf.uni-lj.si

S. Geuens (✉)
Department of Healthcare - Midwifery, PXL University College of Applied Arts and Sciences, Hasselt, Belgium

Outpatient Center for Sexual Health, Saint Franciscus Hospital, Heusden-Zolder, Belgium
e-mail: sam.geuens@pxl.be

© The Author(s) 2023
S. Geuens et al. (eds.), *Midwifery and Sexuality*,
https://doi.org/10.1007/978-3-031-18432-1_28

2. The chapter will address how repeated routine vaginal examinations can impact the woman's feelings of bodily integrity and negatively influence sexual desire and arousability.

Relevant elements of this chapter are context, body integrity, vulnerability, respect, the relationship of the midwife with the couple, and quality of care. That may seem superfluous since most of these are standard healthcare and midwifery training elements. However, it appears that usually, the focus has not been on the implications in the areas of sexuality and intimacy.

We want to clarify that the specific relationship between the professional and the woman or couple is an essential element of optimal care. Research clearly showed that a well-established connection between the woman/couple and the HCP is a vital determining factor in the short-term and long-term development of a positive sexual life [1].

This chapter's message relies much on practical examples.

28.2   Influencing Sexuality and Intimacy

Here, one can discern several lines along which sexuality and intimacy can easily be influenced, both aware and unaware. Some examples:

1. Physical exposure (or nudity), an unavoidable part of pregnancy examination and childbirth, is, for most women, seen as strictly reserved for partner-intimacy. The bare physical routine of pregnancy checks and childbirth can negatively colour the sense of intimacy for both the woman and her partner in the future.
2. There are direct associations between adverse sexual experiences in the past and the possible effects of routine midwifery practice on sexual well-being. For instance, in the sexually abused woman, being naked again, having her breasts touched, or undergoing vaginal penetration during a vaginal examination can easily evoke negative emotions and anxiety.
3. Childbirth can be a traumatic experience, generating long-standing emotional consequences, even when the physical aspects of the entire birthing process go smoothly. The woman still can experience it as traumatic because of too much pain, loss of control, or fear for the baby's health. It can also happen because of poor communication between the HCP and the woman or the couple, or experienced lack of support [2]. Passing through such trauma related to the sexual organs of the body can influence the woman's and partner's sexual well-being.
4. There is the vulnerability of the delicate balance in the intimate relationship between the woman and her partner. The male (or female) partner's presence at childbirth depends on the culture the couple lives in and how the midwife integrates the partner in the care and even the birthing process. The value of the partner's presence depends partly on the couple's relationship. For example, even in countries where the partners are invited to participate in the birth process, women experience the presence of their partner very differently, from very helpful to non-existing or a nuisance. In some couples, what happens during

childbirth can forge a strong bond, whereas, in others, it can negatively impact the couple dyad, creating intimate and sexual distance.

5. There is a connection between how the woman is treated emotionally and how that influences her sexuality and intimacy. In particular, during pregnancy and childbirth care, the consequences of mistreatment, verbal abuse, discrimination, and non-consented procedures (in other words: repeated breaches of her physical and mental integrity), can negatively impact her self-image. At a later moment, such a negative self-image can easily lead to various sexual problems, dysfunctions, and relationship misunderstandings.

This chapter will address these themes with practical examples. Investigative questions will invite the reader to dwell on various automatisms during their standard daily care practices that could negatively impact women's sexual well-being. Aiming to foster reflection on the self-evident daily professional routine, asking, 'Am I providing the best possible care?'

28.3 The Need to Adapt Our Care to the Diversity of the People Entrusted to Us

The great diversity of people keeps our work interesting, but at the same time, it also creates complexity and presents a challenge. One size of care doesn't fit all women and all couples.

1. The situation when a vaginal examination is needed. A few introductory words might suffice for the woman who delivered three children to ensure she knows what to expect. In the young primipara, who has never shown herself in the nude, even not for her husband, the first vaginal examination deserves another approach. A relaxed and precise description of how that is done, reassuring that she remains in control and can always signal discomfort, should ensure experiencing the examination in the best way possible.
2. Before examining the fundal height, a small verbal introduction and gaining consent to touch her will usually be sufficient. The same examination can need extensive preparation for a woman with a physical or sexual abuse history. A traumatic background requires more extensive preparation to instill a sense of safety before being able to undergo routine and seemingly harmless interventions. In that way, we minimise the chance of retraumatisation. With sexual abuse experience, simple, non-intrusive interventions such as measuring blood pressure can create feelings of 'being caught again'. Application of the cuff, especially when it gets under pressure, can resurface frightening memories or even dissociation.
3. For proper repair of an episiotomy or rupture, one needs surgical skills. For some women, that just means 'repairing the body'. For other women, the perineum is the entrance to their sexual garden of pleasure, and that entrance has to look and feel good. They could benefit when the HCP enquires how they think about reparative stitching instead of just stating that the rupture needs stitches. Besides,

the HCP needs good communication skills when asking for consent, answering questions on the why and how, explaining to the woman/couple what one is doing, and adjusting the form and tone of the message to that specific woman and couple.

28.4 Dealing with Body Integrity

Being (partially) naked and being looked at doesn't feel good for nearly all women. Experiencing that can create a temporary loss of the sense of body integrity, potentially influencing the woman's and partner's intimacy. It is a daily reality for maternity professionals to look at or be near vulnerable women and their nakedness. That everyday reality creates the risk that the HCP gradually loses the sense that nearly every woman is vulnerable when in the nude.

Building on this realisation, midwifery practice is loaded with many standard procedures that the pregnant woman easily can experience as a violation of her sense of integrity and physical self.

Here below some significant examples will be described.

28.4.1 Vaginal Examination (VE)

In the setting of reproductive care, physical touch is an inherent part of the daily routine. Vaginal examination (with fingers or ultrasound probe) is such a standard diagnostic procedure that it can make midwives and other HCPs forget that the vagina is, a very intimate area, only touched by the woman herself and sometimes her partner.

For women in labour, an adequately explained and consented VE can be positive and motivating when it confirms that labour is progressing. However, a VE can also be experienced as embarrassing, disturbing, and invasive, especially when explanation or consent is lacking. Women sometimes explicitly remark: *'My vagina has become public property!'*. That will not enhance erotic feelings after the birth. In Dutch research, 35% of women reported a negative experience with VE [3]. Based on that, the researchers recommend that the number of VEs during labour be restricted as much as possible; only be done after the woman's informed consent; and preferably performed by as few different caregivers as possible.

Some points for reflecting on one's own practise of any examination of a woman, including touching, might be the following:

- What do I have to do before any bodily examination? Do I explain why I will do it? Do I ask for permission to do the examination? Is it enough to just announce it? Can I just start the examination because the woman should expect that during antenatal consultations?
- Before performing a vaginal examination, do I ask: *'Do you prefer to have your partner here or in the waiting room?'*.

- The message: *'Please undress, I will be back in a minute!'* can mean a minute gain for the HCP. It can even be a way of fostering privacy during an intimate moment of undressing. But it might also come across as callous and impact the woman's sense of integrity.

28.4.2 Respectful Daily Practice

Being seen, being heard, and being understood are ingredients of the feeling of being respected. To properly treat people with respect, one must understand the impact of feeling vulnerable as a client and what it means to be dependent on people who provide the care you need. This delicate mix of vulnerability and dependence makes it very difficult for clients to comment on or correct the professional's self-evident routine actions.

The following reflective exercise intends to ask oneself and dwell on questions regarding the own clinical practice:

- It is common to have shaved, trimmed, or styled pubic hair in some societies. In other societies, some women don't shave, and both the woman and her partner can be very proud of her pubic hair. With that woman, what will you do when entering the labour ward or preparing to repair an episiotomy or a rupture? Do you ask permission to have the hair shaved? Do you just shave it? Do you only cut it shorter? And how do you communicate the why and how?

  Like nearly any other intervention, shaving should, as much as possible, be tailored to the needs and desires of the client, considering any potential impacts on the client's health and well-being. Research indicates that, regarding this topic, there is no clinical benefit of perineal shaving [4].
- When a woman has to stay in the labour ward for many hours, how many midwives, physicians, students, laboratory staff, and others have, often unannounced, entered that room, and have seen her (partly) naked and/or in distress? Some women experience this as if their body has become public property (which is potentially a problem when trying to reestablish intimacy).
- What is, during childbirth, the bed's position in relation to the door where people enter the delivery room?
- Did you, as an HCP, ever try to lay in that position (even with your panties on)? How did that feel when a colleague entered the room unannounced?
- Even reflecting on the design of rooms and architecture of departments can lead to considerable benefits in daily well-being for women and couples attending the delivery and maternity ward.

Especially in this period of her life, with so many inherent insecurities, not feeling respected can negatively affect a woman's sense of 'being a woman'. That is essential for maintaining a healthy sexual relationship with her partner or re-developing it in postpartum.

In four low- and middle-income countries, they did extensive research on the treatment of women during facility-based childbirth. Physical abuse, verbal abuse, stigma, or discrimination was indicated in 35% of the >2.600 postpartum surveys. There were also direct continuous observations during childbirth. These ill-treatments were directly observed in 41% of the >2000 observations [5]. In 56% of the episiotomies and 10% of the caesarean sections, the women had not given consent.

The way we do things is often central to good practice.

Here below are some examples of a self-reflective exercise on the own practice:

• Non-verbal communication, such as my face and my gaze, can convey important messages of respect or lack of it. How do I react when the next woman entering my office is severely obese?
• How do I react to looking at a woman's perineum who has undergone female genital mutilation? Will my gaze be understanding or inflict shame or even psychological damage!
• After episiotomy or perineal rupture, repairing the damage is needed. When you have prepared everything, the husband positions himself behind you, entirely focusing on the vulva. Will you just ignore this or react to it thoughtfully towards both partners?
• When, in a comparable situation, the husband requests: '*Can you stitch it really tight?*', will you react to that situation? How will you respond without destroying your professional alliance with him whilst caring for her?
• On the day after childbirth, you visit the woman in her private room in the hospital or birth centre. How do you enter the room? Do you just enter? Do you walk in after knocking on the door? Do you wait after knocking and get permission to enter? It could be that the woman is cuddling with her partner. Both could be in tears or engaged in any other behaviour that could confuse them (or you) when you suddenly break the privacy of that moment.

In respectful midwifery practice, small things often make a huge difference.

28.5 Traumatic Experiences

Giving birth can be a traumatic experience. A Dutch study investigated, at 3 years postpartum, recall of the birth experience. In low-risk women, 1 in 6 looked negatively back on childbirth [6]. We may assume that such traumatic experiences could influence sexuality or the intimate relationship, but there is no research confirming or denying that assumption.

In pregnancy and childbirth, traumatic events are sometimes inevitable. An unwanted Caesarean section can suddenly be unavoidable, and babies can even die. This chapter focuses on avoidable aspects. Since the inevitability of what has happened cannot be reversed, it is more important how we deal with it at that moment and afterwards. That includes explaining how this came to be, emotionally comforting the woman/couple, and conveying our heartfelt regret that this has happened.

In a group of nearly 2200 women with traumatic childbirth experiences, the researchers tried to distinguish the various 'causes' attributed to the traumatic experience [2]. In 47%, women indicated communication and lack of explanation caused the traumatic experience. Among the women who lost the baby, 63% mentioned 'a bad outcome' as one of the causes of the traumatic experience, but 37% mainly reported poor communication, lack of respect, and lack of support.

Every childbirth is an important event for the woman and the couple, even more so for a traumatic birth. That affects all segments of a woman's life, including the relationship with her partner, intimacy, and sexuality. Integrating a degree of emotional aftercare and follow-up seems essential.

28.6 Boundaries

In times of worry and insecurity, one can be pleased with a person providing peace and reassurance. Although that role can be gratifying, the HCP should know that being very much appreciated can also have negative consequences. In persons in distress, the feelings for their HCP can become very strong and turn into infatuation. It's not uncommon for women to be ecstatic about their male (and sometimes female) gynaecologist, midwife, paediatrician, or physiotherapist and sometimes develop romantic feelings. In psychotherapy, this process is called transference, based on emotions and unconscious needs that can sometimes be related to the woman's past. In those situations, it will be apparent that psychological help is needed. In a couple with an apparently stable relationship, the midwife can more easily form a good alliance with both partners, a necessary element to deliver good care. When the couple's relationship doesn't seem stable, the midwife should develop a subtle choreography to achieve a good alliance with both partners without creating jealousy or rivalry.

Lastly, midwives and other HCPs are sexual beings too, have sexual feelings, and possibly have a partner. These are all treasures to be cherished.

The midwife's daily practice should not be at the expense of the own sexual pleasure and sexual relationship. Surprisingly, there is very, very little literature on work-related trauma in midwives [7] and on developing sufficient sexual-health-related resilience in the education of young HCPs [8]. We couldn't find anything on work-related influence on the midwife's sexuality.

Just as the traumas in our patients can affect all spheres of their lives, we may assume that traumas in midwives will also affect their intimate life and sexual relationships.

There are two sides to being a midwife or maternity HCP. Witnessing childbirth and the transition to motherhood and parenthood is fulfilling and rewarding. But midwifery also faces sad and traumatic aspects of life. For many, it is difficult to find a good balance between empathising – feeling the patient's pain so that we can provide good care – and not being overwhelmed by it. Not really letting in what is happening sometimes seems necessary to be able to continue working. However, without reflecting on that, it can ultimately cause personal and professional coldness. On the other hand, if we allow trauma and grief to enter too deeply, this could heavily impact our own mental health and well-being.

Several recent studies reported on psychological troubles in midwives. In Swedish midwives, the prevalence of moderate to severe symptoms of depression, anxiety, and stress was between 7–12% [9]. Among UK midwives, 37% scored in the moderate or higher range for stress, 38% for anxiety, and 33% for depression [10]. Among certified US midwives and nurse-midwives, 40% met the criteria for burnout [11]. When falling ill, most HCPs have difficulties stepping out of their professional, caring role and being a patient.

Burnout, stress, anxiety, and depression tend to be accompanied by decreased sexual desire and pleasure, with additional sexual damage when treated with antidepressants (see Chap. 17). In turn, that creates a breeding ground for relationship problems.

How should we react to those figures?

Regarding the care for pregnant women, we dare to guess that the midwife with the above-mentioned psychological disturbances will pay less attention to the sexuality of their clients. But we don't know!

Regarding the care for the midwife, we dare to guess that, with a satisfying sexual life, the midwife will have fewer psychological disturbances and vice versa. Chap. 4 elaborates on the health benefits of sexuality that also apply to midwives and other maternity HCPs.

28.7   Not-Intervening as an Intervention

Although this chapter carries in its name 'Sexual consequences of interventions', we shouldn't forget that omitting interventions also can have negative sexual consequences. Chap. 12 addressed that for high-risk and complicated pregnancies. All sexual information relevant to the woman's or couple's well-being but not mentioned by the HCP reinforces the taboo on addressing sexuality. And as such will increase the risk for sexual disturbances. In situations ripe with uncertainties, we believe that the HCP should pro-actively address and answer the 'not asked questions'.

Chap. 26 gives practical advice on talking about sexuality with clients pro-actively.

28.8   Conclusion and Recommendations

During pregnancy and childbirth, the communication and approach of the midwife (and other HCPs as well) can play an essential role in the further development of the sexual well-being of the woman/couple. A continuous mantra for HCPs should be: *'Our behaviour and communication have (also) sexual consequences!'*.

In daily practice, awareness of the importance of how to address the woman/couple is an essential part of good practice. In midwifery education, we believe that ample time should be allocated to teaching and practising communication skills. Good communication is a prerequisite to delivering high-quality care. A valuable way to stay alert to the impact of one's own practice is by asking for feedback from the woman and her partner throughout the process, especially at the last (postpartum) visit. Experts recommend offering every woman a postpartum visit with the caregiver who assisted her during the delivery for debriefing on the birth process.

Explicitly including sexuality in such an 'exit interview' can be a constructive way to gradually increase the own expertise in sexuality and intimacy.

References

1. Geuens S, Dams H, Jones M, Lefevere G. Back to basics: a solution focused take on using and teaching basic communication skills for health care professionals. J Solut Focus Prac. 2020;4(2):6. https://digitalscholarship.unlv.edu/cgi/viewcontent.cgi?article=1084&context=journalsfp.
2. Hollander MH, van Hastenberg E, van Dillen J, et al. Preventing traumatic childbirth experiences: 2192 women's perceptions and views. Arch Womens Ment Health. 2017;20:515–23.
3. de Klerk HW, Boere E, van Lunsen RH, Bakker JJH. Women's experiences with vaginal examinations during labor in the Netherlands. J Psychosom Obstet Gynaecol. 2018;39:90–5.
4. Basevi V, Lavender T. Routine perineal shaving on admission in labour. Cochrane Database Syst Rev. 2014;2014(11):CD001236.
5. Bohren MA, Mehrtash H, Fawole B, et al. How women are treated during facility-based childbirth in four countries: a cross-sectional study with labour observations and community-based surveys. Lancet. 2019;394(10210):1750–63.
6. Rijnders M, Baston H, Schönbeck Y, et al. Perinatal factors related to negative or positive recall of birth experience in women 3 years postpartum in the Netherlands. Birth. 2008;35:107–16.
7. Aydın R, Aktaş S. Midwives' experiences of traumatic births: a systematic review and meta-synthesis. Eur J Midwifery. 2021;5:31.
8. Kunzler AM, Helmreich I, König J, et al. Psychological interventions to foster resilience in healthcare students. Cochrane Database Syst Rev. 2020;7(7):CD013684.
9. Båtsman A, Fahlbeck H, Hildingsson I. Depression, anxiety and stress in Swedish midwives: a cross-sectional survey. Eur J Midwifery. 2020;4:29.
10. Hunter B, Fenwick J, Sidebotham M, Henley J. Midwives in the United Kingdom: levels of burnout, depression, anxiety and stress and associated predictors. Midwifery. 2019;79:102526.
11. Thumm EB, Smith DC, Squires AP, et al. Burnout of the US midwifery workforce and the role of practice environment. Health Serv Res. 2022;57:351–63.

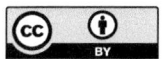

How Sexual Problems are Managed (by Other Professionals)

Patrícia M. Pascoal and Catarina F. Raposo

Midwives are privileged to prevent and detect sexual health problems, concerns, and doubts. In some cases, a referral can seem necessary when they lack the knowledge and skills to tackle the client's issues.

The midwife can detect sexual concerns by listening to the woman and the couple. In that way, she can encounter sexual problems, e.g. existing before pregnancy, triggered or worsened by pregnancy, or childbirth. Furthermore, due to her close contact with the woman and her partner, the midwife may even be elected as a trusted person to share experiences of sexual abuse, neglect, and violence.

Because midwives also contact women who are willing or keen to be involved in clinical interventions to improve their sexual health or eliminate their sexual problems, we will address some basic knowledge on sex therapy. Our goal is to offer information on what sex therapy is about, enabling midwives to refer their clients to sex therapists - whenever that appears needed - with an adequate explanation of what the woman or couple can expect.

Sex therapy was initially developed as a therapeutic approach mainly aimed at changing behaviours and eliminating sexual problems. Currently, it is an integrative therapeutic intervention, utilising different therapeutic methods and tools, aimed at individuals and couples who wish to restore or improve their sexual health and well-being. Sex therapy follows a collaborative model, and people are actively involved in the process. The intervention begins with a clinical evaluation, then therapeutic goals are set together with the client(s), and finally, a personalised intervention plan is made. Sex therapists usually are psychologists, psychotherapists, or physicians of

P. M. Pascoal (✉)
CICPSI, Faculdade de Psicologia, Universidade de Lisboa, Lisbon, Portugal

HEI-Lab: Digital Human-Enviroment Interation Lab, Lusófona University, Lisbon, Portugal

C. F. Raposo
Faculty of Psychology and Education Sciences, University of Porto, Porto, Portugal

Center for Psychology, University of Porto, Porto, Portugal

S. Geuens et al. (eds.), *Midwifery and Sexuality*,
https://doi.org/10.1007/978-3-031-18432-1_29

different specialities who theoretically and practically have been trained in sex therapy. Still, there are other types of health care professionals (HCPs), such as midwives, nurses, physician assistants, and pelvic physiotherapists who, with proper additional training in sexology, can provide support in some cases of sex therapy. These professionals eligible to pursue specialised training may differ across countries, so we recommend consulting the professional sexology associations in each country of interest for more accurate information.

29.1 Context

For several decades, professionals have discussed what constitutes good sexual functioning and a healthy sex life. Clinical psychologists, psychiatrists, and other medical specialists classify sexual dysfunctions in the DSM 5 and the ICD manuals from a clinical perspective. The group of sexual dysfunctions includes a variety of disorders, most of them characterised by sexual distress related to sexual functioning or by problems feeling pleasure. (For a brief overview of when sex isn't working, see Chap. 3. For an overview of the categorisation of sexual dysfunctions according to DSM 5 [1]).

Sexual dysfunction can cause personal and interpersonal distress and can be related to poorer overall well-being, relationship conflict, and lower quality of life. However, one does not need to be eligible to receive a diagnosis of sexual dysfunction to experience the detrimental effects of sexual problems or to benefit from sex therapy.

Even without intense distress, couples might strive for a better sexual life and invest in sex therapy. Midwives are in the privileged position to normalise both the change in sexual experiences during the pregnancy and young parenthood and the need to seek help to promote sexual well-being and prevent sexual dissatisfaction. Sexual problems and sexual difficulties throughout pregnancy can be, for example, due to lack of information, the result of ineffective sexual stimulation in the context of bodily changes or body image concerns throughout pregnancy and after delivery. Referring people who experience sexual distress to a sex therapist with expertise in reproduction-related changes may be adequate as a measure to diminish discomfort but also as a measure that may prevent the development of a serious sexual problem.

29.2 Fundamentals of Sex Therapy

Sex therapy starts from a biopsychosocial understanding of sexuality [2]. The process of sex therapy closely resembles that of general psychotherapy, e.g. the therapeutic process tends to follow the standard steps of the first evaluation, then mutual goal setting followed by collaboratively tailoring interventions with the couple, best suited to help them reach their own goals with regards to their sexual lives. Regarding evaluating sexual problems, the biopsychosocial approach to sexual dysfunctions and problems allows us to understand how physical, psychological, and social variables interact and intricately determine, maintain, and eventually worsen sexual difficulties and dysfunctions. This approach enables a comprehensive assessment of medical, sexual, and psychosocial factors, and their history is considered in both diagnosis and clinical management. So when in sex therapy, the client or couple should expect a proper assessment (with sometimes more than one professional, e.g., gynaecologist and sexologist) to ensure that the relevant physical, psychological, and social factors will be carefully evaluated.

Next to the form of the process, as in all psychotherapeutic approaches, the quality of the therapeutic relationship is a determinant for the success of this type of intervention. An empathic relationship, the validation of concerns and difficulties, motivation, and positive reinforcement, is essential for the success of sex therapy.

Sex therapy is characterised by its focus on a solid therapeutic alliance, multidisciplinary in the stages of evaluation and treatment and prescription of homework assignments designed with the collaboration of patients.

Case Example: Christine
Christine is a heterosexual 40-year-old married primigravid woman pregnant for 7 months. She feels more sexual than ever but feels awkward about these feelings, although she notices her partner is enthusiastic about her renewed interest in sex. Christine thinks she is not normal and that this intense interest in sex is bad. Christine also noticed that reaching orgasm has become much easier for her. Her orgasms are, on the one hand, very pleasurable. But she feels physically depleted afterwards, causing problems because she often orgasms very soon, leaving her unsatisfied partner behind. Christine worries that he will become frustrated by how sex is going and might lose interest. She fears that her sexual interest may diminish after childbirth, causing her partner to feel disappointed. Christine is afraid she will never be as before again, and she has talked with her midwife about her worries.

29.3   Evaluation

Within sex therapy, the first sessions are decisive for establishing a collaborative therapeutic alliance, a clear view of the client's desired outcomes, and possible strategies to achieve those goals. Next to establishing a good working alliance, the first sessions are characterised by the therapist trying to evaluate the client's current situation. Looking at predisposing factors (e.g., poor sex education; negative expectations); precipitating factors related to the events that triggered the onset of the sexual problem (e.g., pain during penetration); and perpetuating factors that maintain the condition (e.g., depression and loss of desire, non-pleasurable sexual activity).

Christine's Case

It would be beneficial to explore Christine's expectations about sexuality during pregnancy, namely the last trimester, and her expectations about postpartum sexuality.

The following questions could be helpful:

"How did you expect your sexual desire to evolve throughout pregnancy?"

"What did you expect to happen in the last trimester and after childbirth?"

"Why would this be a problem in your case?"

The therapist should also evaluate potential triggers for Christine's concerns:

"Did you read about this topic anywhere and did that impact your feelings on the matter?"

"Did your partner express a loss of desire, or did he notice a rise in your desire?"

"Since you started to feel your stronger desire, did you change your behaviour (e.g. checking your partner's level of desire, reading testimonies on the internet about women's desire during pregnancy)?"

"Do you perceive that your partner will be disappointed if your levels of desire diminish after childbirth?"

"How do you feel about the fact that your orgasm comes so quickly?"

"Did you speak to your partner about how this might affect your sex life as a couple?"

In general, the sex therapist will also assess the client's expectations regarding the treatment, the motivation to change the current situation and the belief in the attainability of the set goals. These are considered essential elements for the patient's involvement and the success of the intervention. For example, couples who experience sexual desire discrepancy may expect that sex therapy will 'fix' the person with low desire. Sexual desire discrepancy is, however, a common characteristic of amorous relationships. One cannot avoid changes in desire, and there is no objective standard for the amount of sexual desire of men and women [3].

Christine's Case

It would be important to find out if there is a discrepancy in sexual desire and who is distressed about this: Christine, her partner, or both.

The clinical/sexual interview is an indispensable tool at this stage of the process. The therapist should collect as much information as possible about the nature and development of the problem and factors contributing to its onset and maintenance to establish a differential diagnosis while strengthening the HCP–client relationship. Evaluation in this context could assess different spheres of the individual's life, such as interpersonal aspects (romantic and sexual relationships, family, and friendships), habits and routines, passage through the various stages of life from childhood (e.g., attitudes of parents and significant adults towards sexuality) and adolescence (e.g., sex education and first experiences) to the present (e.g., religious beliefs, sexual practices, attitudes and sexual beliefs), but only when the clinician or the patient deem them relevant. Interpersonal factors (e.g., relational satisfaction, sexual communication) can play a significant role in sexual outcomes (such as sexual satisfaction, pleasure, or distress), and, therefore, in the case of a romantic relationship, the therapist will also try to involve the partner [4]. The therapist will gather information about the current relationship, both partners' ideas on the problem and any information they consider important.

Christine's Case
Questions in this exploration phase could be:
"What messages gave your families, culture, and religion about sexuality in pregnancy?"
How did both internalise those messages?
How has the couple been dealing with Christine's distress?
"Did you show your distress, or are you afraid to tell or show that to your partner?
How has the couple dealt with problems (illness, employment, family of origin) before?
(Previous challenges can indicate strengths and weaknesses relevant to the current situation.)
What are the expectations and fears about her strong sexual desire and her partner's enjoyment? What ideas does that generate?
What changes does Christine expect about motherhood, job, partner roles, et cetera and how that could influence sexuality?

The therapist should always check previous clinical follow-ups, any physical or mental illness, and if the person takes medication. A mental health problem (e.g., depression), a physical condition (e.g., candidiasis), or medication (e.g., hormonal contraception) can be the explanation for the sexual symptoms and signals. Success may come from other interventions rather than just sex therapy in these cases.

Midwives who refer clients to sex therapy can play a crucial role by explaining that sex therapy is not a miracle therapy. Its focus is on sexual response and the emotional experiences linked to sexual activity. But it is not fast and narrowly focused on genital response and deals with knowledge of personal development.

When an organic cause is expected, a medical consultation is needed for a correct diagnosis [5]. In sum, midwives can frame expectations of women experiencing sexual problems by clarifying that the evaluation process in sex therapy uses a comprehensive biopsychosocial approach that takes a developmental look at sexual problems and assumes a multidisciplinary treatment perspective. People can expect that sharing concerns and the therapist's act of collecting information might have a profound positive effect and lead to insight, promoting an atmosphere of trust and even modelling an atmosphere for better sexual communication.

29.4   Treatment

Sex therapy aims to ease anxieties, minimise difficulties, normalise experiences, and look for ways to maximise sexual health and well-being, considering the patient's socio-cultural background and desired sexual outcomes. Over time, sex therapy evolved from a primarily behavioural-oriented approach to an integrative approach that deals with assessment and treatment through a biopsychosocial perspective [6]. Therefore, interventions can also be undertaken in a multidisciplinary clinical context.

Sex therapy is often used as an umbrella concept to refer to many possible effective interventions. Therapeutic interventions are adapted to the needs and uniqueness of the patient and, when in a relationship, to the dynamics in their relationship.

So the midwife can explain that sex therapy deals with increasing good couple communication, broadening their perspective on intimacy and sexuality, and improving how they will experience having sex.

Midwives can explain to their clients that searching for scientifically grounded information in magazines, books, or online can be valuable for couples struggling with sexual worries or problems, especially when sex therapy might not be an option because sex therapists are not available or are too expensive.

Sex therapy will almost always include an amount of behavioural therapy. One's sexuality is expressed through feelings, attitudes, thoughts, and behaviours (alone or in a relational context). So, part of sex therapy often will focus on breaking behavioural patterns and establishing new, more functional, and satisfying ones. When needed, the sharing of information, discussion, and clarification of doubts about aspects of sexual anatomy and physiology often constitute the first sessions of the therapeutic process. Psychoeducation about sexuality is an essential tool in overcoming not-effective sexual concepts and myths that are often at the root and the maintenance of sexual difficulties. Such psychoeducational interventions can be done in individual therapy, couple counselling, or group settings [7]. The partner should preferably be part of this education. Partners tend to share inadequate beliefs and expectations about sexuality.

Through cognitive restructuring, the therapist can address more realistic beliefs. For example, regarding Christine's idea that it is abnormal to feel extra sexual while pregnant, the therapist may address this idea an try to uncover where it comes from, how rigid and how reliable it is.

The most common sexual pitfall is the widespread idea that penile-vaginal intercourse is the only correct way to have sex or the only way for a woman to experience pleasure or orgasm. Such beliefs can keep couples focused on penetrative sex, even during postpartum pain or menopausal lack of lubrication. Such situations need education. For instance, on the clitoris and its function, sexual response changes throughout pregnancy or the physical and sexual effects of menopausal hormonal changes. Part of that education is challenging the couple to think in alternative directions. Such 'cognitive restructuring' may help create room for more sexual variety and experimenting, leading to more pleasurable sexual experiences free from the penile-vaginal penetration pressure.

Christine's Case
The therapist needs to address the beliefs of Christine and her partner about what sexual changes they can expect during pregnancy and postpartum. The therapist will also normalise their solo and their couple experiences (*'That can happen!'*) and call attention to their ongoing rediscovering of sexuality in new ways.

Some midwives will be sufficiently trained to provide couples such 'Limited Information', as in the PLISSIT model, eliminating the need for referral to a sex therapist (or in preparation before referral). For more information on the PLISSIT model, see Chap. 3.

Throughout the sessions, the therapist can indicate new experiences or behavioural patterns to experience at home in between sessions to facilitate change in the currently faltering sexual dynamic. Therapists must ensure that couples clearly understand how to go about these new experiences at home, which sometimes requires detailed behavioural descriptions of intimate or sexual activities. The more the therapist and the couple co-construct these new experiences, the greater the couple's motivation to try them in between sessions and overcome any possible practical and emotional pitfalls when trying out new and sometimes challenging experiences. At the beginning of each consecutive session, the therapist invites the couple to share, in a detailed manner, how they have gone about trying these new experiences so that they can discuss the difficulties and gains to help promote change.

During the consultation, these experiences can be integrated into cognitive tasks (e.g., recording the automatic negative thoughts that appeared during the homework exercises) to work on them. Most people have rigid, repetitive, and limited sexual skills, with interactions generally oriented towards performance and the achievement of specific goals (e.g., reaching orgasm through penile-vaginal intercourse). Such performance-focused attention keeps patients away from concentrating and enjoying pleasurable sensations. In the opposite direction, while experimenting with new ways of sexual interaction, the therapist might advise the couple, when in a sexual encounter, to be aware of the physical sensations without desperately looking for erection, orgasm, or pleasure and, as such, rediscover the wonders of physical intimacy. Therefore, improving the sexual communication skills among partners is another relevant treatment strategy. With better sexual communication, it usually becomes easier to accept differences in desire and preferred sexual scripts by which there will be less reason for tension and guilt.

Those are all aspects of a behavioural approach, focusing on breaking down dysfunctional sexual habits and re-establishing new ones. Besides, therapy sometimes integrates muscle relaxation techniques to enhance levels of relaxation and comfort during homework exercises and new experiences. Occasionally, attention is paid to the surrounding where the homework exercises occur. A comfortable environment can facilitate the gradual development of better sexual interaction through positive associations.

Christine's Case

For Christine and her partner, this could include addressing their habitual way of having sex and challenging their ideas and expectations concerning 'good sex' to create a more flexible set of sexual beliefs, expectations, and practices. In concrete terms, this could mean experimenting with new forms of sexual stimulation that might still be pleasurable to Christine but not bring her to orgasm so quickly.

Christine and her partner could benefit from attention for their feelings. When they can learn to communicate about their fears and anxieties, express themselves positively, and avoid shame and guilt, their sexual relationship will benefit.

Lastly, overcoming uncertainty could be an essential therapeutical goal, as the couple seems to feel distressed about unexpected positive experiences and seems to be distressed by the uncertainty of future events they cannot control.

The idea that women in heterosexual couples are less receptive and hesitant about sex is an example of an almost inevitable message in many sexual scripts. That idea can condition the behaviour of some women and men because women tend to expect the male partner to start sexual interaction. Over time, this internalised message becomes interpersonal, is again and again repeated, and can end up as a pattern in the relationship.

Sex therapy can identify dominant sexual scripts and how they shape and condition the exploration of intimacy and pleasure. That can create room for questioning, co-construction, and exploration of new, different scripts. In the case of Christine and her partner, sexual scripts about what normal sexuality during pregnancy and postpartum should be, may interfere with the enjoyment of the current situation and create negative expectations towards the future. In sex therapy, it is important to address these scripts and clarify that everyone can re-construct new scripts that are not based on dominant representations of sexuality.

The therapist may promote flexible sexual scripts and encourage and stimulate sexual narratives and imagery, exercises for directed masturbation and body exploration, and exercises for reducing performance anxiety and muscle relaxation. Some of these exercises are similar to techniques used in preparation for childbirth, aiming to reconnect the woman with positive body sensations. Relaxation and recognition of body responses and sensations are often used to manage sexual pain, especially when it is associated with a tense pelvic floor (for more details, see Chap. 10).

It is common for clients to have difficulties when they try new experiences at home, that have been co-constructed in the session. This can reflect other difficulties not caused by the sexual problem itself. Personal and interpersonal situations (e.g., fear they might make a bad situation worse, fear of leaving their comfort zone) can obstruct the therapeutic process, sometimes asking for extra consultation.

There is no ideal duration and number of sessions; this aspect is always fluid and continuously adjusted according to the needs and development of each client or couple. It is important to note that there is no physical contact between the therapist and the patient. All co-constructed new experiences are tried out by the client or couple in the privacy of their own home.

As an important final note, we would like to stress that most studies on therapeutic interventions have been done in common, monogamous, heterosexual, non-disabled people. So there is room for broadening knowledge on therapeutic interventions with these client groups [6].

Recently sex therapy has become even more multidisciplinary and has integrated different therapeutic approaches and strategies (e.g., systems therapy, mindfulness), establishing itself as an integrative approach to sexual problems. Also, in recent years the use of internet-delivered sexual interventions has gone up, which may translate into the inclusion of new possibilities for sex therapy, such as reaching people who have more difficulties in enrolling in a face-to-face intervention either due to lack of local resources, or inhibition about approaching sexual issues in a clinical setting.

Midwives can play a pivotal role in referring clients to sex therapy, by educating them about the why and how of sex therapy, explaining that, in the case of a couple, both partners will participate and informing them about the biopsychosocial approach. Besides, midwives should indicate that sex therapy has a more comprehensive focus than only genital stimulation and often includes homework assignments[1].

References

1. Sungur MZ, Gündüz AA. A comparison of DSM-IV-TR and DSM-5 definitions for sexual dysfunctions: critiques and challenges. J Sex Med. 2014;11:364–73.
2. Engel GL. The clinical application of the biopsychosocial model. Am J Psychiatry. 1980;137:535–44. https://doi.org/10.1176/ajp.137.5.535.
3. Dewitte M, Carvallho J, Corona G, et al. Sexual desire discrepancy: a position statement of the European society for sexual medicine. Sex Med. 2020;8:121–31. https://doi.org/10.1016/j.esxm.2020.02.008.

[1]This work is partially funded by national funds from FCT – Fundação para a Ciência e a Tecnologia, I.P, through the Research Center for Psychological Science of the Faculty of Psychology, University of Lisbon (UIDB/04527/2020; UIDP/04527/2020).

4. Pascoal PM, Narciso I, Pereira NM. Emotional intimacy is the best predictor of sexual satisfaction of men and women with sexual arousal problems. Int J Impot Res. 2013;25:51–5. https://doi.org/10.1038/ijir.2012.38.
5. Laan E, Rellini AH, Barnes T. Standard operating procedures for female orgasmic disorder: consensus of the international society for sexual medicine. J Sex Med. 2013;10:74–82. https://doi.org/10.1111/j.1743-6109.2012.02880.x.
6. Hall KS, Binik YM, editors. Principles and practice of sex therapy. 6th ed. New York: Guilford Press; 2020.
7. Smith WJ, Beadle K, Shuster EJ. The impact of a group psychoeducational appointment on women with sexual dysfunction. Am J Obstet Gynecol. 2017;198:697.e1–7. https://doi.org/10.1016/j.ajog.2008.03.028.

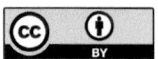

Midwifery of the Future; A Widening Field of Competences

30

Woet L. Gianotten ⓘ, Eva Wendt, and Ana Polona Mivšek ⓘ

30.1 Introduction

In many countries, midwives are considered the professionals who guide uncomplicated pregnancy, childbirth, and the postpartum period. Their independence varies widely around the world. In some countries, midwives manage the first stage of labour and later hand the woman over to the obstetrician. In other countries, midwives supervise the entire process autonomously unless pregnancy or labour complications require an obstetrician referral.

In both cases, midwifery services may be extended to various areas, such as prenatal care, childbirth classes, and family planning. Often this is done without consideration of sexuality and intimacy. That could be called sexuality-insensitive care. This book aims to change that and ensure that midwives and other health care professionals (HCPs) begin to adequately incorporate the topic of intimacy and sexuality into their care. Attention to sexuality and intimacy should be integral to midwifery practice and competencies.

This final chapter of the book takes midwifery to the next level. In the broadest sense, sexuality-positive midwifery creates space for expanding the domains of women's health, with the inclusion of sexual and reproductive health. Sweden is an excellent example of such progressive, sexuality-positive midwifery. While this may sound like midwifery fiction to some parts of the world, this chapter will elaborate on this advanced level and outline visions for the future of midwifery.

W. L. Gianotten (✉)
Department of Gynaecology and Obstetrics, Erasmus University Medical Center,
Rotterdam, The Netherlands
e-mail: woetgia@ziggo.nl

E. Wendt
Halland, Sweden

A. Polona Mivšek
Faculty of Health Studies, University of Ljubljana, Ljubljana, Slovenia
e-mail: polona.mivsek@zf.uni-lj.si

© The Author(s) 2023
S. Geuens et al. (eds.), *Midwifery and Sexuality*,
https://doi.org/10.1007/978-3-031-18432-1_30

30.2 Developing into the Next Level of Sexuality-Positive Midwifery Care

Sometimes, growth and development just happen, and sometimes they are deliberately planned. We are providing examples of possible developments from several perspectives.

30.2.1 The 'Unmet Needs Perspective'

In daily work, the sexuality-positive midwife may become aware of gaps in care. One example is midwife Elena, who saw many young women struggle with unplanned pregnancies. At the local community centre, with the help of local authorities, she set up a weekly contraception and sex education consultation.

Awareness of "unmet needs" can also come from research. That happened, for example, in the midwifery school, where not only pregnant women and women who had recently given birth but also midwifery teachers answered a questionnaire on how to deal with sexuality and intimacy. While most pregnant women said they desperately needed such information, almost none of the teachers talked about this topic to their students or pregnant women. These results shocked the school management and prompted them to add a sexologist to the teaching team and gradually integrate the subject into the curriculum.

30.2.2 The 'Career Perspective'

Midwives who want to expand and develop their competencies in women's health have many essential fields to work within. An example is midwife Mirjam, who, at age 53, changed career, got additional training and continued as a sexuality counsellor with competencies in advising about contraception.

30.2.3 The 'Specialisation Perspective'

Whereas some professionals are pleased with the common daily midwifery challenges, others gradually realise to feel very at home in one of the subareas of the profession, in which they like to invest and develop extra expertise. Such specialisation can be very efficient in group practices with many midwives.

In an extensive urban practice with 17 midwives, Ursula was requested to take care of the antenatal classes. She developed a session for couples entirely devoted to sexuality and intimacy. That session became very well appreciated.

This example calls for a point of attention. When one midwife of a group practice specialises in sexuality, the others are not absolved from the obligation to address sexuality with their own clients.

30.2.4 The 'Curiosity Perspective'

"How about this?" is the fundamental question behind science and the motivation to challenge the usual structures and routines. Janet became interested in sexology when she found that her role as a midwife inspired great confidence in women. With more expertise in sexology, she could also help and support women who had different problems and questions related to sexuality and relationships. Janet's curiosity led to a training in sexology, and she now works for one day a week as a clinical sexologist.

30.2.5 The 'Who Else? Perspective'

When something needs to be done, we usually know which professional should be asked, depending on factors such as skills and knowledge. When it is a task involving people, attitude, confidence, and familiarity with the target population are critical [1]. Midwives seem well equipped for many sexual and reproductive health tasks. They have the essential skills needed for these tasks and work in the right context [2]. The frequent and close contact between the midwife and the woman at a vulnerable stage of life fosters the necessary trust in the midwifery profession, which is essential for promoting healthy sexuality among the women they encounter, fundamental for facilitating healthy sexuality in the long-term [1].

The question "Who else?" may depend on whether other professionals are available. For example, in most affluent countries, there are 20–40 physicians per 10,000 population, while in some low-income countries, there is not even 1 physician per 10,000 population. In these countries, midwives perform tasks that are not fulfilled by other HCPs. In some places in sub-Saharan Africa, midwives with 3 years of additional training in surgery perform caesarean sections to reduce maternal mortality [3].

Consider the management of sexual disorders and dysfunction. In countries where few health professionals have knowledge of sexology or sexual medicine, midwives could fill this gap. Currently, only physicians and psychologists can specialise in sexual medicine. We believe that sexology organisations should recognise that midwives are capable of addressing sexuality. They should either open their courses to midwives or offer courses specific to the midwifery profession. That seems like a win-win situation benefitting clients, midwifery, and sexology.

Women's health can be improved by enhancing the role of midwives [4] and building their basic competencies to include communication about sexuality and sexual health [2]. However, even if women feel comfortable talking to a midwife about sexuality, most women do not start this conversation without being asked or prompted. If a midwife does not proactively approach the topic, women do not get answers to their questions and problems.

Some women feel that sexuality-related questions from health professionals are too personal [1]. While this is not just a matter of trust, a trusting environment increases women's chances of talking about sexuality and intimacy [5]. Creating such opportunities can be critical for many women.

Countries and cultures differ in how they talk about and deal with sexuality. However, although taboos vary, most aspects of love, sexuality, intimacy, hormones, conception, and orgasm are the same worldwide. Some midwives have already taken important steps to incorporate sexuality and intimacy into their daily work. This has happened in Sweden, for example. It could become a model for midwifery profession worldwide.

30.3 The Swedish Experience

Sweden is one of the most affluent countries globally and scores the highest on the European Gender Equality index. Already in 1886, Swedish midwives established the Swedish Association of Midwives. In Sweden, the midwife starts with a bachelor in nursing, followed by 2 years of midwifery. Many continue their education, and 2.5% reach the PhD level, which is one of the indicators of the profession's high professionalism [5].

Swedish midwives work independently and autonomously in basic midwifery care. In addition, they prescribe contraceptives, insert intrauterine devices and implants, and perform medical abortions. They provide over 80% of Sweden's sexual and reproductive healthcare [6].

Below we display, in adapted order, the Swedish list of competencies, specifically mentioned under the umbrella of sexual health [7]. This Swedish list is an addition to the core competencies that the International Confederation of Midwives (ICM) prescribes for midwifery.

The Midwife Has the Competence to:

- perform a gynaecological examination and identify abnormalities,
- inform and give advice on gynaecological conditions and diseases,
- provide care for gynaecological illness and disease.
- provide care in the event of a miscarriage,
- inform about menopause and connected hormonal changes and sexual health,
- inform about treatment for infertility,
- inform and give advice on contraceptive methods and contraceptives,
- inform about sterilisation,
- prescribe contraceptives to healthy women for birth control purposes,
- apply intrauterine and intradermal contraceptives,
- inform about abortion methods,
- provide care in the event of induced abortion,
- identify and provide care in the event of abortion complications,
- perform sampling and counselling regarding sexually transmitted infections (STIs),
- inform about treatment, infection-tracing and laws, and prescribe drugs and treat certain conditions/diagnoses [7].

It is not just the list of competencies that makes the Swedish model an example of quality midwifery care. Also, this model's perception of women's sexual and reproductive rights, their attitude towards clients and their tendency to practice woman-centred midwifery care are important. We realise that various competencies from this list may seem unachievable for many midwives. Neither all midwives are identical nor their cultures. However, one will not advance to a higher level without striving for better.

In the following subchapters, we will elaborate on sexuality education and then on various midwifery skills.

30.4 Sexuality-Positive Midwifery and Sexuality Education

Sexual and reproductive health is essential for people's and society's quality of life. Numerous women die every day because they lack access to various elements of reproductive health care: proper sexuality information, reliable contraception, safe abortion, and adequate maternity care. But also because they lack the power to change their life situation. In many cultures, women lack the right and freedom to decide on their sexuality and cannot choose if and with whom they want to have sex and have children. Among the serious consequences of this lack of rights and power are poverty and poor physical health of women and children.

The WHO describes sexual health as 'a state of physical, emotional, mental and social well-being in relation to sexuality', which not only means the absence of illness and harm. It requires a positive and respectable attitude towards sexuality and sexual relationships and the ability to have pleasurable and safe sexual experiences free from coercion, discrimination, and violence.

The WHO describes reproductive health as 'the possibility of a satisfactory and safe sex life without worries about illness, ability to reproduce and freedom to plan your childbearing'. Women deserve access to effective and acceptable family planning and good healthcare to undergo pregnancy and childbirth safely and be guaranteed the best opportunities to raise healthy children.

Reproductive rights include, among other things, women's right to decide on the number of children and the space between pregnancies. These rights also include access to contraception, education, and sexuality education.

That brings us to the role of the midwife. Midwifery is eminently the profession with several responsibilities in this area.

(a) The midwife should maximally integrate these rights into daily care and practice.
(b) The midwife should integrate this information into all educational activities.
(c) The midwifery profession should proactively promote and practice these rights in society.

To reach these goals, developing skills in counselling and teaching about sexuality and sexual and reproductive health and rights has to be part of the midwifery curriculum; in a basic undergraduate and advanced level. Each of those areas should be integrated into the education of midwives, with a substantial amount of attention directed to sexual pleasure and the wide variety of the normal range of sexual behaviour and a smaller amount focused on sexual problems.

30.4.1 Maximally Integrate Sexual and Reproductive Health and Rights in the Daily Midwifery Care and Practice

Midwives should be competent to support women under their care when they need help or want to talk about sexual pleasure, sexual insecurities, sexual function and dysfunction, orgasm, dyspareunia, sexual desire, and desire differences with their partner. Sexual health also deals with self-respect, with the notion of being mentally, physically, and sexually worthwhile, but also with insecurities nourished by peers, social media and society. Self-respect includes the crucial area of being able to say both 'yes' and 'no' to sex. The midwife can be the ideal person for the woman who wants to talk about intimate relationships and family life in positive aspects but also about negative experiences like various forms of intimate partner violence.

We believe that midwifery should develop adequate interventions to sustain women's health within the woman's reproductive life and empower women for choices tailored to their dreams.

Midwives could also consider couple's groups for sexual and relationship education, just as in prenatal education.

Even if women can feel comfortable having a dialogue with midwives regarding sexuality, many do not raise such questions without being prompted [1]. This means that women experience hindrances in getting answers to their sexual questions and problems. Some women might feel that sexuality-related questions from health professionals are too personal [1]. These women may become comfortable enough to approach the subject in a trusting environment [5]. Creating such opportunities may be crucial for women.

30.4.2 Integrating Sexual and Reproductive Health and Rights Information in All Educational Activities

One may wonder who could be the expert in educating in sexuality. Who gives young people the right and appropriate information at the right moment? In the ideal situation, young people might get information from their parents. However, in many countries, this doesn't happen enough or not at all. The explanation for that is, on the one hand, a combination of religious and cultural taboos and, on the other hand, because many mothers and fathers have never learned such educational skills from their own parents.

The professional knowledge and skills combined with a sexuality-positive approach make the midwife the right professional to educate about sexuality. The midwife's role can be crucial to youngsters who have most of their sexual lives ahead and can benefit from the empowerment created by proper sexuality education and sexual health promotion. When such education (for teenagers of both sexes) includes body integrity, dealing with consent, and saying 'Yes' and 'No' to sexuality, it can prevent many future problems. A small addition to that package can be the integration of 'pelvic floor education' for girls and young women provided by the midwife who has gained such expertise.

Understanding the changes in sexuality over the stages of the woman's life, midwives seem the suitable professionals to educate young girls, and in some situations also their mothers, about physical development, personal hygiene, addressing budding sexuality, sexual pleasure, facts about clitoris, menstruation, tampons etc.

Midwives could be the sexuality educators in the upper years of primary school and in secondary school. Youngsters must navigate cultural messages that, at the same time, idealise and demonise sexual functioning [8]. On the one hand, it is relevant to prevent the apparent risks of sexual behaviour, such as unwanted pregnancy, STIs, and the damage of sexting.[1] However, to develop a healthy sexual future, the benefits of sexual pleasure and sexual behaviour as a basic form of human health and happiness need maybe even more attention. The sexuality-positive midwife pre-eminently appears to be fit for such education.

Potential developments in sexuality education for the midwife of the future:

- Combine sexuality education for mothers and daughters with the potential benefit of enhancing mother-daughter communication.
- After leaving secondary school, youngsters tend to be lost. However, reaching women in this phase for advice concerning contraception, dating, and STIs could have extensive preventive advantages. Midwives could deliver sex education in the workplace or in a community centre. In this phase, preconception health counselling should be an essential element.
- (Group) sexuality enhancement education for divorced/separated women. For re-empowering, re-finding self-respect and re-developing sexuality.
- (Group) sexuality enhancement education for aged/widowed women. For re-developing sexual self-respect and re-balancing sexuality.

30.4.3 Proactively Participating in Advocacy and Promoting Sexual and Reproductive Health and Rights in Society

Midwives should be more involved in the political debate on women's (sexual) health and rights.

The midwifery profession regularly has to go up to the barricades. To prevent their work from drowning in medicalisation and to remain valued as autonomous professionals. In some countries, the midwives have to fight for respect and to be

---

[1] Sexting is the sharing of sexual explicit texts or nude pictures. Although usually intended to share with the partner, in unauthorised forwarding, can cause blaming and shaming usually of the female involved.

able to gradually develop their field in the direction of the above-mentioned Swedish model. Let us call this aspect a struggle of empowering midwifery. In addition, midwives should fight for the empowerment of women and girls. Via private advocacy and through their midwifery associations, midwives should have an influence in creating laws that enable women to practice informed decisions regarding their reproduction, such as freely choosing the place of birth and not being prevented when deciding on safe pregnancy termination.

Few professions can better explain the consequences of insufficient sexual and reproductive laws and the consequences of a society that is unfriendly or unsupportive to women.

30.5   Midwifery and Specialised 'Sexuality-Related Skills'

Here we will elaborate on midwifery possibilities that are both sexuality-positive and progressing. In that imagination, we have used various 'sections'.

30.5.1 The Gynaecology Section

Having extensive knowledge of reproductive hormones, anatomy, and the female mind, the midwife could greatly help in caring for minor gynaecological problems and performing PAP smears. With great skills for education during history-taking and examination, especially at the first vaginal examination, they can have a significant impact on future woman's attitudes towards gynaecological examinations [9, 10].

The vaginal gynaecological or pelvic examination can be a real challenge for girls and women. That procedure is still routinely done in some countries with the introduction of oral contraceptives. One of the drawbacks of that routine is delayed visits for contraception and thereby increased number of undesired pregnancies, especially in women with experiences of intimate partner violence [11]. In many countries, that routine is dropped, focusing on good history-taking and blood pressure checks [12].

When the vaginal examination is needed and performed, the first one can significantly impact the young woman, making her feel safe regarding her body and functions. The examination, and everything surrounding it, needs an intimate atmosphere to feel safe, and the woman needs to feel seen and heard [10]. With models of the vagina, uterus, and clitoris, the girl or the woman can better understand those parts of her body that she cannot see herself. HCPs should not underestimate the importance of the woman's participation in the examination itself. Encouraging her to follow the examination through a mirror while the midwife narrates what they see and explain the anatomy and physiology is a way for women to get in touch with what is imperceptible to them about their genitals. Although not every woman will feel comfortable being examined, or even less via a mirror, the midwife has to consider the individuality of every client. However, encouragement to participate will make most women do so, and in this process of observation and explanation, appreciation can follow with respect and awe for the beauty of her body and its functioning.

30.5.2 Preconception Section

We separate this relatively new area of reproductive healthcare into two parts. On the one hand, preconception deals with the various risk factors that impair future fertility (for instance, smoking, obesity, alcohol, and especially age as a very relevant factor in the affluent Western World) [13, 14]. The midwife can guide fertility awareness and educate or counsel on retaining reproductive abilities when postponing parenthood. Here the importance of communication skills will be obvious.

The other part of preconception deals with the couple that intends to conceive-family planning period. Then the focus is not on fertility but on a smooth process through conception, pregnancy, childbirth, postpartum and healthy parenthood. The sexual aspects of that approach are addressed in Chap. 5. The real challenge here is to reach and 'catch' the couple already half a year before deciding on a pregnancy.

30.5.3 The Menopausal Section

Integral women's health goes from birth to death. Menopause means, next to the start of a low-estrogen life and no more monthly cycles, the end of fertility. Midwives could support women also in this phase of life. Besides, more than the average health care professional, the midwife will understand the sexual implications of hormones, vaginal health, urinary incontinence, and dyspareunia. Some midwives will feel at home in this specific period of the woman's life.

Beyond menopause, there is an era where for many societies, sexuality doesn't seem to exist [15]. Focusing on the ageing women, midwives should draw attention to the fact that aged women are still sexual beings with sexual desire, dreams, questions, and disappointments. Few professional groups seem more appropriate for such care and advocacy than midwives.

30.5.4 The STI: Sexually Transmitted Infections Section

STIs will have a role in everyday practice and sexuality education for the average midwife. In the career of some of them, STI can get a more prominent place. The midwife appears to be an ideal HCP for prevention and education, diagnosis, treatment, and counselling. That will usually take place in the hospital or public health office setting. The more adventurous midwife can be an excellent HCP for education, care and counselling at music festivals, rave parties, and other major public events. The combination of many young people, alcohol, drugs, and exciting music creates situations that can result in STIs (and unplanned pregnancy).

STI care usually has a strong connection with the communities of female, male, and transsexual sex workers. Some midwives will feel at ease in the care for this group, providing contraceptive counselling, STI screening, and, where needed, psychosocial support.

30.5.5 The (in-)Fertility Section

Midwifery communication and skills are needed in subfertility and infertility management. Especially in women with vaginismus or sexual abuse experience, midwifery skills can be precious and welcome when vaginal procedures are required (see Chap. 11). The midwife in a fertility department might be the right person to counsel the patient, the couple, and the staff on fertility treatment's emotional and sexual consequences. Being aware of those sexual implications, the midwife might also be the right professional to recommend considering starting with treatment of the sexual disturbance or the sexual trauma before entering the burdensome fertility trajectory.

30.5.6 The Contraception Section

Every midwife should be familiar with postpartum contraception and more-than-average family planning and child-spacing knowledge. In the Swedish model, the midwife is trained to deal with all phases of fertile life, knows about the sexual implications of various methods, prescribes oral contraceptives, and can also prescribe and insert IUDs or subcutaneous contraceptives.

Every midwife who participates in sexuality education in secondary school or community centres should (be allowed to and) provide emergency contraception and include aftercare and follow-up counselling.

Emergency contraception must be available around the clock ('24/7'). In communities without other emergency health care facilities, the midwife's office could or should offer that service.

Detailed information on emergency contraception is found in Chap. 20.

30.5.7 The Abortion Section

When contraception fails, abortion can be a necessary backup. Globally 30% of all pregnancies end in induced abortion, with >45% considered unsafe and an annual death rate of 26.000 women [16]. The ICM affirms that a woman who seeks or requires abortion-related services is entitled to be provided with such services by midwives [17].

Since oral treatment with 'abortion pills' has simplified the medical aspects, the midwife will, in many countries, be the ideal health care professional for such type of care.

In countries where abortion care is concentrated in specialised 'abortion clinics', the midwife could be an excellent staff member with expertise in history-taking, gynaecological and ultrasound examination, contraception counselling, psychosocial guidance, and aftercare.

Depending on the national jurisdiction, the midwife can even develop the skill to terminate pregnancies with manual or electric vacuum aspiration [18].

30.5.8 The Sexual Abuse and Rape Section

Every midwife should develop enough expertise to deal with pregnancy, childbirth, and breastfeeding, and with the aftermath of sexual abuse (see Chap. 24). With eventually additional expertise when expanding their field of work, some midwives will take that to a much higher level. Her bio-psycho-social skills make the female midwife a perfect partner in a rape crisis centre. She can combine emotional support with practical interventions such as physical examination, STI care, HIV post-exposure prophylaxis, and emergency contraception. The midwife's female gender is especially relevant in direct post-abuse care, applying to 90–95% of situations where the perpetrator was male. In later treatment and trauma processing stages, a male therapist can have additional value for the abused woman to regain confidence in men.

In the 5–10% of cases where the perpetrator was female, it is paramount that a female HCP can be very frightening in immediate post-abuse care [19, 20].

30.5.9 The Midwife-Without-Borders Section

Midwifery is not a profession for the weak. But some jobs ask for midwives with above-average courage and stamina. During natural disasters, armed conflicts and war, midwives are needed to provide quality care to pregnant women. In wartime and among people on the run, girls and women are also at high risk of being raped. Under such conditions, there is emotional trauma and a more-than-average risk for physical trauma, STI and pregnancy. Midwives with several of the above-mentioned additional skills are dearly needed in the medical aid stations or refugee camps and behind the frontline.

30.5.10 The Sexology Section

Sexology can become the main street in a midwife's career. To get there, one needs more-than-average awareness of the importance of sexuality. Given the midwife's healthcare background, it will be logical to focus on those areas where the organic aspects of sexuality play a role. With the widening and professionalisation of sexology, subdisciplines are arising. One of them is 'reproduction sexology', the topic of this book, an area offering a career perspective, particularly suitable for the professional with midwifery insights and skills.

30.6 The Widening Field of Male Midwifery Future

We are aware that part of the midwife's above-mentioned added value lies in her being female. That will create more trust and, in many women, a sense of 'being understood'.

What if we change our perspective and look at the male midwife? A group that in some countries is forbidden by law or barely present. In the UK, they form <1% of the midwifery force, but in Spain and Chile 10%; in Ethiopia 33%; and in Burundi 50% [21]. Let us look at the added value of the male midwife, especially concerning sexuality-positive midwifery. We will give some examples that, in some places, will be a reality, but elsewhere still fiction.

- The male midwife will much better understand the uncertainties of impending fatherhood.
- During childbirth, the male midwife will better understand the male partner's split between being concerned and the fear of showing it.
- The male midwife can be the right person for sexuality and relationship education for boys in puberty and adolescence.
- In case of physical or sexual abuse by men, the male midwife may be less suitable to guide the woman through pregnancy, childbirth, or fertility problems. However, being a male HCP will probably have added value to the 5–10% of women abused by females.
- In STI and contraception, the male midwife might have more 'convincing power' when educating boys and men about contraception, especially condom use and vasectomy.
- In sexuality education, prenatal courses will benefit from the participation of a male midwife in addressing the male partner role(s).
- In educating boys and men on respecting the integrity of women, the male midwife can be very important.
- Within the patriarchal structure of many societies, women (and men) attach more value to what men tell. As long as that is still the reality, it seems sensible to include the male midwife in women's empowerment. His added value seems especially relevant when it comes to how the woman supposes men or her male partner to be and how she interacts with him.

30.7 General Recommendations for the Future

Although there are more ways to integrate the issues of sexuality and intimacy into midwifery practice and core competencies, this chapter used the 'Swedish model' as a starting point to elaborate on the future. We would like to believe that many professional midwifery environments have already deeply incorporated the theme into the standard midwifery management.

Midwifery and midwives can change the attitude toward how society looks at and treats women and girls and, in that way, achieve significant cultural changes in their societies.

We conclude with these recommendations for the future.

- The midwife's approach to sexuality should be woman-centred and holistic, focusing on physical and psychosocial aspects.
- The approach should also be couple-centred for all women with a partner. Since intimacy is an integral part of partner sex, one cannot manage sexuality adequately without addressing and including intimacy.
- Reproductive and sexual health care needs midwives who continue working in pregnancy and childbirth after gaining additional expertise and registration in sexology. That appears to be the ideal situation to become aware of the not-asked reproduction-related questions on sexuality and intimacy.
- New knowledge on sexuality should be disseminated through journals focusing on midwives. For example - Sexual and Reproductive Healthcare is the official journal of the Swedish Association of Midwives, affiliated with other Scandinavian midwifery associations.
- Midwives should be more involved in the political debate on women's health and rights. Via private advocacy and through their midwifery associations, midwives should have an influence in creating laws that enable women to practice informed decisions regarding their reproduction.

References

1. Wendt E, Lidell E, Westersthael A, et al. Young women's sexual health and their views on dialogue with health professionals. Acta Obstet Gynecol Scand. 2007;86:590–5.
2. Mivsek P. Sexology in midwifery. In: Do midwives need sexology in their undergraduate study programme? Study among graduates of midwifery. Rijeka: InTech; 2015. https://doi.org/10.5772/59007.
3. Gianotten WL via personal communication. 2022.
4. Vermeulen J, Luyben A, O'Connell R, et al. Failure or progress?: the current state of the professionalisation of midwifery in Europe. Eur J Midwifery. 2019;3:22.
5. Wendt E, Marklund B, Lidell E, et al. Possibilities for dialogue on sexuality and sexual abuse—midwives' and clinicians' experiences. Midwifery. 2011;27:539–46.
6. https://barnmorskan.se/the-swedish-midwife-barnmorskansar2020/.
7. Kompetensbeskrivning för legitimerad barnmorska (Competence description for the registered midwife). 2019. https://storage.googleapis.com/barnmorskeforbundet-se/uploads/2020/04/Kompetensbeskrivning-for-legitimerad-barnmorska.pdf.
8. Ballonoff Suleiman A, Johnson M, Shirtcliff EA, Galvan A. School-based sex education and neuroscience: what we know about sex, romance, marriage, and adolescent brain development. J School Health. 2015;85:567–74.
9. Wendt E, Fridlund B, Lidell E. Trust and confirmation in a gynecologic examination situation: a critical incident technique analysis. Acta Obstet Gynecol Scand. 2004;83:1208–15.

10. Oscarsson MG, Benzein EG, Wijma BE. The first pelvic examination. J Psychosom Obstet Gynaecol. 2007;28:7–12.
11. Holt HK, Sawaya GF, et al. Delayed visits for contraception due to concerns regarding pelvic examination among women with history of intimate partner violence. J Gen Intern Med. 2021;36:1883–9.
12. Batur P, Berenson AB. Are breast and pelvic exams necessary when prescribing hormonal contraception? Cleve Clin J Med. 2015;82:661–3.
13. Tuomi J. Preconception health and care. 2021. https://webpages.tuni.fi/preco/handbook/.
14. Mivšek P, Rogan N, Petročnik P. From wish to family. In: Darmann-Finck I, Reiber K, editors. Development, implementation and evaluation of curricula in nursing and midwifery education. Cham: Springer; 2021.
15. Radosh A, Simkin L. Acknowledging sexual bereavement: a path out of disenfranchised grief. Reprod Health Matters. 2016;24:25–33.
16. WHO. Abortion care guideline. 2022. https://www.who.int/publications/i/item/9789240039483.
17. ICM. 2018. https://www.internationalmidwives.org/assets/files/statement-files/2018/04/midwives-provision-of-abortion-related-services-eng.pdf.
18. Fullerton J, Butler MM, Aman C, et al. Abortion-related care and the role of the midwife: a global perspective. Int J Women's Health. 2018;10:751–62.
19. Saradjan J. Understanding the prevalence of female-perpetrated sexual abuse and the impact of that abuse on victims. In: Gannon TA, Cortoni F, editors. Female sexual offenders. Theory, assessment and treatment. Hoboken, NJ: Wiley Blackwell; 2010.
20. Munroe C, Shumway M. Female-perpetrated sexual violence: a survey of survivors of female-perpetrated childhood sexual abuse and adult sexual assault. J Interpers Violence. 2022;37(9–10):NP6655–75.
21. Masana S, Sasagawa E, Hikita N, et al. The proportions, regulations, and training plans of male midwives worldwide: a descriptive study of 77 countries. Int J Childbirth. 2019;9:5–18.

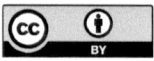

Correction to: Midwifery and Sexuality

Sam Geuens ⑩, Ana Polona Mivšek ⑩,
and Woet L. Gianotten ⑩

Correction to: Sam Geuens et al. (eds.), Midwifery and Sexuality, https://doi.org/10.1007/978-3-031-18432-1

This book was inadvertently published with the following errors, and the errors have been corrected.

On Page 72, footnote 1 for section 6.4.1 has been corrected as "Practical tools on how to effectively 'Talk sexuality' with women and couples can be found in Chap. 26".

On Page ix/FM Contents, the title for chapter 9 has been corrected as "Sexual Aspects of Breast and Lactation".

On Page 51, under Part II Introduction to Module 2: 'Nature Taking Its Course', the title for Chapter 9 has been corrected as "Sexual Aspects of Breast and Lactation".

On Page 99, the title for Chapter 9 has been corrected as "Sexual Aspects of Breast and Lactation".

On Page 147 (under section 12.4.4), in line 1, the word "colonization" has been corrected as "conization".

On Page 181, under section 15.6.1, in the last line, "see Chap 20" has been corrected as "See Chap 17".

On Page 219, under section 19.2, in footnote 3, "see chapter 1.2" has been corrected as "see chapter 1".

On Page 220, under section 19.2, in footnote 4, "see chapter 1.4" has been corrected as "see chapter 3".

On Page 226, footnote for section 19.4.2 has been corrected as "For more information on how to talk about sexuality with clients, see chapter 26 on "Talking Sex".

The updated versions of the chapters can be found at
https://doi.org/10.1007/978-3-031-18432-1
https://doi.org/10.1007/978-3-031-18432-1_6
https://doi.org/10.1007/978-3-031-18432-1_9
https://doi.org/10.1007/978-3-031-18432-1_12
https://doi.org/10.1007/978-3-031-18432-1_15
https://doi.org/10.1007/978-3-031-18432-1_19

S. Geuens et al. (eds.), *Midwifery and Sexuality*,
https://doi.org/10.1007/978-3-031-18432-1_31